Marginal Space Learning for Medical Image Analysis

Yefeng Zheng • Dorin Comaniciu

Marginal Space Learning for Medical Image Analysis

Efficient Detection and Segmentation of Anatomical Structures

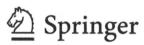 Springer

Yefeng Zheng
Imaging and Computer Vision
Siemens Corporate Technology
Princeton, NJ, USA

Dorin Comaniciu
Imaging and Computer Vision
Siemens Corporate Technology
Princeton, NJ, USA

ISBN 978-1-4939-5575-6 ISBN 978-1-4939-0600-0 (eBook)
DOI 10.1007/978-1-4939-0600-0
Springer New York Heidelberg Dordrecht London

Printed on acid-free paper

Springer is part of Springer Science+Business Media (www.springer.com)

To Muna, Allen, and Amy
– Y. Z.

To my family
– D. C.

Preface

Medical imaging is today an integrated part of the healthcare continuum, supporting early disease detection, diagnosis, therapy, monitoring, and follow-up. Images of the human body help in estimating the organ anatomy and function, reveal clues indicating the presence of disease, or help in guiding treatment and interventions. All these benefits are achieved by extracting and quantifying the medical image content, answering questions such as: "Which part of the 3D image represents the heart and what is the ejection fraction?", "What is the volume of the liver", "Which are the axillary lymph nodes with a diameter larger than 10 mm?", "Is the artificial heart valve being positioned at the right location, with the right angulation?"

With the continuous increase in the spatial and temporal resolution, the informational content of images increases, contributing to new clinical benefits. While most of the content extraction, quantification, and decision making are guided and validated by the clinicians, computer-based image systems benefit from efficient algorithms and exponential increase in computational power. Thus, they play an important role in analyzing the image data, performing tasks such as identifying the anatomy or measuring a certain body function.

Systems based on machine learning have recently opened new ways to extract and interpret the informational content of medical images. Such systems learn from data through a process called training, thus developing the capability to identify, classify, and label the image content.

Learning systems have been initially applied to nonmedical images for two-dimensional (2D) object detection problems such as face detection, pedestrian or vehicle detection in 2D images, and video sequences. In these methods, object detection or localization is formulated as a classification problem: whether an image block contains the target object or not. The robustness of the methods comes from the exhaustive search with the trained classifier during object detection on an input image. The object pose parameter space is first quantized into a set of discrete hypotheses covering the entire space. Each hypothesis is tested by a trained classifier to get a detection score and the hypotheses with the highest score are taken as the detection output. In a typical setting, only three pose parameters are estimated, the position (X and Y) and isotropic scale (S), resulting in a three-dimensional search space and a search problem of relatively low complexity.

On the other hand, most of the medical imaging data used in clinical practice are volumetric and three-dimensional (3D). Computed tomography, C-Arm X-Ray, magnetic resonance, ultrasound, and nuclear imaging create 3D representations of the human body. To accurately localize a 3D object, one needs to estimate nine pose parameters: three for position, three for orientation, and three for anisotropic scaling. However, a straightforward extension of a 2D object detection method to 3D is not practically possible due to the exponential increase in the computation needs attributed to exhaustive search. How do we solve this problem? What kind of learning strategy would help to perform efficient search in a nine-dimensional pose parameter space?

This book presents a generic learning-based method for efficient 3D object detection called Marginal Space Learning (MSL). Instead of exhaustively searching the original nine-dimensional pose parameter space, only low-dimensional marginal spaces are searched in MSL to improve the detection speed.

We split the estimation into three steps: position estimation, position-orientation estimation, and position-orientation-scale estimation. First, we train a position estimator that can tell us if a position hypothesis is a good estimate of the target object position in an input volume. After exhaustively searching for the position marginal space (three-dimensional), we preserve a small number of position candidates with the largest detection scores. Next, we perform joint position-orientation estimation with a trained classifier that answers if a position-orientation hypothesis is a good estimate. The orientation marginal space is exhaustively searched for each position candidate preserved after position estimation. Similarly, we only preserve a limited number of position-orientation candidates after this step. Finally, the scale parameters are searched in the constrained space in a similar way.

Since after each step we only preserve a small number of candidates, a large portion of search space with low posterior probability is pruned efficiently in the early steps. Complexity analysis shows that MSL can reduce the number of testing hypotheses by six orders of magnitude, compared to the exhaustive full space search. Since the learning and detection are performed in a sequence of marginal spaces, we call the method Marginal Space Learning (MSL).

As it will be shown in this book, the MSL has been applied to detect multiple 2D/3D anatomical structures in the major medical imaging modalities. Several key techniques have later been proposed to further improve its detection speed and accuracy: Constrained MSL to exploit the strong correlation existing among pose parameters in the same marginal spaces; Iterated MSL to detect multiple instances of the same object type in a volume; Hierarchical MSL to improve the robustness by performing learning/detection on a volume pyramid; Joint spatio-temporal MSL to detect the trajectory of a landmark in a volume sequence.

With these improvements, we can reliably detect a 3D anatomical structure with a speed of 0.1–0.5 s/volume on an ordinary personal computer (3.2 GHz duo-core processor and 3 GB memory) without the use of special hardware such as graphics processing units.

The MSL can also be applied to generate accurate shape initialization for the segmentation of a nonrigid anatomical structure. To further improve the initialization accuracy, the MSL has been extended to directly estimate the nonrigid deformation parameters in combination with a learning-based boundary detector that guides the boundary evolution.

Several practical anatomy segmentation systems have been built and evaluated at multiple clinical sites. Examples include four-chamber heart segmentation, liver segmentation, and aorta segmentation. At the time of publication they all outperformed the state of the art in both speed and accuracy.

This book is for students, engineers, and researchers with interest in medical image analysis. It can also be used as a reference or supplementary material for related graduate courses. Preliminary knowledge of machine learning and medical imaging is needed to understand the content of the book.

Princeton, NJ, USA   Yefeng Zheng
                                                                              Dorin Comaniciu

Acknowledgements

We owe our gratitude to all colleagues who have made this work possible.

At the beginning, this was a joint project with a former colleague at Siemens Corporate Research, Adrian Barbu. During the summer of 2006 we were looking for an efficient and robust 3D detection method to automatically identify the heart chambers in cardiac computed tomography volumes. Based on our previous experience, we knew machine learning was the right direction; however, we lacked an efficient search method. After a series of systematic investigations, we jointly proposed a simple and elegant method called marginal space learning (MSL) as presented here. We really appreciated Adrian's enthusiasm during this development.

We would also like to thank many other colleagues at Siemens Corporate Research for applying, tuning, and improving the MSL on various 2D/3D object detection and segmentation problems in medical imaging. Bogdan Georgescu and Kevin Zhou contributed to the early development stages of this technology; Zhuowen Tu provided the implementation of the probabilistic boosting-tree and 3D Haar wavelet features; Haibin Ling helped in performing comparison experiments for Constrained MSL and Nonrigid MSL on liver detection; and Xiaoguang Lu and Gustavo Carneiro contributed to the comparison experiments of full space learning and MSL on 2D left ventricle detection in magnetic resonance images. Furthermore, several important improvements of MSL originated from our colleagues' work, including Hierarchical MSL from Michal Sofka and Jingdan Zhang, Iterated MSL from Michael Kelm, and Joint Spatio-Temporal MSL from Razvan Ionasec and Yang Wang.

We thank our colleagues from Siemens Healthcare, especially Michael Scheuering, Fernando Vega-Higuera, Dominik Bernhardt, and Michael Suehling from Computed Tomography; Matthias John, Jan Boese, and Martin Ostermeier from Angiographic and Interventional X-Ray Systems; Arne Littmann, Edgar Mueller, and Berthold Kiefer from Magnetic Resonance; and Helene Houle and Sara Good from Ultrasound. They provided us challenging medical imaging problems so that we had a chance to develop the MSL. They collected data all over the world for us and coordinated the clinical evaluation of the resulting systems. Most importantly, they asked us to continuously improve the detection/segmentation speed and robustness of the algorithms.

We are thankful to the Springer editors, Courtney Clark and Jennifer Evans, for their enthusiasm and support to the project.

Yefeng owes his deepest thanks to his wife, Muna Tang, for allowing him to work overtime, often during the weekends.

Dorin would like to thank his family for being so inspiring and supportive.

Contents

Acronyms

A2C   Apical two chamber view
A3C   Apical three chamber view
A4C   Apical four chamber view
AAM   Active appearance model
AF   Atrial fibrillation
ASM   Active shape model
AV   Aortic valve
CPU   Central processing unit
CT   Computed tomography
CTA   Computed tomography angiography
ED   End-diastole
EF   Ejection fraction
ES   End-systole
FSL   Full space learning
GPU   Graphics processing unit
LA   Left atrium
LAA   Left atrial appendage
LIPV   Left inferior pulmonary vein
LSPV   Left superior pulmonary vein
LV   Left ventricle
LVOT   Left ventricular outflow tract
MRF   Markov random field
MPR   Multi-planar reformatting or multi-planar reconstruction
MRI   Magnetic resonance imaging
MSL   Marginal space learning
MV   Mitral valve
PBT   Probabilistic boosting-tree
PCA   Principal component analysis
PDM   Point distribution model
PV   Pulmonary vein or pulmonary valve
RA   Right atrium

RIPV   Right inferior pulmonary vein
ROI   Region of interest
RSPV   Right superior pulmonary vein
RV   Right ventricle
RVOT   Right ventricular outflow tract
SAX   Short axis view
SNR   Signal-to-noise ratio
SVD   Singular value decomposition
SVM   Support vector machine
TAVI   Transcatheter aortic valve implantation
TAVR   Transcatheter aortic valve replacement
TEE   Transesophageal echocardiography
TPS   Thin-plate spline
TV   Tricuspid valve

Chapter 1
Introduction

The last decade saw tremendous advances in all major medical imaging modalities, with significant improvement in signal-to-noise ratio, sensitivity and specificity, spatial and temporal resolution, and radiation dose reduction. All these developments translated into direct benefits for the quality of care. Most imaging modalities generate now high resolution, isotropic or near-isotropic true 3D volumes, resulting in a large amount of complex data to process. This, however, presents a significant challenge to the already loaded radiologists. As a consequence, intelligent medical image analysis systems are critical to help radiologists to improve accuracy and consistency of diagnosis, increase patient throughput, and optimize daily workflow. The main operations of a computer supported, enhanced reading workflow consist in the detection, segmentation and quantification of various semantic structures in the image data. The quantification of images helps answering questions such as: "Are there inflamed lymph nodes in this volume?", "Does this scan contain bone lesions?", and "Has this lesion decreased following treatment?".

This chapter reviews recent advances in medical imaging and presents some of the new challenges and opportunities for image processing and analysis. We then review applications of automatic detection and segmentation in medical imaging, followed by a literature survey on the existing detection and segmentation methods. A brief introduction to the Marginal Space Learning (MSL) based anatomical structure detection and segmentation is presented, followed by the outline of the book content.

1.1 Advances in Medical Imaging

With the capability of generating images inside a patient's body non-invasively, medical imaging is ubiquitously present in the current clinical practice. It is estimated that about 400 million medical imaging procedures are performed annually in the USA [54]. Although the conventional diagnostic X-ray is still taking a

Y. Zheng and D. Comaniciu, *Marginal Space Learning for Medical Image Analysis:*
Efficient Detection and Segmentation of Anatomical Structures,
DOI 10.1007/978-1-4939-0600-0_1, © Springer Science+Business Media New York 2014

large share, more advanced imaging modalities have significant presence, e.g., 80 million exams annually for diagnostic Ultrasound [41], 27.5 million for Magnetic Resonance Imaging (MRI) [28], and 72 million for Computed Tomography (CT) exams [20].

Most imaging modalities can today generate isotropic or near-isotropic true 3D volumes. For example, earlier CT scanners could only produce a stack of 2D slices with coarse between-slice resolution (large slice thickness), which prevented the true 3D analysis of image data. Introduced in 1998 by several major vendors, Multi-Slice Computed Tomography (MSCT) (also called multi-detector row computed tomography) changed dramatically the field [18]. Dual source CT has further doubled the temporal resolution with the use of two X-Ray tubes. The number of slices increased from 4 to 8, 16, 32, and 64 in just a few years. Now, 640-slice MSCT is available on market with slices as thin as 0.5 mm. The gantry rotation time also reduced steadily, from around 1 s to 0.25 s, with a temporal resolution of about 66 ms.

A decade ago, cardiovascular CT was still an extended target since it demanded high spatial resolution, to distinguish small coronary arteries, and high temporal resolution, to compensate the cardiac and respiratory motion [7, 68]. Multi-segment reconstruction of the heart was necessary, in which the volume was stitched by data captured from several heart beats, and the stair-step artifacts were often present due to irregular heart rate of some patients. Now, cardiovascular CT is a routine practice. With the latest scanners, it is possible to scan the whole heart in one beat.

The radiation dose is a big concern for CT. Previously, a cardiac CT scan imposed about 10–15 mSv dose. With the recent advances in dose management and statistical iterative reconstruction algorithms [17], it is possible to perform a high quality scan for majority of patients with less than 1 mSv dose.

The ultrasonography techniques had also an impressive advance in the last decade. One significant trend is the miniaturization of the ultrasound systems, hand-held devices and wireless probes being available today. An ultrasound probe called Intravascular Ultrasound (IVUS) can be small enough to be attached to the tip of a catheter and inserted into a coronary artery to reveal the existence or nature of the coronary plaque. To visualize in real time the heart valves or the inner lining of the heart, Intracardiac Ultrasound (ICE) has been developed. By the use of a catheter, the ultrasound probe is threaded through the vein in the groin and up into the patient's heart. A less invasive technique is Transesophageal Echocardiogram (TEE) for which the ultrasound probe is inserted through the patient's esophagus. The Transthoracic Echocardiogram (TTE) is non-invasive, assuming the transducer to be placed on the chest wall of the patient.

Early 3D ultrasonography steered the probe mechanically or electrically to generate a set of 2D images (or small volume slabs) and stitch them together to reconstruct a 3D volume. The temporal resolution of such a 3D ultrasound system is limited, being subject to stitching artifacts in the case of organs with rapid motion (e.g., a beating heart). Using matrix arrays, the latest 3D ultrasound scanners can directly capture 3D volumes without stitching, achieving scanning speeds of more than 40 volumes/s.

The same trends are also observed in MRI, with significantly improved signal-to-noise ratio, spatial and temporal resolution. With the higher magnet field of the state-of-the-art MRI scanners, detailed anatomical structures are revealed. The 3-Tesla scanners are now industry standard with wide availability and 7-Tesla scanners are under clinical evaluation. Sparse MRI with compressed sensing [50] and parallel MRI imaging with multi-channel coils [65, 70] significantly accelerate the scanning speed. With all these developments, the current MRI scanners can be used to detect coronary stenosis [22], as an alternative to CT.

With all the focus on performance, the imaging systems are getting more and more complex to operate. As a result, new requirements recognize the need for smarter scanners that make it easier for the operator to perform a high quality scan. For example, to reduce the radiation dose, a CT scanner can dynamically tune the X-ray tube current with respect to the targeted body region. The X-ray tube current is maintained high for large body parts (e.g., abdomen, thorax) to achieve sufficient image quality for diagnosis, while being reduced for a thin body part (e.g., neck), thus achieving a comparable image quality. This process requires the scanner to know which part is currently being scanned. Likewise, a stack of MRI slices often have to be aligned with some standard orientations of the target anatomy (e.g., standard views of the heart). In all these applications, the solution has been usually achieved by scanning in advance a low-resolution image/volume of the anatomy of interest and manually identifying the anatomy or orientation of interest. With the recent developments in the automated image processing such as the methods described in this book, the new scanners provide fully automatic positioning and alignment solutions, thus offering a much simplified clinical workflow.

1.2   Applications of Automatic Detection and Segmentation in Medical Imaging

The improvements in the spatial and temporal resolutions of the main imaging modalities resulted in continuously increasing amounts of data to process, thus presenting a challenge to the radiologists. The average workload of a radiologist grew by 34 % from 1991–1992 to 2006–2007 [4], reaching 14,900 studies annually for a full-time job, about 70 cases per day. This represents indeed an important and tedious effort especially when we consider the inherent complexity of the imaging content. For example, it is time consuming for a physician to identify in a volumetric scan small target anatomies such as nodules in the lung or breast. Methods that automatically or semi-automatically detect, segment (delineate), and measure specific structures in the data are therefore critical to optimize the clinical workflow.

As it will be shown, using the Marginal Space Learning (MSL) method, the mean shape aligned with the estimated position, orientation, and anisotropic scales is often very close to the true object boundary. It is also possible to estimate a few nonrigid deformation parameters using the MSL principle to further improve the accuracy of the shape estimate. For such an approach, the border between automated detection and segmentation is blurred, since after object detection we get a quite accurate initial segmentation.

In [8], Carneiro et al. presented an application of automatic detection and measurement in obstetric ultrasonography. During such exam, the sonographer estimates the gestational age of a fetus by measuring the size of a few anatomical structures, including the bi-parietal diameter, head circumference, abdominal circumference, femur length, humerus length, and crown rump length. Accurate estimation of gestational age is important to assess the fetal size, monitor fetal growth, and estimate the expected delivery date. Without automated processing, the clinical workflow requires sonographers to perform those measurements manually, resulting in the following potential issues: (1) The quality of the measurements are user dependent; (2) Exams can take more than 30 min; and (3) Sonographers may suffer from repetitive stress injury (RSI) due to the multiple keystrokes needed to perform the measurements. Therefore, the automation of ultrasound measurements has the potential of improving everyday workflow, increasing patient throughput, improving accuracy of measurements, bringing expert-like consistency to every exam, and reducing the risk of RSI to specialists.

Automatic detection and segmentation is especially useful for interventional cardiology, where the image/volume is captured in real time and needs to be processed as fast as possible. For example, in minimally invasive Transcatheter Aortic Valve Implantation (TAVI), a C-arm CT volume of the aorta is captured during the intervention [31]. The aorta and aortic valve landmarks need to be detected/segmented and overlaid to a real-time 2D fluoroscopic image sequence to provide visual guidance to physicians during the positioning of the prosthetic valve. It may take more than 10 minutes to manually segment the aorta in 3D and specify the valve landmarks. In addition, it is difficult for the physicians at the side of the surgery table to have access to the computer keyboard and mouse in a sterile environment. Therefore, a dedicated technician needs to be available in the workstation room to perform the manual segmentation. During that period, the whole surgery team (including interventional cardiologists or cardiac surgeons, nurses, and technicians) may be halted, waiting for the segmentation result, while the patient is lying on the table under general anesthesia, with multiple inserted medical devices (e.g., a TEE probe and various catheters). This is clearly not an ideal scenario. It would be highly beneficial to reduce the image segmentation time, therefore reduce the intervention time and associated risk. An automatic detection/segmentation system designed by us using the methods presented in this book has been developed for this application [85, 86]. It takes only 1–2 s to get an accurate 3D model for the overlay and the system has been successfully tested in real clinical practice at multiple hospitals on thousands of procedures. The physicians can hardly notice the processing delay since the resulting system is so fast, thus contributing to the shortening of the procedure duration.

A few years ago, before the introduction of 3D echocardiography, the sonographers exclusively used 2D echocardiography to evaluate the function of the heart. A few standard 2D cardiac views, e.g., the apical two-chamber view, apical four-chamber view, parasternal long-axis and parasternal short-axis views, were captured and all recommended measurements were performed on these 2D views. More recently, 3D echocardiography started to gradually enter the clinical practice. A large amount of information became available in the 3D volumes and multiple new 3D measurements could be extracted from this data, thus contributing to a richer diagnosis of the patient's heart condition. However, it has been shown that the sonographer might get quickly lost in the multi-planar reconstruction (MPR) views due to information overload. To increase the acceptability of 3D echocardiography, there was a need to automatically identify in a 3D volume the standard 2D cardiac views that the physicians and sonographers were used to [48]. The automatically detected views helped extracting the traditional 2D measurements and therefore, accelerating the acceptance of 3D echocardiography in clinical practice.

In medical imaging, it often takes tremendous time to train junior physicians such as residents or fellows to have sufficient proficiency to work independently, especially if the task is challenging, e.g., detecting coronary stenosis [37, 64]. Clinical experiments show that an automatic coronary stenosis detection system helps to improve the diagnosis accuracy of junior physicians [1]. Moreover, a computer assisted diagnosis system such as lung nodule detection [51] or colon polyp detection [47, 71], also provides a second opinion that has the potential to improve the diagnosis sensitivity of the expert.

A different need for automation comes from the use of a topogram, which is a 2D X-ray image captured as a scout image to plan the CT exam. A human operator has to manually define the Region of Interest (ROI) of the target organ (e.g., the liver) on this topogram to determine the extent of the desired axial/helical scan (3D). Nevertheless, an automatic algorithm can detect the organs reliably on the topogram, therefore save time and improve consistency/repeatability, especially for follow-up studies of the same patient or for cross-patient comparison [60].

Scout images are also used to plan MRI exams. An MRI scanner has the capability to capture an image with any orientation, however, the between-slice resolution is normally lower than the in-slice resolution. To exam an organ, we often want to align the slice stack properly. For example, in a spinal exam, the task is to align the imaging plane with the target intervertebral disk [13, 35, 36]. Therefore, during exam planning, a low resolution scout volume is captured first. After the detection of the target vertebra disk, the imaging plane orientation and field of view can be automatically determined and the scanning can be triggered using the proper setting. By eliminating user interaction as much as possible, such smart scanner can reduce the cost to train a technician, while increasing the patient throughput. In addition, an automatically determined scanning protocol is especially useful for the follow-up exams to improve the consistency across time.

In summary, the automatic detection and segmentation of anatomical structures in 2D/3D medical images have the following potential benefits in clinical practice:

1. Reduce the repetitive stress injury.
2. Reduce the exam time, therefore increase the patient throughput.

3. Reduce the cost of personnel training, by making the scanner and software more automated and intelligent.
4. Increase consistency and reproducibility of the exam.
5. Increase diagnosis accuracy of an expert.
6. Act as a training tool for junior physicians.

1.3   Previous Work on Automatic Object Detection in Medical Images

The capability to detect an object robustly and efficiently in a cluttered environment is an amazing feature of the human visual system. Automatic object detection received a lot of attention in computer vision, a prominent example being face detection from video [25, 77, 78]. In medical imaging, ad-hoc methods were often proposed to detect a specific anatomy in a specific imaging modality. For example, in [19], the barycenter of the voxels weighted by intensity was used as a rough estimate of the heart center in a cardiac CT volume. Such solution is not robust since it is based on a strong assumption of the imaging protocol: the heart is at the center of the volume and well contrasted.

A limited number of theoretically motivated, generic object detection methods were proposed in the literature. The Hough transform, originally proposed to detect straight lines [26], is a well known technique to detect an object based on its edges. It converts the global pattern detection problem in the image space to a local pattern (ideally a point) detection problem in a transformed parameter space. To detect a straight line, each pixel in an image space is transformed into a sinusoidal curve in the Hough parameter space. After the transformation, collinear points in the image space intersect at a point in the Hough parameter space. Therefore, a peak in the transformed space provides strong evidence that a corresponding straight line exists in the image. It is straightforward to extend the Hough transform to detect other analytic shapes, such as circles and ellipses. Later on, the Hough transform method was extended to detect arbitrary shapes [2]. In the training phase, the complete specification of the exact shape of the target object is pre-computed in the form of the r-table. In the detection phase, the r-table is used to vote for the presence of the target object. The generalized Hough transform has been applied in medical imaging to detect the heart chamber center in [3, 15, 16, 44, 45, 67]. Although it may work well for a rigid object, one drawback of this method is the lack of robustness to detect nonrigid objects.

Unlike the generalized Hough transform that was originated in the computer vision community, the atlas based method [32, 46, 56, 61, 62, 66] was first proposed in the medical imaging community and it is almost a standard method for brain segmentation [52]. Suppose we have a training volume with the target organ delineated (i.e., we know which voxels belong to the target organ). Given an input volume, we do volume registration to align the input volume to the training volume.

We can achieve segmentation by transferring the voxel label from the training volume to the corresponding voxel in the input volume. However, due to the large variation of the nonrigid shape and imaging intensity, the result is not robust using only one training volume.

Using multiple training volumes, we can build a statistical atlas. First, we align all training volumes under either affine transformation or nonrigid transformation. We then build two atlases after the alignment, one for a probabilistic atlas where the intensity of each voxel represents its probability belonging to the target organ, and the other for a gray-level atlas where a voxel takes the mean intensity of the corresponding voxels in the aligned training volumes. Given an input volume, we do volume registration to align it with the gray-level atlas. By transforming from the corresponding probabilistic atlas, we know the probability for each voxel of the input volume belonging to the target organ. Initial segmentation can be extracted from this probability map by simple thresholding. However, more accurate segmentation results can be achieved by boundary evolution using active contours, level set, or active shape models.

An atlas based method combines the object detection and rough segmentation into one step, through the volume registration. A major drawback of this method is that volume registration is a hard problem itself, may be even harder than object detection/segmentation it is solving. This is the motivation of some recent work trying to use automatically detected landmarks to initialize the volume registration. Another drawback is that volume registration is computationally expensive, especially for nonrigid volume registration.

Machine learning based methods represent an important class of algorithms for object detection. They are popular and dominate some 2D object detection applications in computer vision, e.g., face detection, after Viola and Jones' influential work [72]. They leverage the recent advances in discriminative machine learning.

In these methods, object detection or localization is formulated as a classification problem: whether an image block contains the target object or not (see Fig. 1.1a). The object pose parameter space is quantized into a large set of discrete hypotheses. Each hypothesis is tested by the trained classifier to get a detection score. The hypothesis with the highest score is taken as the final detection result (see Fig. 1.1b). This search strategy is quite different from other parameter estimation approaches, such as deformable models, where an initial estimate is adjusted (e.g., using the gradient descent technique) to optimize a predefined objective function. To accurately estimate the object pose, all combinations of translation, rotation, and scaling need to be tested, as shown in Fig. 1.2. However, due to computational power constraints, only three pose parameters (namely 2D translation plus isotropic scaling) are estimated in almost all applications of these techniques. These methods are often called "sliding window" methods since the object position is detected by sliding a window over the whole image and testing each window position.

Exhaustive search makes the system robust under local optima, however there are two challenges to extend the learning based approaches to 3D. First, the number of hypotheses increases exponentially with respect to the dimensionality of the parameter space. For example, there are nine degrees of freedom for the

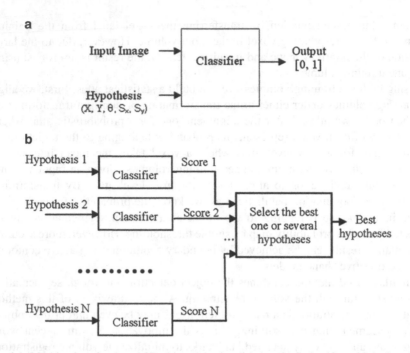

Fig. 1.1 Machine learning based 2D object detection. (**a**) A trained classifier with its input and output. (**b**) Use of the classifier for object detection. ©2008 IEEE. Reprinted, with permission, from Zheng, Y., Barbu, A., Georgescu, B., Scheuering, M., Comaniciu, D.: Four-chamber heart modeling and automatic segmentation for 3D cardiac CT volumes using marginal space learning and steerable features. *IEEE Trans. Medical Imaging* **27**(11), 1668–1681 (2008)

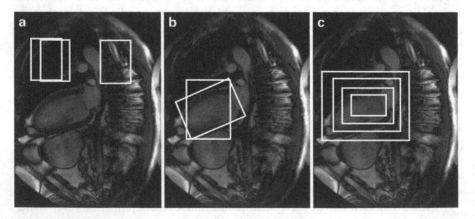

Fig. 1.2 All combinations of the (**a**) translations, (**b**) rotations, and (**c**) scaling need to be tested to detect an object (demonstrated on left ventricle detection in a 2D magnetic resonance image)

3D anisotropic similarity transformation, namely three translation parameters, three rotation angles, and three scales. Note that the ordinary similarity transformation allows only isotropic scaling. In this work, we search for anisotropic scales to cope with the nonrigid deformation of the object. Suppose each dimension is quantized to n discrete values, the total number of hypotheses is n^9 (for very coarse estimation with a small $n = 10$, $n^9 = 1,000,000,000!$). The computational demands are too high for the capabilities of the current desktop computers.

The second challenge is that we need efficient features to search the orientation spaces. To estimate the object orientation, one has to rotate either the feature templates or the volume. The widely used Haar wavelet features can be efficiently computed under translation and scaling [58, 72], but no efficient ways are available to rotate the Haar wavelet feature templates. Previously, time-consuming image/volume rotation has been performed to estimate the object orientation [71].

1.4   Previous Work on Medical Image Segmentation

After the region of interest is specified for the target anatomical structure (either manually or automatically detected), we often need to segment it from the background (delineating its boundary). In the following, we review a few popular segmentation methods. A complete review of the previous work on medical image segmentation is out of the scope of this book. Interested readers are referred to the dedicated survey papers [23, 27, 42, 53, 55, 57, 63].

Medical image segmentation methods range from simple thresholding, region growing, watershed, to more complicated approaches, e.g., deformable models, level set, graph cuts, and random walker. Depending on the application, a simple approach may meet the requirement. For example, thresholding followed by connected component analysis may be enough to segment a healthy lung in a CT scan, due to its typical dark appearance. However, in general, more sophisticated methods are often demanded to make a better use of the boundary and region information during segmentation.

Deformable models are a category of popular segmentation methods. For example, as a typical deformable model, the active contour [34] minimizes a predefined energy function to keep the balance between the external force (fitting the contour to the object boundary) and internal force (keeping the contour smooth). The active contour method is likely to get stuck in a local optimum and many variations have been proposed to improve its robustness, e.g., gradient vector flow (GVF) [75] and active balloons [9]. Refer to [53, 74] for more comprehensive reviews of the applications of deformable models to medical image segmentation.

The level set method [59] is closely related to the deformable models, however it has no explicit boundary representation. Instead, the boundary is embedded in an implicit function, which has negative values inside of the object, positive values outside, and a zero value for the object boundary. As an advantage over the active contour, the level set method can handle structural changes (splitting or merging of regions) during the boundary evolution.

Graph cuts are often employed to efficiently solve some global energy minimization problems, therefore have a wide variety of applications in computer vision since many problems can be formulated via energy minimization, e.g., image smoothing, stereo correspondence, and image segmentation. In a typical graph cuts based segmentation [5] we need to specify seed points inside the target object and some seeds outside. The optimal partition of all other pixels is achieved by a minimal-energy cut of the graph that separates the graph into unconnected foreground (target object) and background sets. Different to the deformable models and level set, graph cuts can achieve the global minimum of the energy function. However, the type of energy function that can be solved via graph cuts is limited [39]; therefore the global minimum often does not correspond to the best segmentation of the image from the clinical point of view.

The random walker algorithm [21] also needs some seed points with known labels (foreground or background). At each unlabeled pixel, we can imagine that a random walker is released and walks around according to an underlying probability distribution. If the random walker has a higher probability to first arrive a foreground seed point, this unlabeled pixel is assigned to foreground; otherwise, it is a background pixel. Similar to graph cuts, the random walker algorithm can also be formulated as a graph optimization problem.

All the above methods have difficulty to incorporate prior shape information, which is a major difference between medical image segmentation and general image segmentation. Note that there were a few attempts to incorporate the prior shape information in the deformable models [12] and level set [38]. However, there are still some limitations in these new algorithms.

In multiple clinical applications, there is often the need of a dedicated segmentation system for one specific organ scanned with a particular imaging protocol. There is a rich domain information (e.g., shape and appearance) available in such applications to improve the segmentation accuracy. The Active Shape Model (ASM) [11] is an elegant method to enforce prior shape constraints during boundary evolution. A statistical shape model is built during the training of the ASM, which generates a shape subspace spanned by a few major deformation modes. The boundary evolution is composed of a two-step iterative process: (1) adjusting the shape to fit the image boundary and (2) projecting the shape into the shape subspace to enforce the prior shape constraints. The Active Appearance Model (AAM) [10] is an extension of the ASM by incorporating the prior appearance constraints into the statistical model.

Note that all segmentation methods reviewed here need an accurate shape initialization either to avoid getting stuck in a local optimum (e.g., deformable models, level set, active shape models, and active appearance models) or to provide the initial seed points of the foreground and background (e.g., the graph cuts and random walker).

1.5   Marginal Space Learning

To accurately localize a 3D object, we need to estimate nine pose parameters: three
for position, three for orientation, and three for anisotropic scaling. As discussed
in Sect. 1.3, a straightforward extension of a 2D object detection method to 3D is
not possible due to the exponential increase in the computations, corresponding to
the exhaustive search. In this section we introduce the Marginal Space Learning
(MSL) [80, 81] as a generic learning based method for efficient 3D object detection.
Instead of exhaustively searching the original nine-dimensional pose parameter
space, only low-dimensional marginal spaces are searched in MSL, to improve the
detection speed.

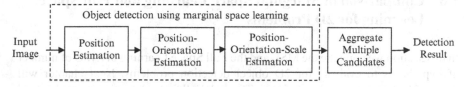

Fig. 1.3 Diagram for object detection using marginal space learning

The parameter estimation process is split into three steps, each with its own
set of classifiers: position estimation, position-orientation estimation, and position-
orientation-scale estimation (Fig. 1.3). First, we train a position estimator that is
testing if a certain location is a good estimate of the target object position in
an input volume. After exhaustively searching the three dimensional marginal
space of the position, we preserve a small number of position candidates with
the largest detection scores. Next, we perform joint position-orientation estimation
with a trained classifier that is testing if a position-orientation hypothesis is a
good estimate. The orientation marginal space is exhaustively searched for each
position candidate preserved after position estimation. Similarly, we only preserve
a limited number of position-orientation candidates after this step. Finally, the scale
parameters are searched in the constrained space in a similar way. Since after each
step, we only preserve a small number of candidates, a large portion of search space
with low posterior probability is pruned efficiently in the early steps. Due to this
pruning, MSL reduces the number of testing hypotheses by six orders of magnitude,
compared to the exhaustive full space search. The name "Marginal Space Learning"
is due to the learning and detection performed in a sequence of marginal spaces.

An efficient learning based detection method always comes with efficient image
features. Global features such as Haar wavelet features are effective to capture
the global information (e.g., orientation and scale) of an object. To capture the
orientation information of a hypothesis, we should rotate either the volume or the
feature templates. However, it is time consuming to rotate a 3D volume and there
are no efficient ways to rotate the Haar wavelet feature templates. Local features
are fast to evaluate but lose the global information of the whole object. We will

later on introduce a special set of features, called steerable features, which can capture the orientation and scale of the object and at the same time being efficient. In steerable features, we sample a few points from the volume under a sampling pattern. We then extract a few local features at each sampling point (e.g., voxel intensity and gradient). The novelty of our steerable features is that we embed the orientation and scale information into the distribution of the sampling points, while each individual feature is locally defined. Instead of aligning the volume to the hypothesized orientation, we steer the sampling pattern. In this way, we can combine the advantages of both global and local features. This is where the name "steerable features" comes from.

1.6 Comparison of Marginal Space Learning and Full Space Learning for 2D Problems

In this section we compare the MSL and the Full Space Learning in terms of number of hypotheses to evaluate for 2D object detection problems. Next chapter will discuss 3D detection and comparisons. Through Full Space Learning we understand exhaustive search, similarly to [72], the training and detection being performed in the full pose parameter space.

For 2D object detection, the degrees of freedom are five: two for location, two for scale and one for rotation. It is possible to create hypotheses in the full parameter space using a coarse-to-fine strategy. First, a coarse search step is used for each parameter to limit the number of hypotheses to a tractable level. Let us take a cardiac MRI example with a typical size of 300×200 pixels and define the problem of left ventricle (LV) detection. The search step for position can be set to as large as eight pixels to generate around 1,000 hypothesis for translation and the orientation search step is set to 20 degrees to generate 18 hypotheses for the whole orientation range. If we take about 10 hypotheses for each scale, the total number of resulting coarse hypotheses reaches 1.8 million. During the fine search step, we search around each candidate using a smaller search step, typically reduced by half with respect to the previous stage. This refinement procedure can be iterated several times until the search step is small enough.

In [87] we performed a thorough comparison for the task of LV detection in MRI. Experiments showed the MSL significantly outperforming the FSL on both training and test sets. The MSL was about eight times faster than the FSL, reducing the LV bounding box detection error by 78 %.

1.7 Constrained Marginal Space Learning

In terms of computational efficiency, the MSL can be improved since the lower dimension marginal spaces are still exhaustively searched.

The first improvement option is to use the training set to determine the distribution range of a parameter. During searching, each parameter is uniformly sampled within that range to generate testing hypotheses. Due to the heterogeneity in the capture range of the scanning protocols, the position of an organ may vary significantly in a volume. Nevertheless, the center of an organ cannot be arbitrarily close to the volume border. Using this observation, we can safely skip those hypotheses around volume border during object position estimation.

The second improvement is about exploiting the correlations existent among parameters in the same marginal space. For example, a larger object, like the heart of an adult, will probably have larger values in all dimensions when compared to a smaller object, like the heart of a baby. Independent sampling of each parameter will result in much more testing hypotheses than necessary. Because the detection speed is roughly proportional to the number of hypotheses, reducing the size of the testing hypothesis set can speed up the system. To constrain the number of hypotheses, we should only sample regions with large probabilities in the joint parameter space, using the information provided by the training set. It is, however, difficult to estimate the joint distribution since usually only a limited number of positive training samples (couple of hundreds) are available. To solve this problem and generate testing hypotheses, we use uniform kernels in the joint parameter space centered around the training samples, a process called *example-based sampling*. We first uniformly sample the marginal space to get a large set, S_u. For each training sample, we add its neighboring hypotheses in S_u to the test set S_t. Repeating the above process for all training samples and removing redundant hypotheses from S_t, we end up with a test set S_t much smaller than S_u.

Using the constrained marginal space learning with the changes discussed above, we can further improve the detection speed by order of magnitude [83]. Besides the speed-up, constraining the search to a small valid region can reduce the likelihood of detection outliers, thus improving the detection accuracy.

Finally, let us discuss the sampling of the orientation space. In the first version of MSL we used three Euler angles to represent the 3D orientation space [81]. This formulations has a number of limitations: (1) There are multiple configurations of the Euler angles that can yield the same orientation, leading to a fundamental ambiguity. (2) Although the Euclidean distance in the Euler angle space was used in [81] as the distance measurement between two orientations, the mapping from Euler angles to orientation space is not distance-preserving. In other words, uniform sampling in the Euler angle space is not uniform in the orientation space [40], this effect introducing degradations in the overall method [33].

In constrained MSL, we introduced the use of *quaternions* [33] to overcome the Euler angle limitations. Quaternions provide an elegant conceptual framework, handling simply and efficiently the problem of rotation and the distance between two orientations.

1.8   Marginal Space Learning for Nonrigid Object Detection

The MSL is often applied to provide an accurate initial shape estimate for nonrigid object segmentation in medical imaging. In this section, we discuss a couple of techniques to improve the shape initialization accuracy.

1.8.1   Optimal Mean Shape

After MSL based object pose estimation, we align the mean shape (which is trained on a set of example shapes) with the estimated translation, rotation, and scales as an initial shape. This initialization needs to be accurate; otherwise, the final boundary evolution may get stuck in a local minimum due to the complexity of the data.

The mean shape is generally calculated as the average of the normalized shapes in an object-oriented coordinate system. Therefore, the mean shape depends on the definition of the object-oriented coordinate system, which is often set heuristically. For example, in facial feature detection and face recognition, the face coordinate system is often determined by setting the left and right eyes to a normalized position [79]. In [81], the orientation of a heart chamber is defined by its long axis. The chamber center and scales are determined by the bounding box of the chamber surface mesh. Although working well in applications with relatively small shape variations, the mean shape derived using a heuristic object-oriented coordinate system is not optimal.

A better solution is to formulate the optimal mean shape $\bar{\mathbf{m}}$ according to generalized Procrustes analysis [14, 84, 85]. Let us define a group of training shapes, $\mathbf{M}_1, \mathbf{M}_2, \ldots, \mathbf{M}_N$, each shape being represented by J points $\mathbf{M}_i^j, j = 1, 2, \ldots, J$ with built-in point correspondence. The optimal mean shape $\bar{\mathbf{m}}$ should minimizes the residual errors after alignment,

$$\bar{\mathbf{m}} = arg\min_{\mathbf{m}} \sum_{i=1}^{N} \| \mathcal{T}_i(\mathbf{m}) - \mathbf{M}_i \|^2$$

$$= arg\min_{\mathbf{m}} \sum_{i=1}^{N} \sum_{j=1}^{J} \left\| \mathcal{T}_i(\mathbf{m}^j) - \mathbf{M}_i^j \right\|^2. \tag{1.1}$$

Here, $\mathcal{T}_i$ is the corresponding transformation from the mean shape $\bar{\mathbf{m}}$ to each individual shape $\mathbf{M}_i$. An iterative approach can be used to search for the optimal solution. First, we randomly pick an example shape as a mean shape. We then align each shape to the current mean shape. The average of the aligned shapes (the simple average of the corresponding points) is calculated as a new mean shape. The iterative procedure converges to a local optimal solution after a few iterations.

We use an anisotropic similarity transformation $\mathcal{T}$ to represent the transformation between two shapes. Since there are no closed-form solutions for estimating

$\mathscr{T}$ we designed a two-step iterative approach to search for the optimal transformation [84]. First, we calculate the isotropic similarity transformation using a closed-form solution [14]. In the second step, assuming that the isotropic similarity transformation is given, we estimate the optimal anisotropic ratios, for which we can derive a closed-form solution. The above two steps are iterated a few times. Experiments show that the optimal mean shape can reduce the initialization error by 17 % in segmenting the whole heart surface (see Chap. 6), compared to the bounding box based mean shape. Besides the optimal mean shape, the optimal alignment $\mathscr{T}$ from the mean shape to each training shape is also obtained. The transformation parameters of the optimal alignment provide the pose ground truth that the MSL can learn to estimate.

1.8.2 Direct Estimation of Nonrigid Deformation Parameters

The original MSL was proposed to estimate the rigid transformation (translation, rotation, and scaling) of an object [81]. To better localize a nonrigid object, we may need to further estimate its nonrigid deformation. The marginal space learning principle can be extended to directly estimate the nonrigid deformation parameters [82].

Using the statistical shape model, a nonrigid shape can be represented parametrically as $(\mathbf{T}, \mathbf{R}, \mathbf{S}, c_1, \ldots, c_K, \bar{\mathbf{m}}, \mathbf{e})$, where $\mathbf{T}, \mathbf{R}$, and $\mathbf{S}$ represent the translation, rotation, and scaling to transfer a nonrigid shape in the aligned shape space back to the world coordinate system; $c_1, \ldots, c_K$ are coefficients of the major deformation modes; $\bar{\mathbf{m}}$ is the mean shape calculated from a training set and is fixed during shape detection; $\mathbf{e}$ is the residual error and is sufficiently small if K is large enough (e.g., with enough training shapes). With this representation, we can convert the segmentation or boundary delineation problem to a parameter estimation problem. Among all these parameters, we only need to estimate $(\mathbf{T}, \mathbf{R}, \mathbf{S}, c_1, \ldots, c_K)$ by ignoring the small residual error $\mathbf{e}$. The original MSL only estimates the rigid part $(\mathbf{T}, \mathbf{R}, \mathbf{S})$ of the transformation. Here, we extend MSL to directly estimate the parameters of nonrigid deformation $(c_1, \ldots, c_K)$. Given a hypothesis $(\mathbf{T}, \mathbf{R}, \mathbf{S}, c_1, \ldots, c_K)$, we train a classifier based on a set of image features to distinguish a correct hypothesis from a wrong one. The image features should be a function of the hypothesis, $\mathscr{F} = \mathscr{F}(\mathbf{T}, \mathbf{R}, \mathbf{S}, c_1, \ldots, c_K)$, to incorporate sufficient information for classification.

Let us revisit now the steerable features. Their basic idea is to steer (translate, rotate, and scale) a sampling pattern w.r.t. the testing hypothesis. At each sampling point, a few local image features (e.g., intensity and gradient) are extracted. A regular sampling pattern was used in [81] to embed the object pose parameters $(\mathbf{T}, \mathbf{R}, \mathbf{S})$. Here, we need to also embed the nonrigid shape parameters $c_i, i = 1, \ldots, K$, into the sampling pattern. For this purpose, we use a sampling pattern based on the synthesized nonrigid shape. Each hypothesis $(\mathbf{T}, \mathbf{R}, \mathbf{S}, c_1, \ldots, c_K)$ corresponds to a nonrigid shape using the statistical shape model. We use this synthesized shape as the sampling pattern and extract the local image features at the deformed mesh points. If the shape is represented with J points and at each point we extract F features, we get a feature pool with $J \times F$ features. If the hypothesis is close to the ground truth, the sampling points should be close to the true object boundary. The image features (e.g., gradient of the image intensity) extracted on these sampling points can help us to distinguish it from a wrong hypothesis where the sampling points are far from the object boundary and likely to lie in a smooth region.

Experiments on liver detection demonstrated the effectiveness of the nonrigid MSL. Combined with constrained MSL, it reduced the shape initialization error by 11 % [82].

1.9   Other Extensions of Marginal Space Learning

The MSL is a generic approach and can be applied to detect different anatomical structures in various medical imaging modalities. It is also an open framework and multiple improvements can be incorporated to make it faster and more robust. In this section we discuss a few other extensions of the MSL.

The MSL is good at detecting a single object instance in an image since the pose candidates are likely concentrated on the most salient region. If we directly apply MSL to detect multiple instances of the same object type, for example detecting the spinal intervertebral disks, it may miss some true instances, especially when the number of instances are large, say, in the tens. For example, after position detection, if we keep 500 candidates, they might not be evenly distributed across disks. Some disks get more candidates than the others. After joint position-orientation estimation, we find that the candidates concentrated more on a few salient disks and some true disks have fewer or no detection hypotheses. Similarly, after joint position-orientation-scale estimation, the candidates can become even more skewed towards a few salient samples. This is the so-called *sample concentration* problem.

One straightforward solution is to increase the number of preserved candidates after each step. However, such approach contributes to an increase in the computational cost, which is proportional to the number of preserved candidates. To solve the sample concentration problem during the detection of multiple objects of the same type, we developed the iterated MSL [35,36]. After the position detection, we keep P candidates and only the top $N \ll P$ candidates are propagated to the MSL detection pipeline. We then use the detected instances (with all estimated parameters) to prune the original P position candidates by removing those candidates close to the already detected instances. The process is continued with a second iteration, by selecting the next top N remaining position candidates, which are propagated to detect more object instances. The iterations continue until there are no more preserved position candidates. It can be easily inferred that the iterated MSL overcomes the sample concentration issue of the original MSL, while keeping its efficiency.

A different setting is hierarchical MSL, where we perform learning and detection at different resolutions of a pyramid [69]. This strategy has been efficient for the detection of small and ambiguous objects, like the brain structures in fetal ultrasound volumes. There are many possible combinations to combine the MSL detection pipeline across the pyramid resolutions. For example, we can perform position detection at 4 mm resolution and keep a small number of candidates. These position candidates can be propagated to a higher resolution, e.g., 2 mm. If necessary, we train a classifier at 2 mm to verify the propagated candidates from a lower resolution. We then can do a joint position-orientation detection at 2 mm. Similarly, the final joint position-orientation-scale detection can be performed at an even higher resolution (e.g., 1 mm). Alternatively, the whole MSL detection pipeline can be performed at two different resolutions independently and be combined together to get the final detection score of a pose hypothesis.

Classifier ensemble is an active research topic in machine learning, being effective to increase the classification accuracy. The random forests classifier [6] is a known example in this class. It trains multiple decision trees with randomly selected training samples and randomly selected features. Using simple majority voting, the ensemble of decision trees can achieve significantly higher classification accuracy than each individual tree classifier. The robustness of hierarchical MSL can be explained due to its similarity to ensemble learning.

Let us now discuss object detection in spatio-temporal sequences. Multiple imaging modalities can capture dynamic sequences of an anatomical structure, e.g., a beating heart in a 3D ultrasound sequence. It is often required to detect/segment such anatomical structure in the whole sequence. We can process each frame independently or we perform detection in the first frame followed by tracking techniques to track the structure's motion along the sequence in the subsequent frames. However, such traditional methods are not optimal in using temporal information. In joint spatio-temporal MSL, we perform joint detection of the structure in the whole sequence [29, 30]. Unlike the independent detection method, we consider the temporal context of the anatomy. And, unlike the tracking method, all frames are equally treated.

The spatio-temporal MSL has been applied to the trajectory detection of a 3D anatomical landmark (of a heart valve) in a sequence. Due to repetitive nature of motion, we first perform Fourier analysis of the trajectory of the 3D landmark. The first a few frequency components can explain main course of the motion and approximate the trajectory. This is similar to nonrigid MSL, where we use the statistical shape model to concentrate the variations to a few major deformation modes, applying the MSL principle to estimate the corresponding deformation coefficients directly. In spatio-temporal MSL, we use the MSL principle to estimate the Fourier coefficients. Similarly to the nonrigid MSL, the steerable features framework is extended by the spatio-temporal MSL to capture the motion information.

1.10 Nonrigid Object Segmentation

In multiple applications, the ultimate goal is segmenting an anatomical structure. Although the MSL plays a key role in automatic object pose estimation and shape initialization, there are several other important components in building a robust segmentation system such as the accurate modeling of the anatomical structure and establishing mesh point correspondence to train an active shape model [11].

Let us take the heart chamber segmentation in cardiac CT as an example to illustrate the steps of the detection/segmentation framework. We employ a model based segmentation such that the anatomical information (e.g., landmarks) can be extracted from the model, after segmentation. To this end, we first need to build an anatomically accurate model to represent the target anatomy. If the shape is simple, we define a closed mesh to enclose the whole structure. If the shape is complex, like the right ventricle and heart valves, it might take some effort to build an accurate, part based mesh model. We also need a tool to annotate a sufficient number of training datasets, at least 50 for the beginning. After that, we establish the mesh point correspondence across volumes. This is necessary to calculate the mean shape and train the statistical shape model to enforce the prior shape constraint during the subsequent boundary evolution. For a few geometrically simple shapes (e.g., a tube, a parabola, and other rotation symmetric shapes), we use a mesh resampling technique to establish the mesh correspondence. In the case of a more complicated shape, we build a part based mesh model, by splitting the shape into a few parts, each one defined by a geometrically simple shape. For example, the right ventricle in our four-chamber heart model is split into three parts: the main body, inflow tract, and outflow tract [81].

During the automatic detection/segmentation, we first use MSL to estimate the pose of the target structure. We then align the mean shape with the estimated position, orientation, and scale (also a few major nonrigid deformation parameters estimated by nonrigid MSL, if applicable) as an initial estimate of the shape. We use the active shape model (ASM) [11] for the final refinement. However, we found that in many applications, the original non-learning based boundary detector in the ASM does not work well due to the potential weak boundary, noise, and artifacts. To compensate, we use a learning based boundary detector trained with the steerable features to guide the boundary evolution.

1.11 Applications of Marginal Space Learning

The MSL based detection and segmentation method is general and we have extensively tested it on multiple challenging 2D/3D tasks in medical imaging. Examples are interventional devices in fluoroscopy [24, 73], ileocecal valve [47] and liver [43] in abdominal CT, brain structures [69] in ultrasound, and heart chambers in CT [80], MRI [49], and ultrasound [48, 76]. In Chap. 8, we review the published work on MSL applications. In some applications, variants of the MSL are developed to further improve the detection speed and robustness. In others, the MSL is only a component, providing an estimate of the bounding box of an anatomical structure, and the contributions might cover other tasks, such as the segmentation and tracking of the target structure. We include such work in the review to illustrate the generalization capability of the MSL. Interested readers are referred to the corresponding publications for more details.

1.12 Organization of this Book

The basic idea of MSL is presented in Chap. 2 and a quantitative comparison between MSL and full space learning (FSL) is shown in Chap. 3. Chapter 4 presents the constrained MSL, which can significantly improve the method's efficiency by exploiting the correlation among pose parameters. Chapter 5 presents several part-based detection schemes that benefit from the fact that an object part is typically subject to less variability than the whole object. Technologies to improve the shape initialization accuracy for nonrigid object segmentation are described in Chap. 6. In Chap. 7, we present a generic automatic detection and segmentation framework, demonstrated on four-chamber heart segmentation in cardiac CT volumes. A comprehensive review of published applications of MSL is available in Chap. 8. Finally, in Chap. 9 we present a brief summary of our contributions and discuss the future work.

References

1. Arnoldi, E., Gebregziabher, M., Schoepf, U.J., Goldenberg, R., Ramos-Duran, L., Zwerner, P.L., Nikolaou, K., Reiser, M.F., Costello, P., Thilo, C.: Automated computer-aided stenosis detection at coronary CT angiography: Initial experience. European Radiology **20**(5), 1160–1167 (2009)
2. Ballard, D.H.: Generalizing the Hough transform to detect arbitrary shapes. Pattern Recognition **13**(2), 111–122 (1981)
3. von Berg, J., Lorenz, C.: Multi-surface cardiac modelling, segmentation, and tracking. In: Proc. Functional Imaging and Modeling of the Heart, pp. 1–11 (2005)
4. Bhargavan, M., Kaye, A.H., Forman, H.P., Sunshine, J.H.: Workload of radiologists in United States in 2006–2007 and trends since 1991–1992. Radiology **252**(2), 458–467 (2009)
5. Boykov, Y.Y., Jolly, M.P.: Interactive graph cuts for optimal boundary and region segmentation of objects in N-D images. In: Proc. Int'l Conf. Computer Vision, pp. 105–112 (2001)
6. Breiman, L.: Random forests. Machine Learning **45**(1), 5–32 (2001)
7. Budoff, M.J., Shinbane, J.S. (eds.): Cardiac CT Imaging: Diagnosis of Cardiovascular Disease, 2nd edn. Springer (2010)
8. Carneiro, G., Georgescu, B., Good, S., Comaniciu, D.: Detection of fetal anatomies from ultrasound images using a constrained probabilistic boosting tree. IEEE Trans. Medical Imaging **27**(9), 1342–1355 (2008)
9. Cohen, L.D.: On active contour models and balloons. CVGIP: Image Understanding **53**(2), 211–218 (1991)
10. Cootes, T.F., Edwards, G.J., Taylor, C.J.: Active appearance models. IEEE Trans. Pattern Anal. Machine Intell. **23**(6), 681–685 (2001)
11. Cootes, T.F., Taylor, C.J., Cooper, D.H., Graham, J.: Active shape models—their training and application. Computer Vision and Image Understanding **61**(1), 38–59 (1995)
12. Cremers, D., Tischhäuser, F., Weickert, J., Schnörr, C.: Diffusion snakes: Introducing statistical shape knowledge into the Mumford-Shah functional. Int. J. Computer Vision **50**, 295–313 (2002)
13. Dewan, M., Zhan, Y., Peng, Z., Zhou, X.S.: Robust algorithms for anatomic plane primitive detection in MR. In: Proc. of SPIE Medical Imaging, pp. 1–5 (2009)
14. Dryden, I.L., Mardia, K.V.: Statistical Shape Analysis. John Wiley, Chichester (1998)

15. Ecabert, O., Peters, J., H. Schramm et al.: Automatic model-based segmentation of the heart in CT images. IEEE Trans. Medical Imaging **27**(9), 1189–1201 (2008)
16. Ecabert, O., Peters, J., Weese, J.: Modeling shape variability for full heart segmentation in cardiac computed-tomography images. In: Proc. of SPIE Medical Imaging, pp. 1199–1210 (2006)
17. Fleischmann, D., Boas, F.E.: Computed tomography — old ideas and new technology. European Radiology **21**(3), 510–517 (2011)
18. Flohr, T.G., Schaller, S., Stierstorfer, K., Bruder, H., Ohnesorge, B.M., Schoepf, U.J.: Multi-detector row CT systems and image-reconstruction techniques. Radiology **235**(3), 756–773 (2005)
19. Funka-Lea, G., Boykov, Y., Florin, C., Jolly, M.P., Moreau-Gobard, R., Ramaraj, R., Rinck, D.: Automatic heart isolation for CT coronary visualization using graph-cuts. In: Proc. IEEE Int'l Sym. Biomedical Imaging, pp. 614–617 (2006)
20. de González, A.B., Mahesh, M., Kim, K.P., Bhargavan, M., Lewis, R., Mettler, F., Land, C.: Projected cancer risks from computed tomographic scans performed in the United States in 2007. Archives of Internal Medicine **169**(22), 2071–2077 (2009)
21. Grady, L.: Random walks for image segmentation. IEEE Trans. Pattern Anal. Machine Intell. **28**(11), 1768–1783 (2006)
22. Hamdan, A., Asbach, P., Wellnhofer, E., Klein, C., Gebker, R., Kelle, S., Kilian, H., Huppertz, A., Fleck, E.: A prospective study for comparison of MR and CT imaging for detection of coronary artery stenosis. JACC: Cardiovascular Imaging **4**(1), 50–61 (2011)
23. Heimann, T., Meinzer, H.P.: Statistical shape models for 3D medical image segmentation: A review. Medical Image Analysis **13**(4), 543–563 (2009)
24. Heimann, T., Mountney, P., John, M., Ionasec, R.: Learning without labeling: Domain adaptation for ultrasound transducer localization. In: Proc. Int'l Conf. Medical Image Computing and Computer Assisted Intervention, vol. 3, pp. 49–56 (2013)
25. Hjelmasa, E., Lowb, B.K.: Face detection: A survey. Computer Vision and Image Understanding **83**(3), 236–274 (2001)
26. Hough, P.V.C.: Machine analysis of bubble chamber pictures. In: Int'l Conf. High Energy Accelerators and Instrumentation, pp. 554–558 (1959)
27. Hu, Y.C., Grossberg, M., Mageras, G.: Survey of recent volumetric medical image segmentation techniques. In: C.A.B. de Mello (ed.) Biomedical Engineering, pp. 321–346. InTech (2009)
28. Hundley, W.G., Bluemke, D.A., Finn, J.P., Flamm, S.D., Fogel, M.A., Friedrich, M.G., Ho, V.B., Jerosch-Herold, M., Kramer, C.M., Manning, W.J., Patel, M., Pohost, G.M., Stillman, A.E., White, R.D., Woodard, P.K.: ACCF/ACR/AHA/NASCI/SCMR 2010 expert consensus document on cardiovascular magnetic resonance: A report of the American College of Cardiology Foundation Task Force on Expert Consensus Documents. Circulation **121**, 2462–2508 (2010)
29. Ionasec, R.I., Voigt, I., Georgescu, B., Wang, Y., Houle, H., Vega-Higuera, F., Navab, N., Comaniciu, D.: Patient-specific modeling and quantification of the aortic and mitral valves from 4D cardiac CT and TEE. IEEE Trans. Medical Imaging **29**(9), 1636–1651 (2010)
30. Ionasec, R.I., Wang, Y., Georgescu, B., Voigt, I., Navab, N., Comaniciu, D.: Robust motion estimation using trajectory spectrum learning: Application to aortic and mitral valve modeling from 4D TEE. In: Proc. Int'l Conf. Computer Vision, pp. 1601–1608 (2009)
31. John, M., Liao, R., Zheng, Y., Nottling, A., Boese, J., Kirschstein, U., Kempfert, J., Walther, T.: System to guide transcatheter aortic valve implantations based on interventional 3D C-arm CT imaging. In: Proc. Int'l Conf. Medical Image Computing and Computer Assisted Intervention, vol. 1, pp. 375–382 (2010)
32. Kalinic, K.: Atlas-based image segmentation: A survey. Technical Report (2008). URL http://bib.irb.hr/datoteka/435355.jnrl.pdf
33. Karney, C.F.F.: Quaternions in molecular modeling. Journal of Molecular Graphics and Modeling **25**(5), 595–604 (2007)

34. Kass, M., Witkin, A., Terzopoulos, D.: Snakes: Active contour models. Int. J. Computer Vision 1(4), 321–331 (1988)
35. Kelm, B.M., Wels, M., Zhou, S.K., Seifert, S., Suehling, M., Zheng, Y., Comaniciu, D.: Spine detection in CT and MR using iterated marginal space learning. Medical Image Analysis 17(8), 1283–1292 (2013)
36. Kelm, B.M., Zhou, S.K., Suehling, M., Zheng, Y., Wels, M., Comaniciu, D.: Detection of 3D spinal geometry using iterated marginal space learning. In: Proc. MICCAI Workshop Medical Computer Vision — Recognition Techniques and Applications in Medical Imaging, pp. 96–105 (2010)
37. Kelm, M., Mittal, S., Zheng, Y., Funka-Lea, G., Bernhardt, D., Vega-Higuera, F., Comaniciu, D.: Detection, grading and classification of coronary stenoses in computed tomography angiography. In: Proc. Int'l Conf. Medical Image Computing and Computer Assisted Intervention, vol. 3, pp. 25–32 (2011)
38. Kohlberger, T., Uzunbas, M.G., Alvino, C.V., Kadir, T., Slosman, D.O., Funka-Lea, G.: Organ segmentation with level sets using local shape and appearance priors. In: Proc. Int'l Conf. Medical Image Computing and Computer Assisted Intervention, vol. 2, pp. 34–42 (2009)
39. Kolmogorov, V., Zabih, R.: What energy functions can be minimized via graph cuts? IEEE Trans. Pattern Anal. Machine Intell. 26(2), 147–159 (2004)
40. Kuffner, J.J.: Effective sampling and distance metrics for 3D rigid body path planning. In: Proc. IEEE Int'l Conf. Robotics and Automation, pp. 3993–3998 (2004)
41. Kurtz, A.B.: The AIUM celebrates 50 years of excellence. Journal of Ultrasound in Medicine 22(6), 545–548 (2003)
42. Lenkiewicz, P., Pereira, M., Freire, M.M., Fernandes, J.: Techniques for medical image segmentation: Review of the most popular approaches. In: M. Pereira, M. Freire (eds.) Biomedical Diagnostics and Clinical Technologies: Applying High-Performance Cluster and Grid Computing, pp. 1–33. IGI Global (2011)
43. Ling, H., Zhou, S.K., Zheng, Y., Georgescu, B., Suehling, M., Comaniciu, D.: Hierarchical, learning-based automatic liver segmentation. In: Proc. IEEE Conf. Computer Vision and Pattern Recognition, pp. 1–8 (2008)
44. Lorenz, C., von Berg, J.: Towards a comprehensive geometric model of the heart. In: Proc. Functional Imaging and Modeling of the Heart, pp. 102–112 (2005)
45. Lorenz, C., von Berg, J.: A comprehensive shape model of the heart. Medical Image Analysis 10(4), 657–670 (2006)
46. Lorenzo-Valdés, M., Sanchez-Ortiz, G.I., Mohiaddin, R., Rueckert, D.: Atlas-based segmentation and tracking of 3D cardiac MR images using non-rigid registration. In: Proc. Int'l Conf. Medical Image Computing and Computer Assisted Intervention, vol. 1, pp. 642–650 (2002)
47. Lu, L., Barbu, A., Wolf, M., Liang, J., Salganicoff, M., Comaniciu, D.: Accurate polyp segmentation for 3D CT colonography using multi-staged probabilistic binary learning and compositional model. In: Proc. IEEE Conf. Computer Vision and Pattern Recognition, pp. 1–8 (2008)
48. Lu, X., Georgescu, B., Zheng, Y., Otsuki, J., Bennett, R., Comaniciu, D.: AutoMPR: Automatic detection of standard planes from three dimensional echocardiographic data. In: Proc. IEEE Int'l Sym. Biomedical Imaging, pp. 1279–1282 (2008)
49. Lu, X., Wang, Y., Georgescu, B., Littmann, A., Comaniciu, D.: Automatic delineation of left and right ventricles in cardiac MRI sequences using a joint ventricular model. In: Proc. Functional Imaging and Modeling of the Heart, pp. 250–258 (2011)
50. Lustig, M., Donoho, D., Pauly, J.M.: Sparse MRI: The application of compressed sensing for rapid MR imaging. Magnetic Resonance in Medicine 58(6), 1182–1195 (2007)
51. Matsumoto, T., Yoshimura, H., Giger, M.L., Doi, K., MacMahon, H., Montner, S.M., Nakanishi, T.: Potential usefulness of computerized nodule detection in screening programs for lung cancer. Invest. Radiol. 27(6), 471–475 (1992)
52. Mazziotta, J., Toga, A., A. Evans et al.: A probabilistic atlas and reference system for the human brain: International Consortium for Brain Mapping (ICBM). Phil. Tans. R. Soc. Lond. B 356, 1293–1322 (2001)

53. McInerney, T., Terzopoulos, D.: Deformable models in medical image analysis: A survey. Medical Image Analysis **1**(2), 91–108 (1996)
54. Mettler, F.A., Thomadsen, B.R., Bhargavan, M., Gilley, D.B., Gray, J.E., Lipoti, J.A., McCrohan, J., Yoshizumi, T.T., Mahesh, M.: Medical radiation exposure in the U.S. in 2006: Preliminary results. Health Physics **95**(5), 502–507 (2008)
55. Noble, J.A., Boukerroui, D.: Ultrasound image segmentation: A survey. IEEE Trans. Medical Imaging **25**(8), 987–1010 (2006)
56. Okada, T., Shimada, R., Sato, Y., Hori, M., Yokota, K., Nakamoto, M., Chen, Y.W., Nakamura, H., Tamura, S.: Automated segmentation of the liver from 3D CT images using probabilistic atlas and multi-level statistical shape model. In: Proc. Int'l Conf. Medical Image Computing and Computer Assisted Intervention, vol. 1, p. 86–93 (2007)
57. Olabarriaga, S., Smeulders, A.W.M.: Interaction in the segmentation of medical images: A survey. Medical Image Analysis **5**(2), 127–142 (2001)
58. Oren, M., Papageorgiou, C., Sinha, P., Osuna, E., Poggio, T.: Pedestrian detection using wavelet templates. In: Proc. IEEE Conf. Computer Vision and Pattern Recognition, pp. 193–199 (1997)
59. Osher, S., Fedkiw, R.: Level Set Methods and Dynamic Implicit Surfaces. Springer (2003)
60. Peng, Z., Zhan, Y., Zhou, X.S., Krishnan, A.: Robust anatomy detection from CT topograms. In: Proc. of SPIE Medical Imaging, pp. 1–8 (2009)
61. Perperidis, D., Lorenzo-Valdes, M., Chandrashekara, R., Rao, A., Mohiaddin, R., Sanchez-Ortiz, G.I., Rueckert, D.: Building a 4D atlas of the cardiac anatomy and motion using MR imaging. In: Proc. IEEE Int'l Sym. Biomedical Imaging, pp. 412–415 (2004)
62. Perperidis, D., Mohiaddin, R., Rueckert, D.: Construction of a 4D statistical atlas of the cardiac anatomy and its use in classification. In: Proc. Int'l Conf. Medical Image Computing and Computer Assisted Intervention, vol. 2, pp. 402–410 (2005)
63. Pham, D.L., Xu, C., Prince, J.L.: Current methods in medical image segmentation. Annual Review of Biomedical Engineering **2**, 315–337 (2000)
64. Pugliese, F., Hunink, M.G.M., Gruszczynska, K., Alberghina, F., Malago, R., van Pelt, N., Mollet, N.R., Cademartiri, F., Weustink, A.C., Meijboom, W.B., Witteman, C.L.M., de Feyter, P.J., Krestin, G.P.: Learning curve for coronary CT angiography: What constitutes sufficient training? Radiology **251**(2), 359–368 (2009)
65. Riederer, S.J.: New advances in MRI. In: Proc. Int'l Workshop Medical Imaging and Augmented Reality, pp. 1–9 (2004)
66. van Rikxoort, E.M., Isgum, I., Staring, M., Klein, S., van Ginneken, B.: Adaptive local multi-atlas segmentation: Application to heart segmentation in chest CT scans. In: Proc. of SPIE Medical Imaging, pp. 1–6 (2008)
67. Schramm, H., Ecabert, O., Peters, J., Philomin, V., Weese, J.: Towards fully automatic object detection and segmentation. In: Proc. of SPIE Medical Imaging, pp. 11–20 (2006)
68. Shoenhagen, P., White, R.D., Stillman, A.E., Halliburton, S.S.: Atlas and manual of cardiovascular multidetector computed tomography. Taylor and Francis (2005)
69. Sofka, M., Zhang, J., Zhou, S.K., Comaniciu, D.: Multiple object detection by sequential Monte Carlo and hierarchical detection network. In: Proc. IEEE Conf. Computer Vision and Pattern Recognition, pp. 1735–1742 (2010)
70. Steckner, M.: Advances in MRI equipment design, software, and imaging procedures. In: Proc. Annual Meeting AAPM, pp. 1–9 (2006)
71. Tu, Z., Zhou, X.S., Barbu, A., Bogoni, L., Comaniciu, D.: Probabilistic 3D polyp detection in CT images: The role of sample alignment. In: Proc. IEEE Conf. Computer Vision and Pattern Recognition, pp. 1544–1551 (2006)
72. Viola, P., Jones, M.: Rapid object detection using a boosted cascade of simple features. In: Proc. IEEE Conf. Computer Vision and Pattern Recognition, pp. 511–518 (2001)
73. Wang, P., Zheng, Y., John, M., Comaniciu, D.: Catheter tracking via online learning for dynamic motion compensation in transcatheter aortic valve implantation. In: Proc. Int'l Conf. Medical Image Computing and Computer Assisted Intervention, vol. 2, pp. 17–24 (2012)

74. Xu, C., Pham, D.L., Prince, J.L.: Medical image segmentation using deformable models. In: J. Fitzpatrick, M. Sonka (eds.) SPIE Handbook on Medical Imaging – Volume III: Medical Image Analysis, vol. 2, pp. 129–174. SPIE (2000)

75. Xu, C., Prince, J.L.: Snakes, shapes, and gradient vector flow,. IEEE Trans. Image Processing **7**(3), 359–369 (1998)

76. Yang, L., Georgescu, B., Zheng, Y., Meer, P., Comaniciu, D.: 3D ultrasound tracking of the left ventricles using one-step forward prediction and data fusion of collaborative trackers. In: Proc. IEEE Conf. Computer Vision and Pattern Recognition, pp. 1–8 (2008)

77. Yang, M.H., Kriegman, D., Ahuja, N.: Detecting faces in images: A survey. IEEE Trans. Pattern Anal. Machine Intell. **24**(1), 34–58 (2002)

78. Zhang, C., Zhang, Z.: A survey of recent advances in face detection. Technical Report MSR-TR-2010-66 (2010)

79. Zhao, W., Chellappa, R., Phillips, J., Rosenfeld, A.: Face recognition: A literature survey. ACM Computing Surveys **35**(4), 399–458 (2003)

80. Zheng, Y., Barbu, A., Georgescu, B., Scheuering, M., Comaniciu, D.: Fast automatic heart chamber segmentation from 3D CT data using marginal space learning and steerable features. In: Proc. Int'l Conf. Computer Vision, pp. 1–8 (2007)

81. Zheng, Y., Barbu, A., Georgescu, B., Scheuering, M., Comaniciu, D.: Four-chamber heart modeling and automatic segmentation for 3D cardiac CT volumes using marginal space learning and steerable features. IEEE Trans. Medical Imaging **27**(11), 1668–1681 (2008)

82. Zheng, Y., Georgescu, B., Comaniciu, D.: Marginal space learning for efficient detection of 2D/3D anatomical structures in medical images. In: Proc. Information Processing in Medical Imaging, pp. 411–422 (2009)

83. Zheng, Y., Georgescu, B., Ling, H., Zhou, S.K., Scheuering, M., Comaniciu, D.: Constrained marginal space learning for efficient 3D anatomical structure detection in medical images. In: Proc. IEEE Conf. Computer Vision and Pattern Recognition, pp. 194–201 (2009)

84. Zheng, Y., Georgescu, B., Vega-Higuera, F., Zhou, S.K., Comaniciu, D.: Fast and automatic heart isolation in 3D CT volumes: Optimal shape initialization. In: Proc. MICCAI Workshop Machine Learning in Medical Imaging, pp. 84–91 (2010)

85. Zheng, Y., John, M., Liao, R., Boese, J., Kirschstein, U., Georgescu, B., Zhou, S.K., Kempfert, J., Walther, T., Brockmann, G., Comaniciu, D.: Automatic aorta segmentation and valve landmark detection in C-arm CT: Application to aortic valve implantation. In: Proc. Int'l Conf. Medical Image Computing and Computer Assisted Intervention, vol. 1, pp. 476–483 (2010)

86. Zheng, Y., John, M., Liao, R., Nottling, A., Boese, J., Kempfert, J., Walther, T., Brockmann, G., Comaniciu, D.: Automatic aorta segmentation and valve landmark detection in C-arm CT for transcatheter aortic valve implantation. IEEE Trans. Medical Imaging **31**(12), 2307–2321 (2012)

87. Zheng, Y., Lu, X., Georgescu, B., Littmann, A., Mueller, E., Comaniciu, D.: Robust object detection using marginal space learning and ranking-based multi-detector aggregation: Application to automatic left ventricle detection in 2D MRI images. In: Proc. IEEE Conf. Computer Vision and Pattern Recognition, pp. 1343–1350 (2009)

Chapter 2
Marginal Space Learning

2.1 Introduction

Automatic detection of an anatomical structure (object) in medical images is a prerequisite for subsequent tasks such as recognition, segmentation, measurement, or motion tracking, and therefore has numerous applications. The goal of the detection is to estimate the position, orientation, and size of the target anatomical structure. The pose parameters can be represented as an oriented bounding box (to distinguish from an axis-aligned bounding box).

Recently, discriminative learning based approaches have been proved to be efficient and robust to detect 2D objects [14,31]. In these methods, object detection is formulated as a classification problem: whether an image window contains the target object or not [31]. During object detection, the pose parameter space is quantized into a large set of discrete hypotheses and each hypothesis is tested by a trained classifier to get a detection score. The hypotheses with the highest score are taken as the detection results. Exhaustive search for the best hypothesis makes the system robust under local optima. This search strategy is quite different from other parameter estimation approaches, such as deformable models, where an initial estimate is adjusted using the gradient descent techniques to optimize a predefined objective function.

There are two challenges to extend learning based object detection approaches to 3D. First, the number of hypotheses increases exponentially with respect to the dimensionality of the parameter space. Although the dimensionality of the image space only increases by one from 2D to 3D, the dimensionality of the pose parameter space increases from 5 to 9. For 2D object detection, there are five unknown parameters to be estimated or searched for from an input image, namely, translation in two directions, one rotation angle, and two scales. For 3D object detection, there are nine degrees of freedom for the anisotropic similarity transformation, namely three translation parameters, three rotation angles, and three scales. Note that the ordinary similarity transformation defines only isotropic scaling, corresponding to one scale parameter. However, to better cope with nonrigid deformations of the

Y. Zheng and D. Comaniciu, *Marginal Space Learning for Medical Image Analysis: Efficient Detection and Segmentation of Anatomical Structures,* DOI 10.1007/978-1-4939-0600-0_2, © Springer Science+Business Media New York 2014

target object, we use anisotropic scales. The number of hypotheses is an exponential function of the dimensionality of the pose parameter space. If each dimension is quantized to n discrete values, the number of hypotheses is n^9. For a very coarse estimation with $n = 10$, $n^9 = 1,000,000,000$ for 3D instead of $n^5 = 100,000$ for 2D. As a result, the computational demands for the 3D case present a challenge to the current desktop computers, to provide the testing results in a reasonable time. Even a five dimensional pose parameter space for a 2D object is already too large to achieve real-time performance. Note that for the 2D face detection example in [31], they only searched a three dimensional pose parameter space, two dimensions for position and one dimension for isotropic scaling, by constraining the face in an up-straight front view with a fixed aspect ratio.

The second challenge of extending the learning based object detection to 3D is that we need efficient features to search the orientation space. To perform a classification to an orientation hypothesis, the image features should be a function of the orientation hypothesis. Since we want to explicitly estimate the orientation of an object, rotation invariant features cannot be applied. There are two ways to embed the orientation information into image features, rotating either the feature template or the volume. Haar wavelet features can be efficiently computed under translation and scaling using the integral images [24, 31], but no efficient ways are available to rotate the Haar wavelet features. For 2D object detection, there is only one degree of freedom in rotation. It is possible to discretize orientation into a small number of categories, e.g., $10°$ of incremental rotation in $[0, 360°)$, resulting in 36 orientations. The input image is rotated accordingly for each orientation category to generate a set of rotated images. A detector is trained under one fixed orientation and is applied to all the rotated images to detect an object with different orientations [8]. However, a 3D volume contains much more data; therefore, it is very time consuming to rotate the volume. The computation time to rotate a volume with $512 \times 512 \times 512$ voxels is equivalent to rotate 512 images each with 512×512 pixels. Furthermore, there are three degrees of freedom in 3D rotations. To cover the full orientation space with a sampling resolution of $9.72°$, we need 7416 discrete orientation hypotheses [18]. Since volume rotation is time consuming, it is impractical to perform thousands of volume rotations for orientation estimation.

This chapter presents solutions to the two challenges discussed above. First, it introduces an efficient 3D learning-based object detection method, called Marginal Space Learning (MSL). The idea of MSL is to avoid learning in the full similarity transformation space by incrementally learning classifiers in marginal spaces of lower dimensions. The estimation of an object's pose is split into three problems: position estimation, position-orientation estimation, and position-orientation-scale estimation. This incremental learning approach contributes to a highly efficient object detection paradigm. Second, we introduce the steerable features, as a mechanism to search the orientation space, thus avoiding expensive volume/image rotations. The idea is to sample points (voxels) from a given volume under a sampling pattern that embeds the position, orientation, and scale information of a pose hypothesis. Each sample point is associated with a set of local features such as local intensity and gradient. The efficiency of steerable features comes from the fact that much fewer points (defined by the sampling pattern) are needed for manipulation, in comparison to the whole volume.

The remainder of this chapter is organized as follows. In Sect. 2.2, we present the whole MSL workflow, including the derivation of the pose parameter ground truth from a training set with annotated meshes, training of each individual pose parameter estimator, and aggregation of multiple pose candidates to achieve a consolidated estimate of the object. We then discuss implementation details, introducing 3D image features in Sect. 2.3 and the Probabilistic Boosting-Tree (PBT) classifier in Sect. 2.4. In Sect. 2.5, we use automatic 3D heart chamber detection in CT volumes as an example to demonstrate the efficiency and robustness of MSL. In Sect. 2.6, we extend the MSL principle to directly estimate nonrigid deformation parameters to further improve the shape initialization accuracy for nonrigid object segmentation. In Sect. 2.7, we provide theoretical justifications of MSL and link it to the shortest path computation in graph search. The MSL is shown to be an efficient breadth-first beam search in the posterior probability of the pose parameter space. This chapter concludes with Sect. 2.8.

2.2 3D Object Detection Using Marginal Space Learning

For an in-depth understanding of this section, we refer the reader to earlier learning based object detection publications [14, 29, 31].

2.2.1 Derivation of Object Pose Ground Truth From Mesh

To train object detection classifiers, we need a set of 3D volumes, called the training set. The volumes in the training set are typically converted to a low isotropic resolution (e.g., 3 mm). For each volume, we need a nine dimensional vector of the ground truth about the position, orientation, and size of the target object in the volume. These nine pose parameters can be visually represented as a bounding box of the object. In some applications, the pose parameters are readily available from the annotation of the image data. This is especially common for 2D object detection since it is easy to draw a bounding box of the target object. However, drawing a 3D bounding box aligned with the orientation of the 3D object is not trivial. It is more convenient to annotate a few landmarks of the object and derive a box from the landmarks. Alternatively, since in many applications, the accurate object segmentation is the ultimate goal, a 3D surface mesh is annotated by experts for each volume in the training set, either manually or semi-automatically. In the following, we present an ad-hoc method to derive the 3D pose parameters/bounding box of a surface mesh. This is an intuitive solution, but by no means optimal.

In Chap. 6, we present a more theoretically founded solution to derive optimal nine pose parameters from a set of 3D meshes to minimize the mesh initialization error after pose estimation.

The object orientation cannot be easily derived from a 3D mesh. Different methods are often demanded to define the orientation of different target objects. Many anatomies have an intrinsic, well-accepted orientation definition. For example, the orientation of the heart chambers, defined by the long axis and short axis, is documented in detail by the echocardiography community [17]. In the heart chamber segmentation application [33, 34], we use the long axis of a chamber as the z axis. The perpendicular direction from a predefined anchor point to the long axis defines axis x. For different chambers, we have freedom to select the anchor point, as long as it is consistent. For example, for the left ventricle, we can use the aortic valve center as the anchor point. The third axis y is the cross-product of axes z and x. A 3×3 rotation matrix $\mathbf{R}$ is determined using the x, y, and z axis as the first, second, and last column of $\mathbf{R}$, respectively. An orientation hypothesis is represented as three Euler angles, ψ^t, ϕ^t, and θ^t, which can be derived from the rotation matrix $\mathbf{R}$ using the following relationship

$$\mathbf{R} = \begin{bmatrix} \cos\psi\cos\phi - \cos\theta\sin\phi\sin\psi & \cos\psi\sin\phi + \cos\theta\cos\phi\sin\psi & \sin\psi\sin\theta \\ -\sin\psi\cos\phi - \cos\theta\sin\phi\cos\psi & -\sin\psi\sin\phi + \cos\theta\cos\phi\cos\psi & \cos\psi\sin\theta \\ \sin\theta\sin\phi & -\sin\theta\cos\phi & \cos\theta \end{bmatrix}. \quad (2.1)$$

We then calculate a bounding box aligned with the object-oriented local coordinate system for the mesh points. The bounding box center gives us the position ground truth X^t, Y^t, and Z^t, and the box size along each side defines the ground truth of scaling S_x^t, S_y^t, and S_z^t, respectively.

For object segmentation, we also need to calculate the mean shape from the training set so that after object pose estimation we can align the mean shape to get an initial estimate of the true shape. For a target object, using the above bounding box based method, we calculate its position ($\mathbf{T} = [X, Y, Z]'$), orientation (represented as a rotation matrix $\mathbf{R}$), and anisotropic scaling ($\mathbf{S} = [S_x, S_y, S_z]'$). We then transform each point from the world coordinate system, $\mathbf{M}_{world}$, to the object-oriented coordinate system, $\mathbf{m}_{object}$, and calculate the average over the whole training set to get a mean shape. Here, we assume that the training shapes have intrinsic mesh point correspondence, namely, each mesh has the same number of points and the same point index in different meshes corresponds to the same anatomy. The transformation between $\mathbf{M}_{world}$ and $\mathbf{m}_{object}$ is

$$\mathbf{M}_{world} = \mathbf{R} \begin{bmatrix} S_x & 0 & 0 \\ 0 & S_y & 0 \\ 0 & 0 & S_z \end{bmatrix} \mathbf{m}_{object} + \mathbf{T}. \quad (2.2)$$

Reversing the transformation, we can calculate the position in the object-oriented coordinate system as

$$\mathbf{m}_{object} = \begin{bmatrix} \frac{1}{S_x} & 0 & 0 \\ 0 & \frac{1}{S_y} & 0 \\ 0 & 0 & \frac{1}{S_z} \end{bmatrix} \mathbf{R}^{-1} \left(\mathbf{M}_{world} - \mathbf{T} \right). \tag{2.3}$$

The mean shape is the average over the whole training set

$$\bar{\mathbf{m}} = \frac{1}{N} \sum_{i=1}^{N} \mathbf{m}_{object}^{i}, \tag{2.4}$$

where N is the number of training samples.

2.2.2 Principle of Marginal Space Learning

Figure 2.1 shows the basic idea of machine learning based 3D object detection. First, we train a classifier, which assigns a score in the range [0, 1] to each input hypothesis about the object pose. We then quantize the full pose parameter space into a large number of hypotheses. Depending on the quantization resolution, the number of hypotheses can easily reach an order over 1 billion. Each hypothesis is tested with the classifier to get a score. Based on the classification scores, we select the best one or several hypotheses. We may need to aggregate multiple best hypotheses into a final single detection result. Unlike the gradient based search in deformable models or Active Appearance Models (AAM) [4], the classifier in this framework acts as a black box without an explicit closed-form objective function.

As we discussed, one drawback of the learning based approach is that the number of hypotheses increases exponentially with respect to the dimensionality of the parameter space. Nevertheless, in many applications, the posterior distribution is clustered in a small region in the high dimensional parameter space. Therefore, the uniform and exhaustive search is not necessary and wastes the computational power.

The MSL is an efficient method to partition such parameter space, by gradually increasing the dimensionality of the search space. Let Ω be the space where the solution to the given problem exists and let P_Ω be the true probability distribution that needs to be learned. The learning and computation are performed in a sequence of marginal spaces

$$\Omega_1 \subset \Omega_2 \subset \ldots \subset \Omega_n = \Omega \tag{2.5}$$

such that Ω_1 is a low dimensional space (e.g., three-dimensional translation instead of nine-dimensional similarity transformation), and for each k, $\dim(\Omega_k) - \dim(\Omega_{k-1})$ is small. A search in the marginal space Ω_1 using the learned probability model finds a subspace $\Pi_1 \subset \Omega_1$ containing the most probable values and discards the rest of the space. The restricted marginal space Π_1 is then extended to $\Pi_1^e = \Pi_1 \times X_1 \subset \Omega_2$. Another stage of learning and testing is performed on Π_1^e obtaining

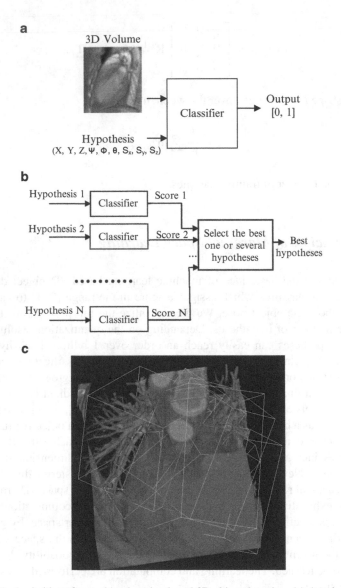

Fig. 2.1 The basic idea of a machine learning based 3D object detection. (**a**) A trained classifier assigns a score to a pose hypothesis. (**b**) The pose parameter space is quantized into a large number of discrete hypotheses and the classifier is used to select the best hypotheses through exhaustive search. (**c**) A few pose hypotheses of the left ventricle (represented as boxes) embedded in a CT volume. ©2008 IEEE. Reprinted, with permission, from Zheng, Y., Barbu, A., Georgescu, B., Scheuering, M., Comaniciu, D.: Four-chamber heart modeling and automatic segmentation for 3D cardiac CT volumes using marginal space learning and steerable features. *IEEE Trans. Medical Imaging* **27**(11), 1668–1681 (2008)

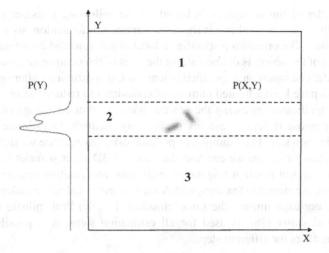

Fig. 2.2 Marginal space learning to search the peaks of the joint distribution $p(x,y)$. A classifier trained on a marginal distribution $p(y)$ can quickly eliminate a large portion (regions 1 and 3) of the search space. Another classifier is then trained on a restricted space (region 2) for the joint distribution $p(x,y)$. ©2008 IEEE. Reprinted, with permission, from Zheng, Y., Barbu, A., Georgescu, B., Scheuering, M., Comaniciu, D.: Four-chamber heart modeling and automatic segmentation for 3D cardiac CT volumes using marginal space learning and steerable features. *IEEE Trans. Medical Imaging* **27**(11), 1668–1681 (2008)

a restricted marginal space $\Pi_2 \subset \Omega_2$ and the procedure is repeated until the full space Ω is reached. At each step, the restricted space Π_k is one or two orders of magnitude smaller than $\Pi_{k-1} \times X_k$. This results in a very efficient algorithm with minimal loss in performance.

Figure 2.2 illustrates a simple example for 2D space search. A classifier trained on $p(y)$ can quickly eliminate a large portion of the search space. We can then train a classifier in a much smaller region (region 2 in Fig. 2.2) for the joint distribution $p(x,y)$. Note that MSL is significantly different from a classifier cascade [31]. In a cascade the learning and search are performed in the same space while for MSL the learning and search space is gradually increased.

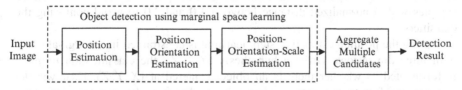

Fig. 2.3 Diagram for 3D object detection using marginal space learning

Let us describe now the general idea of the MSL for 3D object detection. As shown in Fig. 2.3, we split 3D object detection into three steps: position estimation, position-orientation estimation, and position-orientation-scale estimation. The searching order of the subspaces is based on the following considerations. The position of the object in a volume is the most important information, so it should be determined first. The orientation specifies a local object-oriented coordinate system and the scale of the object is defined along the axes of the coordinate system. Since the scale is defined based on a specified orientation, it is estimated after orientation. After each step we keep a limited number of candidates to reduce the search space.

Besides significantly reducing the search space, another advantage of the MSL is that we can use different features or learning methods to estimate the pose parameters in each step. For example, in position estimation, since we treat rotation as an intra-class variation, we can use the efficient 3D Haar wavelet features. In the following steps of position-orientation estimation and position-orientation-scale estimation, we use steerable features, which are efficient to calculate under rotations. Although in our experiments, the same classifier, i.e., the Probabilistic Boosting-Tree (PBT) classifier [28], is used for all estimation steps, it is possible to use different classifiers for different steps.

2.2.3 Training of Position Estimator

To train a classifier, we need to split hypotheses into two groups, positive and negative, based on their distance to the ground truth. The error in object position and scale estimation is not comparable with that of orientation estimation. Therefore, a search-step-normalized distance measure is defined by normalizing the error in each dimension to the corresponding search step size,

$$E = \max_{i=1,\ldots,D} |P_i^e - P_i^t|/\text{SearchStep}_i, \qquad (2.6)$$

where P_i^e is the estimated value for parameter i; P_i^t is the corresponding ground truth; and D is the dimension of the parameter space. For 3D similarity transformation estimation, the pose parameter space is nine dimensional, $D = 9$. A sample is regarded as a positive one if $E \leq 1.0$ or a negative one if $E > 2.0$. The distance from a hypothesis to the ground truth takes a continuous value. It is difficult to draw a clear line to separate positive and negative samples. We intentionally discard samples with a normalized distance between 1.0 and 2.0 to avoid confusing the classifiers.

During the position estimation step, learning is constrained in a marginal space with three dimensions. Given a hypothesis (X, Y, Z), the classification problem is formulated as whether there is an object centered at (X, Y, Z). Haar wavelet features are fast to compute and have been shown to be effective for many applications [24, 31]. Therefore, we extended the Haar wavelet features to 3D to be used for learning in this step. Please refer to Sect. 2.3.1 for more information about Haar wavelet features. Note that we tried a position estimator using steerable features and its performance was slightly worse than the Haar wavelet features on some applications, an expected result.

The search step for position estimation is one voxel. According to Eq. (2.6), a positive sample (X, Y, Z) should satisfy

$$\max\{|X - X^t|, |Y - Y^t|, |Z - Z^t|\} \leq 1 \text{ voxel}, \tag{2.7}$$

where (X^t, Y^t, Z^t) is the ground truth of the object center. Normally, there are $2^3 = 8$ position candidates for each training volume satisfying Eq. (2.7) if the position ground truth X^t, Y^t, and Z^t are not on the imaging grid (e.g., $X^t = 45.2$ voxels). If the ground truth is lying on the imaging grid (e.g., $X^t = 45$ voxels), we may have up to $3^3 = 27$ positive position hypotheses for each training volume.

A negative sample is one with

$$\max\{|X - X^t|, |Y - Y^t|, |Z - Z^t|\} > 2 \text{ voxels}. \tag{2.8}$$

Normally, we have far more negative samples than positive ones. The classifier should have the capability to handle such a significantly skewed distribution of positive and negative samples; otherwise, we have to randomly sample roughly the same number of negative samples to match the positive samples.

The Probabilistic Boosting-Tree (PBT) [28] classifier used in most of our experiments has no difficulty to handle uneven distributions of positive and negative samples; therefore, it does not impose constraints on the cardinality of the sample sets.

However, in some applications we still have to subsample the negative samples because of the memory constraints of a desktop computer. On a 32-bit Windows operating system, the maximum amount of memory a program can use is bounded to 2 GB and can be increased to 3 GB with a special setting of Windows, which still limits the number of negative samples that can be loaded into memory. Normally, we train the classifiers on a 64-bit Windows systems with sufficient amount of memory (we tried up to 72 GB of memory). In addition, the memory constraint can be further alleviated by using a computer cluster or a connection to a cloud system.

We often set an upper limit for negative samples (e.g., 10 million) since we need a reasonable speed for the training process. Our training software first gets a rough estimate of the total number of negative samples. If the result is smaller than the upper limit, no sub-sampling is applied; otherwise, we randomly subsample the negative samples to match that limit. We found through experiments that increasing the number of positive samples by adding more training datasets improves substantially the generalization capability of the trained classifiers. Increasing the number of negative samples also helps, however, after a certain level, no further improvement is observed; therefore, random sub-sampling of the negative samples with our current setting (10 million) does not deteriorate the performance of the classifiers.

Given a set of positive and negative training samples, we extract 3D Haar wavelet features and train a classifier (e.g., the PBT). After that, we test each voxel in a volume one by one as a hypothesis of the object position using the trained classifier.

As shown in Fig. 2.1a, the classifier assigns each hypothesis a score, and we preserve a small number of candidates (100 in our experiments) with the highest detection score for each volume.

There are various ways to select candidates for the following steps. The first approach is based on the detection score: we keep those candidates with a detection score larger than a threshold. One problem with this approach is that the number of candidates retained varies from volume to volume with a fixed threshold. For a volume with bad image quality, we may find no candidates with a detection score larger than a preset threshold. In many applications, we know there is one and only one target anatomy in a volume. Thus, we select a fixed number of candidates that have the highest detection probability. This approach is more robust and the overall detection speed is consistent from volume to volume.

Sometimes, there may be multiple hypotheses ranking around the cutoff line. For example, if we want to keep 100 hypotheses, we may get five hypotheses with the same score ranking at the 100th. Randomly selecting one from these five hypotheses may introduce randomness in the final detection results, while selecting with a fixed heuristic rule (e.g., selecting the one with the smallest z position) may introduce bias. In our work, we keep all hypotheses ranking around the cutoff line; therefore, the actual number of retained candidates may be slightly larger.

2.2.4   Training of Position-Orientation Estimator

In this step, the task is to jointly estimate the position and orientation. The classification problem is formulated as whether there is an object centered at (X, Y, Z) with orientation (ψ, ϕ, θ). After object position estimation, we preserve the top 100 candidates, (X_i, Y_i, Z_i), $i = 1, \ldots, 100$. Since we want to estimate both the position and orientation, we need to augment the dimension of candidates. For each position candidate, we quantize the orientation space uniformly to generate hypotheses. In the experiments on heart chamber detection (see Sect. 2.5), the orientation is represented as three Euler angles in the ZXZ convention, ψ, ϕ, and θ. The distribution range of an Euler angle is estimated from the training data. Each Euler angle is quantized within the range using a step size of 0.2 radians (11 degrees). For each position candidate (X_i, Y_i, Z_i), we augment it with N (about 1,000) hypotheses of orientation, $(X_i, Y_i, Z_i, \psi_j, \phi_j, \theta_j)$, $j = 1, \ldots, N$. Some position-orientation hypotheses are close to the ground truth (positive) and others are far away (negative).

The learning goal is to distinguish the positive and negative samples using a trained classifier. Using the normalized distance measure of Eq. (2.6), a hypothesis $(X, Y, Z, \psi, \phi, \theta)$ is regarded as a positive sample if it satisfies both Eqs. (2.7) and

$$\max\{|\psi - \psi^t|, |\phi - \phi^t|, |\theta - \theta^t|\} \le 0.2, \qquad (2.9)$$

where $(\psi^t, \phi^t, \theta^t)$ represent the orientation ground truth. A negative sample has either a large position error, satisfying Eq. (2.8), or a large orientation error,

$$\max\{|\psi - \psi^t|, |\phi - \phi^t|, |\theta - \theta^t|\} > 0.4. \tag{2.10}$$

To capture the orientation information, we have to rotate either the volume or feature templates. We use the steerable features (refer to Sect. 2.3.2), which are efficient to extract under rotation. Similarly, the PBT is used for training and the trained classifier is used to prune the hypotheses to preserve only a few candidates (50 in our experiments).

In the above procedure, the positive/negative training samples of the position-orientation classifier are generated from the augmented position candidates. On some datasets, a couple of good position hypotheses that satisfy Eq. (2.7) may be missed after position estimation. We could add them back to generate more position-orientation hypotheses. However, through comparison experiments, we did not find noticeable improvement in the generalization capability of the trained position-orientation estimator. Therefore, the missed good position candidates are not added back during training. Generally, how the classifier is trained should match how the classifier is used. It is preferable to have the same pose hypothesis generation scheme for both the training and testing procedures since during the testing on an unseen volume, we cannot add missed good position candidates back to generate position-orientation hypotheses.

2.2.5   Training of Position-Orientation-Scale Estimator

The training of the position-orientation-scale estimator is analogous to that of the position-orientation estimator except learning is performed in the full nine dimensional similarity transformation space. The dimension of each retained position-orientation candidate is augmented by searching the scale subspace uniformly and exhaustively. The scale search step is set to two voxels. That means a hypothesis $(X, Y, Z, \psi, \phi, \theta, S_x, S_y, S_z)$ is regarded as a positive sample if, in addition to Eqs. (2.7) and (2.9), it satisfies

$$\max\{|S_x - S_x^t|, |S_y - S_y^t|, |S_z - S_z^t|\} \leq 2 \text{ voxels}, \tag{2.11}$$

where (S_x^t, S_y^t, S_z^t) represent the scale ground truth. A negative sample has a large error in position (Eq. (2.8)), orientation (Eq. (2.10)), or scale

$$\max\{|S_x - S_x^t|, |S_y - S_y^t|, |S_z - S_z^t|\} > 4 \text{ voxels}. \tag{2.12}$$

2.2.6 Aggregation of Pose Candidates

The goal of object detection is to obtain a single aggregated estimate of the pose parameters of the object. Multiple detections usually occur around the true object pose since the MSL detectors are insensitive to small changes in the pose parameters. Occasionally, false positives may appear. Some false positives are scattered sparsely, while others may be concentrated around a region that appears similar to the target object.

Intuitively, cluster analysis might help to remove sparsely distributed false positives. However, it is very difficult to perform cluster analysis on a small set of top candidates (e.g., 100) in a nine dimensional pose parameter space. Furthermore, the orientation is represented in a completely different space to the position and scale. To perform clustering we need a distance measurement combining the distances in different marginal spaces. The orientation distance measure needs to be weighted properly to be combined with the position and scale distances. Through experiments, we found that clustering did not improve the accuracy, compared to a simple averaging of the top K $(K = 100)$ candidates.

Since each pose candidate has a classification score given by the PBT classifier, we tried a weighted average scheme by assigning a larger weight to a pose candidate with a higher classification score. However, we did not find significant difference to a simple unweighted average.

The robustness of the aggregation with simple averaging is partially explained by the fact that there are far more good pose hypotheses in 3D than 2D. An exponential increase of pose hypotheses for 3D objection detection also comes with a lot of good hypotheses. For example, there are at least $2^9 = 512$ hypotheses within one search step size from the ground truth. If we include hypotheses within an error of two search step sizes, the total number of good hypotheses increases dramatically to $4^9 = 262,144$. By exploiting the rich image information in a 3D volume and the state-of-the-art learning algorithms, our MSL detectors perform quite well. Most of the preserved top 100 pose candidates are good and the small portion of outliers does not affect too much the detection accuracy after averaging.

Note that the average based aggregation only works if we know a priori that there is only a single instance of the object in the volume. If there might be multiple instances of the same object type (e.g., intervertebral disks of the spine), cluster analysis should be used to select multiple final detection results [19, 20]. To avoid the sparse-sample issue in a high dimensional space, clustering is often performed only for the position component of the pose candidates.

2.2.7 Object Detection in Unseen Volume

This section provides a summary of the testing procedure on an unseen volume. The input volume is first converted to a low isotropic resolution (e.g., 3 mm) matching the volumes in the training set. All voxels are tested using the trained position estimator and the top 100 candidates, (X_i, Y_i, Z_i), $i = 1,\ldots,100$, are kept. Each candidate is augmented with N (about 1,000) hypotheses of orientation, $(X_i, Y_i, Z_i, \psi_j, \phi_j, \theta_j)$, $j = 1,\ldots,N$. Next, the trained position-orientation classifier is used to prune these $100 \times N$ hypotheses and the top 50 candidates are retained, $(\hat{X}_i, \hat{Y}_i, \hat{Z}_i, \hat{\psi}_i, \hat{\phi}_i, \hat{\theta}_i)$, $i = 1,\ldots,50$. Similarly, we augment each candidate with M (also about 1,000) hypotheses of scaling and use the trained position-orientation-scale classifier to rank these $50 \times M$ hypotheses. The average of the top K ($K = 100$) candidates is taken as the final aggregated estimate.

In the following, we analyze the computational complexity of heart chamber detection from a cardiac CT volume [34]. For position estimation, all voxels (about 260,000 voxels for a small volume with $64 \times 64 \times 64$ voxels at the 3 mm resolution) are tested for possible object position. There are about 1,000 hypotheses for orientation and scale each. If the parameter space is searched uniformly and exhaustively, there are about 2.6×10^{11} hypotheses to be tested! However, using MSL, we only test about $260,000 + 100 \times 1,000 + 50 \times 1,000 = 4.1 \times 10^5$ hypotheses and reduce the testing by almost six orders of magnitude.

In practice, an irrelevant volume might be fed into the automatic detection and segmentation system due to mis-labeling. For example, the input data to a heart chamber segmentation system may be an abdominal scan without the heart in the volume at all. There are different strategies to handle such situation.

One is the "garbage-in garbage-out" principle, in which the algorithm just tries its best to produce the best segmentation it can achieve. All segmentation results will eventually be double checked by a physician and a non-meaningful segmentation result on a wrong input data can be easily identified and discarded. In the second strategy, the automatic segmentation algorithm is expected to intelligently tell if a target anatomy is present in the data or not. Depending on the presence or absence of the target anatomy, different processing workflows may be invoked later on. In such scenario, a threshold can be set to reject a wrong input. For example, we check the maximum detection score of the preserved position candidates. If it is less than a preset threshold, the data is rejected. Normally, we set the threshold very low to avoid rejecting a good input data. Wrong results can later be rejected in the subsequent detection pipelines, e.g., position-orientation estimation and position-orientation-scale estimation.

2.3 3D Image Features

The MSL is an open and flexible object detection framework. Any image features can be integrated into the framework as long as they can provide some information to discriminate between positive and negative hypotheses. In this section, we present two kinds of 3D image features used in a specific implementation of MSL for heart chamber detection in cardiac CT volumes (as presented in Sect. 2.5). The Haar wavelet features are used for object position estimation and the steerable features, capable of encoding the orientation hypothesis, are used for position-orientation estimation and position-orientation-scale estimation. In fact, these two kinds of features work well on multiple object detection problems in major imaging modalities, including ultrasound data.

2.3.1 3D Haar Wavelet Features

Haar wavelet features were first proposed for object detection by Oren et al. [24]. Figure 2.4a shows a few Haar feature templates, where the value of the feature is calculated by subtracting the sum of pixel intensity inside the dark boxes from the sum of pixel intensity of the bright boxes. Different to the Haar wavelet basis

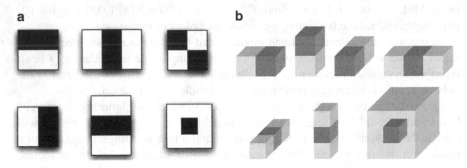

Fig. 2.4 Haar wavelet features are calculated by subtracting the sum of pixel intensity inside the dark boxes from the sum of pixel intensity of the bright boxes. (**a**) A few 2D Haar feature templates. (**b**) A few 3D Haar feature templates

functions, Haar features are an open feature family and basically any configuration of the dark and bright boxes can be used, e.g., two-box, three-box, and four-box feature templates as shown in Fig. 2.4a. By translating and scaling the feature templates over the image, we can generate a huge number of image features. Therefore, Haar features are often over-complete and not restricted to the complete linearly-independent Haar wavelet basis functions. Haar features were made popular by [31] with introduction of the integral image, which contributed to a fast computation of Haar features. Using the integral image, the computation of the sum of pixel intensity inside a rectangle at any position and size only involves addition or subtraction of four elements of the integral image (as shown in Fig. 2.5). The computation time is constant no matter how large the rectangle is.

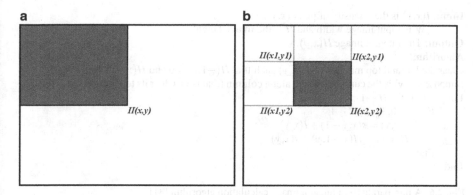

Fig. 2.5 2D integral image for efficient calculation of the sum of intensity of pixels inside a box. (**a**) Each element $II(x,y)$ of an integral image indicates the sum of intensity of pixels inside the box formed by the origin (the top-left corner) and position (x,y). (**b**) Calculating the sum of intensity of any axis-aligned box only involves addition/subtraction of four elements

We reported the first extension of Haar features to 3D in [29]. Figure 2.4b shows a few 3D Haar feature templates. Suppose $I(x,y,z)$ is the intensity of voxel (x,y,z). The 3D integral image $II(x,y,z)$ is defined as

$$II(x,y,z) = \sum_{u=0}^{x} \sum_{v=0}^{y} \sum_{w=0}^{z} I(u,v,w). \qquad (2.13)$$

The sum of voxel intensity inside a box of $x \in [x_1,x_2]$, $y \in [y_1,y_2]$, and $z \in [z_1,z_2]$ is

$$S_{x_1,y_1,z_1}^{x_2,y_2,z_2} = II(x_2,y_2,z_2) - II(x_1,y_2,z_2) - II(x_2,y_1,z_2) - II(x_2,y_2,z_1) +$$
$$II(x_2,y_1,z_1) + II(x_1,y_2,z_1) + II(x_1,y_1,z_2) - II(x_1,y_1,z_1), \quad (2.14)$$

which involves the addition/subtraction of eight elements of the integral image.

The integral image can be calculated by passing original image once using the algorithm described in [31], as shown in Fig. 2.6. This algorithm can be directly extended to 3D; however, the resulting computation is sub-optimal since it does not benefit from the existence of multiple Central Processing Units (CPU). For example, sequential integral image calculations take about 0.6 s for a brain MRI volume of 1.35 mm resolution with $192 \times 192 \times 149$ voxels. Since the overall MSL-based detection is approaching a sub-second speed, the integral image calculation becomes a computational bottleneck.

Note that almost all up-to-date personal computers have multiple CPUs and therefore it is advantageous to use parallel computing to make full use of all CPUs. Here, we present a 2D integral image calculation method, which is suited for parallel computation (as shown in Fig. 2.7). We pass the image twice to calculate the cumulative sum along rows and columns, respectively. Since each row is processed independently when we calculate the row sums, the computation can be parallelized.

Input: $I(x,y)$ is the intensity of pixel (x,y).
           W is input image width and H is the image height.
Output: The integral image $II(x,y)$.
Algorithm:
Clear the left and top margins of $II(x,y)$ such that $II(-1,:) = 0$ and $II(:,-1) = 0$.
Suppose $s(x,y)$ is the cumulative sum along column (that is y). Clear its top margin $s(:,-1) = 0$.
For $y = 0,1,\ldots,H-1$
      For $x = 0,1,\ldots,W-1$
           $s(x,y) = s(x,y-1) + I(x,y)$
           $II(x,y) = II(x-1,y) + s(x,y)$
      End
End

Fig. 2.6 A non-parallelized integral image calculation algorithm [31]

Input: $I(x,y)$ is the intensity of pixel (x,y).
           W is input image width and H is the image height.
Output: The integral image $II(x,y)$.
Algorithm:
Clear the left and top margins of $II(x,y)$ such that $II(-1,:) = 0$ and $II(:,-1) = 0$.
/* Calculate the cumulative sum for each row, which can be done with multiple threads independently. */
For $y = 0,1,\ldots,H-1$ /* This loop can be parallelized. */
      For $x = 0,1,\ldots,W-1$
           $II(x,y) = II(x-1,y) + I(x,y)$
      End
End
/* Calculate the cumulative sum for each column, which can be done with multiple threads independently. */
For $x = 0,1,\ldots,W-1$ /* This loop can be parallelized. */
      For $y = 0,1,\ldots,H-1$
           $II(x,y) = II(x,y-1) + I(x,y)$
      End
End

Fig. 2.7 An integral image calculation algorithm suitable for parallel computation

The same applies to the calculation of the cumulative sums along columns. Our parallel algorithm does not consume extra memory. Compared to the sequential algorithm we need to pass the image twice; however, the number of mathematical operations (additions) is the same. When the parallel algorithm is implemented on a single CPU, it is as efficient as the sequential algorithm [31]. However, when casted into multi-threading computation, it can make full use of the multiple CPU cores with little overhead in synchronizing multiple threads.

The parallel algorithm can be extended to 3D in a straightforward way. We first calculate the integral image for each slice independently using parallel computation. We then calculate the cumulative sums along the slices (the z axis), which can also be computed independently for each (x,y). The computation threads only need to synchronize once to wait for the 2D integral images of all slices to be generated before calculating the cumulative sums along the z direction. On a computer with quad-core CPUs, after using multi-threading, the integral image calculation time is reduced to one third, from 601 to 194 ms, for a brain MRI volume with $192 \times 192 \times 149$ voxels.

2.3.2 Steerable Features

Global features, such as 3D Haar wavelet features, are effective to capture the global information (e.g., scale) of an object. To capture the orientation information of a hypothesis, we should rotate either the volume or the feature templates. However, it is time consuming to rotate a 3D volume and there is no efficient way to rotate the Haar wavelet feature templates. Local features are fast to evaluate but they lose the global information of the whole object.

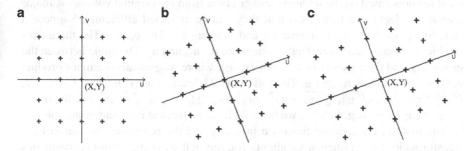

Fig. 2.8 Using a regular sampling pattern to incorporate a hypothesis (X, Y, ψ, S_x, S_y) about a 2D object pose. The sampling points are indicated as '+'. (**a**) Move the pattern center to (X, Y). (**b**) Align the pattern to the orientation ψ. (**c**) The final aligned sampling pattern after scaling along each axis, proportionally to (S_x, S_y). ©2008 IEEE. Reprinted, with permission, from Zheng, Y., Barbu, A., Georgescu, B., Scheuering, M., Comaniciu, D.: Four-chamber heart modeling and automatic segmentation for 3D cardiac CT volumes using marginal space learning and steerable features. *IEEE Trans. Medical Imaging* **27**(11), 1668–1681 (2008)

As a solution, we introduced the steerable features, which can capture the global position, orientation, and scale of the object and at the same time can be efficiently computed. To define steerable features, we sample a few points from the volume under a sampling pattern. We then extract a few local features at each sampling point (e.g., voxel intensity and gradient). The novelty is that we embed the global position, orientation, and scale information into the distribution of sampling points, while each individual feature is locally defined. Instead of aligning the volume to the hypothesized orientation, we steer the sampling pattern. This is where the name "steerable features" comes from. In this way, we combine the advantages of both global and local features.

Figure 2.8 shows how to embed a pose hypothesis in steerable features using a regular sampling pattern (illustrated for a 2D case for clearance in visualization). Suppose we want to test if hypothesis $(X, Y, Z, \psi, \phi, \theta, S_x, S_y, S_z)$ is a good estimate of the similarity transformation of the object. A local coordinate system is defined to be centered at position (X, Y, Z) (Fig. 2.8a) and the axes are aligned with the hypothesized orientation (ψ, ϕ, θ) (Fig. 2.8b). A few points (represented as '+' in Fig. 2.8) are uniformly sampled along each coordinate axis inside a rectangular region. The size of the rectangular region along an axis is proportional to the scale of the shape in that direction (S_x, S_y, or S_z) to incorporate the scale information (Fig. 2.8c).

Note that the steerable features are also used for position-orientation estimation and at that stage there are no hypotheses about the scales yet. We use the mean scale values calculated from the training set to resize the sampling pattern. The steerable features constitute a general framework, in which different sampling patterns can be defined. Please refer to Fig. 2.16b for another sampling pattern which can incorporate the nonrigid deformation parameters.

Let us discuss now the local features. At each sampling point, we extract a few local features based on the intensity and gradient from the original volume. A major reason to select these features is that they can be extracted efficiently. Suppose a sampling point (x, y, z) has intensity I and gradient $\mathbf{g} = (g_x, g_y, g_z)$. The three axes of object-oriented local coordinate system are $\mathbf{n}_x$, $\mathbf{n}_y$, and $\mathbf{n}_z$. The angle between the gradient g and the z axis is $\alpha = arccos(\mathbf{n}_z.\mathbf{g})$, where $\mathbf{n}_z.\mathbf{g}$ means the inner product between two vectors $\mathbf{n}_z$ and $\mathbf{g}$. The following 24 features are extracted: I, $\sqrt{I}$, $\sqrt[3]{I}$, I^2, I^3, $\log I$, $\|\mathbf{g}\|$, $\sqrt{\|\mathbf{g}\|}$, $\sqrt[3]{\|\mathbf{g}\|}$, $\|\mathbf{g}\|^2$, $\|\mathbf{g}\|^3$, $\log\|\mathbf{g}\|$, α, $\sqrt{\alpha}$, $\sqrt[3]{\alpha}$, α^2, α^3, $\log\alpha$, g_x, g_y, g_z, $\mathbf{n}_x.\mathbf{g}$, $\mathbf{n}_y.\mathbf{g}$, $\mathbf{n}_z.\mathbf{g}$. In total, we have 24 local features at each sampling point.

The first six features are based on intensity and the remaining 18 features are transformations of gradients. Gradients roughly tell us if the sampling point lies on a boundary and they can also be calculated very fast. Feature transformation, a technique often used in pattern classification, is a process through which a new set of features is created [21]. We use it to enhance the feature set by adding a few transformations of an individual feature. Suppose there are P sampling points, we get a feature pool containing $24 \times P$ features. In our case, a $5 \times 5 \times 5$ regular sampling pattern is used for object detection, resulting in $P = 125$ sampling points.

Steerable features can be computed at different levels of an image pyramid and then put together to get a bigger feature pool. For example, a total of $n \times 24 \times P$ features can be extracted on a pyramid with n levels. Computing steerable features in a low resolution volume makes the local features more stable. At a low resolution, the image intensity of a voxel actually corresponds to the average intensity in a small block at a high resolution. In this case, for example, an image intensity feature is less affected by the pepper-and-salt noise and the spectral noise in ultrasound. The gradient can also be calculated more reliably in a smoothed low resolution volume. However, the image pyramid has also limitations. For example, a small object (e.g., a coronary artery) may be smoothed out in a low resolution volume. Furthermore, it may be time consuming to build a pyramid for a large volume. Therefore, it really depends on the application what type of image pyramid is employed, if any. For the experiments on heart chamber detection (see Sect. 2.5), the steerable features are calculated on a pyramid with three levels (3, 6, and 12 mm, respectively).

By extracting steerable features on a pyramid with three levels, we create a feature pool with a total of $3 \times 24 \times 125 = 9{,}000$ features. These features are used to train histogram-based weak classifiers [26] and we apply the PBT [28] to combine the selected weak classifiers to achieve a strong classifier. Here are some statistics concerning the selected features by the boosting algorithm, as part of the experiments on heart chamber detection in cardiac CT volumes, as presented in Sect. 2.5. Overall, there are 3,696 features selected by all object detection classifiers. We found that each feature type was selected at least once. The intensity features, I, $\sqrt{I}$, $\sqrt[3]{I}$, I^2, I^3, and $\log I$, counted about 26 % of the selected features, while the following four gradient-based features, g_x, g_y, g_z, and $\|\mathbf{g}\|$, counted about 34 %.

2.4 Classifiers

The MSL is not bounded to a particular classifier and any state-of-the-art learning algorithms can be used to train its classifiers. We employ the Probabilistic Boosting-Tree (PBT) [28] as a default classifier in MSL due to its classification efficiency and capability to deal with unbalanced training samples. The efficiency of the PBT is further improved by adaptively combining it with the classifier cascade [31].

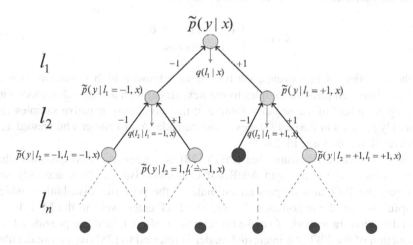

Fig. 2.9 The probabilistic boosting-tree. The dark nodes are the leaf nodes. Each tree node is a strong classifier. Each level of the tree corresponds to an augmented variable l_i. Image courtesy of Zhuowen Tu. ©2005 IEEE. Reprinted, with permission, from Tu, Z.: Probabilistic boosting-tree: Learning discriminative methods for classification, recognition, and clustering. In: Proc. Int'l Conf. Computer Vision, pp. 1589–1596 (2005)

2.4.1   Probabilistic Boosting-Tree

Since a large weak feature pool (in the order of 100,000+ features) can be computed from image data, a process of feature reduction or feature selection is needed for training a classifier. This process is required as a preprocessing step for classifiers such as the Support Vector Machine (SVM) [30], or it is intrinsic to boosting based classifiers [11, 26] and random forests [2]. Classifiers with intrinsic feature selection can train directly on a large feature pool with weak features and this explains the popularity of boosting and random forests. Increased classifier efficiency can be obtained through cascading of classifiers (e.g., AdaBoost [31]) to efficiently detect rare events, e.g., much fewer positive samples than the negatives.

An AdaBoost classifier is an implementation of the boosting technique for a binary classification problem. The final classification decision is based on weighted average of the classification results of the selected weak classifiers

$$H(x) = \sum_{i=1}^{K} w_i h_i(x), \tag{2.15}$$

where $h_i(x)$ is the classification result (+1 for positive output and -1 for negative output) of a weak classifier; w_i is the weight of each weak classifier, which is determined by the boosting technique. The final output of the class label $C(x)$ is positive if $H(x) > 0$; otherwise, it is negative. An additional threshold θ can be used to tune the performance of an AdaBoost classifier,

$$C(x) = \begin{cases} 1 & \text{if } H(x) > \theta \\ -1 & \text{otherwise} \end{cases}. \tag{2.16}$$

For the detection of rare events, we tune θ to achieve a high sensitivity (which can pass almost all positive samples to the next stage) with a reasonable specificity (e.g., rejecting half of the negative samples); therefore, easy negative samples can be quickly rejected in the early stages of the cascade. A cascade can be viewed as a degenerated decision tree [3, 25].

The Probabilistic Boosting-Tree (PBT) [28] is a tree-structured classifier, that combines the decision tree and AdaBoost classifiers. Besides high accuracy and efficiency, the PBT also outputs an estimate of the posterior distribution, which is helpful to rank the hypotheses. We use the PBT extensively in the MSL based object detection framework. To make this chapter self-contained, we provide a brief introduction of the PBT. An interested reader is referred to [28] for a more detailed description of the algorithm.

As shown in Fig. 2.9, the PBT shares the same tree structure as the decision tree. However, different to the decision tree, each node in the PBT is an AdaBoost strong classifier, instead of a simple weak classifier. Another difference is that the PBT can output an estimate of the posterior distribution $p(y|x)$, instead of just a classification label. Here, x is an observed sample and y is its class label (+1 or -1). In MSL, we need to rank the hypotheses to preserve a small number of top hypotheses after each MSL classification stage. Therefore, the capability to compute the discriminative probability is very important.

A number of learning algorithms can generate a classification score in addition to the class label. Empirically, the classification score can be normalized to the range [0, 1] to mimic the posterior distribution $p(y|x)$. However, such an ad hoc approach lacks theoretical foundation. In practice, many classifiers are only sensitive to the region around the boundary between positive and negative samples. In other words, the performance is tuned at a specific point (with a normalized classification score of 0.5) on the Receiver-Operating-Characteristic (ROC) curve. Therefore, their performance on other regions is not optimal. From this view, the PBT has an advantage over other learning algorithms such as the decision trees.

Friedman et al. [12] have shown that AdaBoost is approximating logistic regression. The probability computed from an AdaBoost classifier

$$q(+1|x) = \frac{e^{2H(x)}}{1 + e^{2H(x)}}, \tag{2.17}$$

is a good estimate of the posterior probability. Here, $H(x)$ is the weighted sum of the weak classifier responses in AdaBoost, Eq. (2.15). In many real applications, the posterior probability may be very complicated, therefore difficult to estimate accurately. Many weak classifiers (often a few hundred) need to be integrated to approximate the posterior probability well.

The PBT approaches the target posterior probability by data augmentation (tree expansion) through a divide-and-conquer strategy. Figure 2.9 is an illustration of the PBT, where the tree level l_i is an augmented variable. At the top of the tree node, it gathers the information from its descendants and reports an overall posterior probability,

$$\tilde{p}(y|x) = \sum_{l_1} \tilde{p}(y|l_1, x)q(l_1|x)$$

$$= \tilde{p}(y|l_1 = 1, x)q(l_1 = 1|x) + \tilde{p}(y|l_1 = -1, x)q(l_1 = -1|x). \tag{2.18}$$

Here, $q(l_1|x)$ as defined in Eq. (2.17) is the posterior probability estimated by the root AdaBoost classifier. We can expand the posterior probability estimate of a PBT with a depth of $n+1$ levels as

$$\tilde{p}(y|x) = \sum_{l_1} \tilde{p}(y|l_1, x)q(l_1|x)$$

$$= \sum_{l_1, l_2} \tilde{p}(y|l_2, l_1, x)q(l_2|l_1, x)q(l_1|x)$$

$$\cdots$$

$$= \sum_{l_1, \ldots, l_n} \tilde{p}(y|l_n, \ldots, l_1, x)\cdots q(l_2|l_1, x)q(l_1|x). \tag{2.19}$$

At a tree leaf node, $\tilde{p}(y|l_n,\dots,l_1,x)$ is the posterior probability estimated at that node for class y

$$\tilde{p}(y|l_n,\dots,l_1,x) = \sum_{l_{n+1}} \delta(y = l_{n+1}) q(l_{n+1}|l_n,\dots,l_1,x), \qquad (2.20)$$

where $\delta(.)$ is the Dirac delta function.

Different weak classifiers can be used to train the AdaBoost strong classifiers in the PBT. To increase the efficiency, a weak classifier is normally trained on one feature. The decision stump is a very popular weak classifier, which makes a prediction by comparing the value of a single input feature with a threshold [26]. Depending on the polarity, the decision stump may output a positive or negative class label if the feature value is larger than the threshold. Therefore, a decision stump has only two free parameters to train, the polarity (a boolean variable) and the threshold (a real variable). This weak classifier works well to separate unimodal distributions, however, in most typical applications we encounter distributions with multiple modes.

Fig. 2.10 Histogram based weak classifier

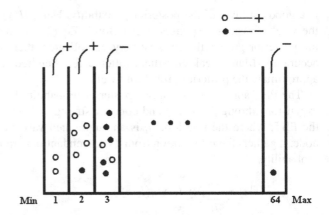

To deal with this challenge, the MSL uses by default a histogram based classifier [26], more flexible than a decision stump. Given a weak feature, we calculate its minimum and maximum values from a training set. The distribution range is then uniformly split into a number of bins (64 bins as used throughout our experiments), as shown in Fig. 2.10. In each bin, we count the total weight of positive and negative samples, respectively, that fall inside the bin. Note that the weight of a sample is adjusted by the AdaBoost algorithm at each iteration to assign a higher weight to the previously mis-classified samples. If the total weight of positive samples is larger than that of the negatives in a bin, the bin polarity is set to be positive; otherwise, it is a negative bin. During classification, a sample falling in a positive bin will get a positive class label. Similarly, a sample in a negative bin is classified as negative. The histogram based weak classifier has more parameters (minimum and maximum feature values, polarity of each bin) that can be adapted to the training set; therefore, it is more powerful than a decision stump. It has capability to separate distributions with multiple modes.

In Sect. 2.3.2, we use feature transformation to enhance the steerable features. For example, for the intensity feature I extracted at a sampling point, we add a few more transformations, including $\sqrt{I}$, $\sqrt[3]{I}$, I^2, I^3, and $\log I$. Such a monotonic feature transformation does not change the classification result of a decision stump. However, it may provide additional classification power to a histogram based weak classifier since a feature after a nonlinear transformation has a different histogram.

As mentioned in Sect. 2.2.3, the distribution of positive and negative samples is skewed. There are far more negative samples (may be up to 10 million in our default setting) than positive samples (often in the order of tens of thousand or less). A classifier should have the capability to handle such a significantly skewed distribution. In the PBT, to train a classification node, we randomly select a small set of positive/negative samples (e.g., 5,000). After training the AdaBoost classifier for a classification node, all available samples at that node are classified. The threshold of the AdaBoost classifier is tuned on all available samples (not the selected subsamples) to achieve the minimum classification error. All samples that are classified as positive (including both true positives and false positives) are passed to the left child of this node and other samples are passed to the right child node. In addition, samples with ambiguity (with a classification score in [0.4, 0.6]) are passed to both the left and right children nodes to enrich the training samples of the children nodes.

2.4.2   Combining Classifier Cascade and Tree

Table 2.1 Comparison between probabilistic boosting-tree [28] and classifier cascade [31]

	Probabilistic Boosting-Tree	Cascade
Pros	(1) More powerful for hard classification problems	(1) Efficient for detection of rare events
		(2) Faster to train
		(3) Less likely to over-fit
Cons	(1) More likely to over-fit	(1) Less powerful for hard problems
	(2) More time-consuming for detection	
	(3) More time-consuming for training	

The classifier cascade [31] is a widely used structure to combine multiple classifiers to efficiently detect rare events (Fig. 2.11a). In a cascade, a threshold is picked at each classification stage to achieve a perfect or near perfect detection rate for positive samples. Most negative samples can be screened out in the first several stages. However, achieving a near perfect detection rate for positives may cause a high false positive rate, specially when the positives and negatives are hard to separate.

The PBT is more powerful to classify hard samples using a divide-and-conquer strategy of the decision tree [3, 25]. Starting from the tree root, the training samples are split along the tree, level by level. If the tree is very deep, at a leaf node, the number of positive and negative samples is small; therefore, it is almost always possible to separate positive and negative samples using a big weak feature pool. That means, a PBT has potential to over-fit the training data if the tree is fully expanded. In practice, the over-fitting issue is mitigated by limiting the tree depth (e.g., to 5 or 6 levels). Furthermore, a tree node is not trained and further expanded if the number of positive/negative samples falling on this node is small (e.g., less than 100 samples).

In a decision tree, a sample goes from the tree root to a leaf node. The path is determined by the classification result at each node, and the number of classifications is the level of the tree. However, in a PBT, an unknown sample should be classified by all nodes in the tree, and the probabilities given by all nodes are combined to get the final estimate of the posterior probability of a class label, Eq. (2.20). The number of nodes of a PBT is an exponential function of the tree depth. Suppose, a tree has n levels. The number of nodes of a full tree is $2^0 + 2^1 + \cdots + 2^{n-1} = 2^n - 1$ (Fig. 2.11b). For comparison, the number of nodes of a cascade with n levels is n. With more nodes, a PBT may consume more training and detection time than a cascade. In the original PBT [28], a heuristic rule is used to reduce the number of probability evaluations. Only samples with an ambiguous classification score (in the range of [0.4, 0.6]) are sent to both left and right children nodes for further evaluation. If the classification score is larger than 0.6, the sample is sent only to the left child note by assuming the estimated probability from the right child note is $q(+1|x) = 0$. The same approximation is applied to a sample with sufficient confidence to be negative (classification score less than 0.4). Such an ad hoc solution makes the probability estimate less reliable. Table 2.1 highlights the pros and cons of a PBT and a cascade classifier.

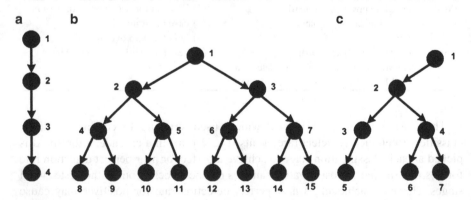

Fig. 2.11 Different structures to combine multiple classifiers. (**a**) Cascade. (**b**) Tree. (**c**) A mixed structure of the cascade and tree

It is possible to combine the advantages of both a cascade and tree. For example, we can put a few levels of cascade before a PBT [29]. The cascade helps to efficiently screen out a large percentage of easy negative samples (e.g., 90 % of negative samples may be filtered by the first two cascades). Since the remaining samples are harder to separate, we can then switch to a tree structure to train more powerful classifiers. However, there are still several issues of this approach. First, we need to manually tune a critical parameter, the number of cascade nodes. If the problem is easy, we should use more cascade nodes to claim the advantage of fast detection speed of the cascade. In addition, for some applications in which a high detection rate is achieved with a high false positive rate, a cascade cannot effectively screen out negatives.

A better approach to combine the advantages of both trees and cascades is to use cascades inside the PBT structure. At each node, we train a strong AdaBoost classifier. After that, we evaluate the trained classifier on all available training samples to this node. If we can achieve a high detection rate (e.g., higher than 97 %) and a low false positive rate (e.g., lower than 50 %), we use the cascade structure. That means we push almost all positive samples to the left child node. The right child node is composed almost purely of negative samples, and it is not necessary to train further. In this way, the structure of the tree is adaptively tuned based on the current training performance. Compared to the naive cascade-before-tree integration, we do not need to manually tune the number of cascade nodes to be appended before a PBT. We only need to set the target detection rate and false positive rate to switch a tree structure to a cascade structure. Figure 2.11c shows a mixed classifier structure with a cascade and tree. During training, after evaluating the classifier node 1, we find its performance can meet the required detection rate and false positive rate. A cascade structure is selected and the right child node of node 1 is not trained. At node 2, we find the classification problem difficult and the trained classifier cannot meet the required accuracy; therefore, a tree structure is used by adding two children nodes to 2. Inside the tree structure, if we find the classification problem becoming easy again, a cascade structure can still be adaptively invoked, e.g., for node 3 in Fig. 2.11c.

2.5 Experiments on Heart Chamber Detection in CT Volumes

In this section, we evaluate MSL on heart chamber detection in cardiac CT volumes. The heart is a complex organ, composed of four chambers, the Left Ventricle (LV), the Right Ventricle (RV), the Left Atrium (LA), and the Right Atrium (RA). We develop a comprehensive four-chamber heart model (refer to Chap. 7), as shown in Fig. 2.12, to provide accurate representation of the anatomies. Our heart model includes the endocardium of all four chambers. In addition, since the epicardium of the left ventricle is clearly visible in a cardiac CT volume, it is also integrated into the heart model.

Under the guidance of cardiologists, we manually annotated all four chambers in 323 cardiac CT volumes (with various cardiac phases) from 137 patients with cardiovascular diseases. Since the LV is clinically more important than other chambers, to improve the system performance on LV detection and segmentation, we annotated extra 134 volumes. In total, we have 457 volumes from 186 patients for the LV. The imaging protocols are heterogeneous with different capture ranges and resolutions. A volume may contain 80–350 slices, while the size of each slice is the same with 512×512 pixels. The resolution inside a slice is isotropic and varies from 0.28 to 0.74 mm for different volumes. The slice thickness (distance between neighboring slices) is larger than the in-slice resolution and varies from 0.4 to 2.0 mm for different volumes.

We use fourfold cross-validation to evaluate the detection algorithm. The whole dataset is randomly split into four roughly equal sets. Three sets are used to train the

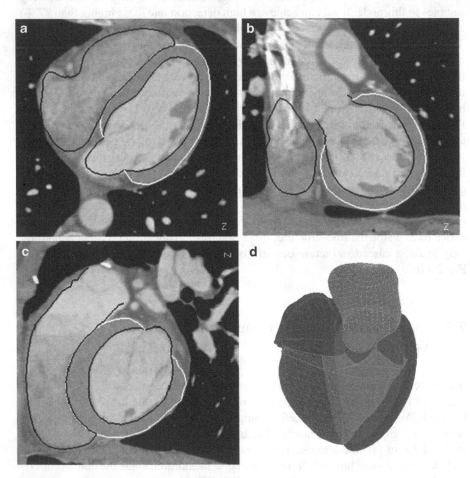

Fig. 2.12 A four-chamber heart model with (**a**) transaxial view, (**b**) coronal view, (**c**) sagittal view, and (**d**) 3D visualization of the mesh model

system and the remaining set is reserved for testing. The configuration is rotated, until each set has been tested once. Data from the same patient may have similar shapes and image characteristics since they are often captured on the same CT scanner with the same scanning parameters. If such data appear in both the training and test sets during cross-validation, the result is biased toward a lower detection error. To remove such bias, we enforce the constraint during cross-validation that the volumes from the same patient can only appear in either the training or test set, but not in both.

The search-step-normalized error as defined in Eq. (2.6) is used to evaluate the heart chamber detection accuracy since we can easily distinguish optimal and non-optimal estimates using this error measurement, but not for other error measures such as the weighted Euclidean distance. The optimal estimate is upper-bounded by 0.5 search steps under any search grid. However, a non-optimal estimate has an error larger than 0.5.

The efficiency of MSL comes from the fact that we prune the search space after each step. One concern is that since the space is not fully explored, the MSL might miss the optimal solution at an early stage. In the following, we show that pruning deteriorates only slightly the accuracy in MSL. Figure 2.13 shows the error of the best candidate after each step with respect to the number of candidates preserved. The curves are calculated on all volumes based on cross-validation. The dotted lines at the bottom show the error of the optimal solution under the search grid. As shown in Fig. 2.13a for position estimation, if we keep only one candidate, the average error may be as large as 3.5 voxels. However, by retaining more candidates, the minimum errors have a fast decrease. We have a high probability to keep the optimal solution when 100 candidates are preserved. We observed the same trend in different marginal spaces, such as the position-orientation space as shown in Fig. 2.13b. Based on the trade-off between accuracy and speed, we preserve 50 candidates after position-orientation estimation. After full similarity transformation estimation, the best candidates we get have an error ranging from 1.0 to 1.4 search steps as shown in Fig. 2.13c.

As discussed before, the unweighted averaging of the top candidates into a final estimate achieves the best results. As shown in Fig. 2.14a, the errors decrease quickly with more candidates for averaging until 100 and after that they saturate. Using the average of the top 100 candidates as the final single estimate, we achieve an error of about 1.5–2.0 search steps for different chambers. Figure 2.14b shows the cumulative distribution of errors on all volumes. The LV and LA have smaller errors than the RV and RA since the contrast of the blood pool in the left side of a heart is consistently higher than the right side due to the using of contrast agent (as shown in Figs. 2.12 and 2.15). Compared to the LA, the LV detection error is even smaller because the LV is larger in size and we have more LV training data to cover various cardiovascular diseases. Our approach is robust and we did not observe any major failures. For comparison, the heart detection modules in both [10] and [13] fail on about 10 % volumes. The conclusion of these experiments is that only a small number of candidates are necessary to be preserved after each step, without deteriorating the accuracy of the final estimate.

Fig. 2.13 The searching-step-normalized error, defined in Eq. (2.6), of the best candidate with respect to the number of candidates preserved after each step. (**a**) Position estimation. (**b**) Position-orientation estimation. (**c**) Position-orientation-scale estimation. The dotted lines at bottom show the lower bound of the detection error. ©2008 IEEE. Reprinted, with permission, from Zheng, Y., Barbu, A., Georgescu, B., Scheuering, M., Comaniciu, D.: Four-chamber heart modeling and automatic segmentation for 3D cardiac CT volumes using marginal space learning and steerable features. *IEEE Trans. Medical Imaging* **27**(11), 1668–1681 (2008)

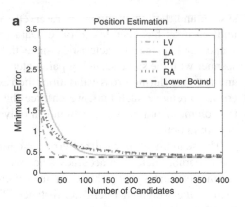

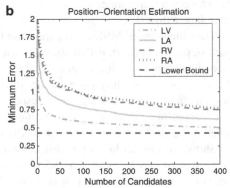

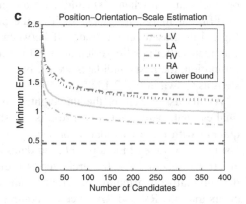

We also evaluated the mesh initialization errors after aligning the mean shape with respect to the automatically estimated pose. As a widely used criterion [10, 13, 22], the symmetric point-to-mesh distance, E_{p2m}, is exploited to measure the accuracy in surface boundary delineation. For each point on a mesh, we search for the closest point (not necessarily a mesh triangle vertex) on the other mesh to calculate the minimum Euclidean distance. We calculate the point-to-mesh distance from the detected mesh to the ground truth and vice versa to make the measurement

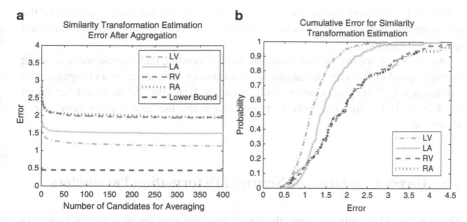

Fig. 2.14 Final similarity transformation estimation error after aggregating multiple candidates using un-weighted average. (a) Error vs. the number of candidates for averaging. (b) Cumulative distribution of errors on all test datasets using 100 candidates for aggregation

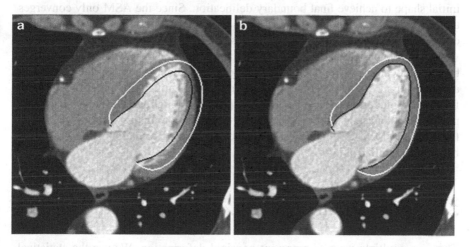

Fig. 2.15 Segmentation of the left ventricle in a cardiac CT volume with a black contour for the endocardium and a white contour for the epicardium. (a) Aligned mean shape with respect to the automatically estimated pose. (b) Final segmentation

symmetric. In our experiments, we estimate the pose of each chamber separately. The mean E_{p2m} error after heart detection is 3.17 mm for the LV endocardium, 2.51 mm for the LV epicardium, 2.78 mm for the LA, 2.93 mm for the RV, and 3.09 mm for the RA.

Figure 2.15a shows the aligned mean shape of the left ventricle (including both the endocardium and epicardium) with the estimated pose. As we can see, the initial shape is already quite close to the true boundary. After nonrigid deformation estimation of the mesh points, the final segmentation error ranges from 0.84 to

1.57 mm for different chambers. Figure 2.15b shows the final segmentation of the left ventricle. Please refer to Chap. 7 for more details on the nonrigid deformation estimation method.

After code optimization and using the multi-threading techniques, we achieve an average speed of 0.5 s for the automatic detection of a chamber on a computer with a dual-core 3.2 GHz processor and 3 GB memory. Boundary delineation takes about 0.5 s more. If all four chambers are to be segmented, the total computation time is about 4 s.

2.6   Direct Estimation of Nonrigid Deformation Parameters

The standard MSL only estimates the rigid transformation for object localization. In many cases, we want to delineate the boundary of a nonrigid organ. For this purpose, the mean shape is aligned with the estimated object pose as an initial rough estimate of the shape. The Active Shape Model (ASM) [5] is then exploited to deform the initial shape to achieve final boundary delineation. Since the ASM only converges to a local optimum, the initial shape needs to be close to the true object boundary; otherwise, the deformation is likely to get stuck in a suboptimal solution.

This problem is typical for liver segmentation since the liver is the largest organ in human body and is surrounded by several other anatomies: heart, kidney, stomach, and diaphragm. As a soft organ, the liver deforms significantly under the pressure from the neighboring organs. As noted in [16], for a highly deformable shape, the pose estimation can be improved by further initialization. In this section, we present the Nonrigid MSL to directly estimate the nonrigid deformation of an object for better shape initialization.

2.6.1   Nonrigid Marginal Space Learning

There are multiple ways to represent nonrigid deformation. We use the statistical shape model or the so-called Point Distribution Model (PDM) [5] since it can capture the major deformation modes with a few parameters. To build a statistical shape model, we need N shapes, each being represented by M points with anatomical correspondence. By stacking the 3D coordinates of these M points, we get a $3M$-dimensional vector $\mathbf{x}$ to represent a shape. To remove the relative translation, rotation, and scaling, we first jointly align all shapes using generalized Procrustes analysis (as presented in Sect. 6.3), obtaining the aligned shapes $\mathbf{x}_i, i = 1, 2, \ldots, N$. The mean shape $\bar{\mathbf{x}}$ is calculated as the simple average of the aligned shapes, $\bar{\mathbf{x}} = \frac{1}{N} \sum_{i=1}^{N} \mathbf{x}_i$. The shape space spanned by these N aligned shapes can be represented as a linear space with $K = \min\{3M - 1, N - 1\}$ eigen vectors, $\mathbf{V}_1, \ldots, \mathbf{V}_K$, based on Principal Component Analysis (PCA) [5]. A new shape $\mathbf{y}$ in the aligned shape space can be represented as

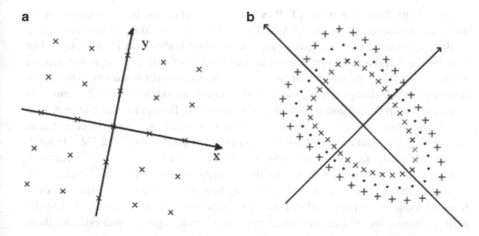

Fig. 2.16 Sampling patterns in steerable features for rigid and nonrigid deformation estimation. (a) Regular sampling pattern for estimating translation, rotation, and scaling. (b) Sampling pattern based on a synthesized shape for estimating nonrigid deformation parameters

$$y = \bar{x} + \sum_{j=1}^{K} c_j V_j + e, \qquad (2.21)$$

where c_i the so-called PCA coefficient and e is a $3M$-dimensional vector for the residual error. Using the statistical shape model, a nonrigid shape can be represented parametrically as $(T, R, S, c_1, \ldots, c_K, \bar{x}, e)$, where T, R, S represent the translation, rotation, and scaling to transfer a nonrigid shape in the aligned shape space back to the world coordinate system.

With this representation, we convert a segmentation (or boundary delineation) problem to a parameter estimation problem. Among all these parameters, $\bar{x}$ is fixed and e is sufficiently small if K is large enough (e.g., with enough training shapes). The standard MSL only estimates the rigid part (T, R, S) of the transformation. Here, we extend MSL to directly estimate the parameters for nonrigid deformation $(c_1, \ldots, c_K)$.

Given a hypothesis $(T, R, S, c_1, \ldots, c_K)$, we train a classifier based on a set of image features F to distinguish a positive hypothesis from a negative one. The image features should be a function of the hypothesis, $F = F(T, R, S, c_1, \ldots, c_K)$ and incorporate sufficient information for classification. The steerable features presented in Sect. 2.3.2 of Chap. 2 help to efficiently embed the object pose information into the feature set by steering (translate, rotate, and scale) a sampling pattern with respect to the testing hypothesis. In the original MSL estimation of the rigid transformation, we extract at each sampling point 24 local image features, using a regular sampling pattern to embed the object pose parameters (T, R, S). For the Nonrigid MSL, we need to also embed the nonrigid shape parameters $c_j, j = 1, \ldots, K$, and achieve this through a new sampling pattern based on the synthesized nonrigid shape (as shown in Fig. 2.16b). Each hypothesis $(\mathbf{T}, \mathbf{R}, \mathbf{S}, c_1, \ldots, c_K)$ corresponds to a nonrigid shape using the statistical shape model (see Eq. (2.21)). We use this synthesized shape as the sampling pattern and extract the local image features on its M points. The dots in Fig. 2.16b are the synthesized shape. If a hypothesis is close to the ground truth, the sampling points should be close to the true object boundary. The image features based on image intensity and local gradient are extracted on these sampling points and help distinguishing the object's boundary. To capture more information for classification, we also sample a layer of points inside the shape (represented as 'x' in Fig. 2.16b) and a layer of points outside the shape ('+' in Fig. 2.16b). In total, we get $3M$ sampling points, resulting in a feature pool with $24 \times 3 \times M$ features. Similarly to the standard MSL, we use the boosting technique to learn the classifier.

Due to the exponential increase of testing hypotheses, we cannot train a monolithic classifier to estimate all deformation parameters simultaneously. Using the MSL principle, we split the deformation parameters into groups and estimate them sequentially. To be specific, after position-orientation-scale estimation, we train a classifier in the marginal space of $(\mathbf{T}, \mathbf{R}, \mathbf{S}, c_1, c_2, c_3)$, where (c_1, c_2, c_3) correspond to the top three deformation modes. Given a small set of candidates after position-orientation-scale estimation, we augment them with all possible combinations of (c_1, c_2, c_3) and use the trained nonrigid MSL classifier to select the best hypotheses. In theory, we can apply the MSL principle to estimate more and more nonrigid deformation parameters sequentially. In practice, we find that with the increase of the dimensionality of the marginal spaces, the classifier is more likely to over-fit the data due to the limited number of training samples. No significant improvement has been observed by estimating more than three nonrigid deformation parameters.

2.6.2 Experiments on Liver Detection in 3D CT Volumes

Table 2.2 Comparison of the standard, rigid MSL and Nonrigid MSL on liver detection in 226 CT volumes. Average point-to-mesh error E_{p2m} (in millimeters) of the initialized shape is used for evaluation

	Mean	Std Dev	Median
MSL	7.44	2.26	6.99
Nonrigid MSL	6.65	1.96	6.25

In this experiment, we compare Nonrigid MSL against the standard, rigid MSL on liver detection in 226 3D CT volumes. The dataset is very challenging, including both contrasted and non-contrasted scans, with volumes coming from different clinical sites, generated by different protocols. After object localization, we align the mean shape (a surface mesh) to the estimated transformation. The accuracy of the initial shape estimate is measured with the symmetric point-to-mesh distance E_{p2m}. The initial mesh is then deformed through a subsequent nonrigid estimation step, to fit the image boundary and further reduce the error.

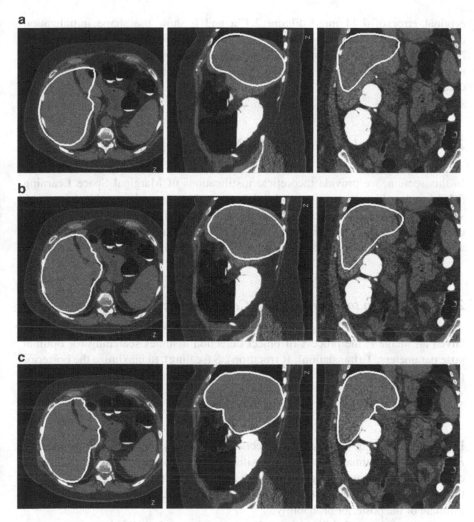

Fig. 2.17 Liver segmentation result on a CT volume. (**a**) Initialization with the mean shape aligned to the translation, orientation, and scale estimated by standard, rigid MSL. (**b**) Initialization by estimating additional three principal components of nonrigid deformation using nonrigid MSL. (**c**) Final segmentation result. From left to right: transaxial, sagittal, and coronal views

Since the focus of this section is to compare the errors corresponding to rigid and nonrigid MSL estimation for object localization, in the following we only measure the error after the MSL estimation. A threefold cross-validation is performed to evaluate the algorithm. As shown in Table 2.2, the rigid MSL achieves a mean initialization error of 7.44 mm and a median error of 6.99 mm after pose estimation. By estimating three more nonrigid deformation parameters (top three PCA coefficients), as shown in the last row of Table 2.2, we can further reduce the average E_{p2m} to 6.65 mm, about 11 % improvement compared to the original error of 7.44 mm.[1] Figure 2.17a and b show the shape initialization of liver segmentation with baseline MSL and Nonrigid MSL, highlighting that Nonrigid MSL can generate more accurate initial shape. Figure 2.17c shows the final segmentation results obtained by adding the ASM and a learning based boundary detector.

2.7 Theoretical Foundations of Marginal Space Learning

In this section, we provide theoretical justifications of Marginal Space Learning (MSL) and make a connection to the shortest path computation problem in graph search and to particle filtering. The analysis is focused on the standard MSL for estimating the anisotropic similarity transformation parameters of a target object in a 3D volume, although it can be extended to cover Nonrigid MSL.

2.7.1 Relation to Shortest Path Computation

Given an image I, the process of object detection assumes searching for optimal pose parameters, $\hat{\mathbf{T}}$ (translation), $\hat{\mathbf{R}}$ (rotation), $\hat{\mathbf{S}}$ (scaling), to maximize the posterior probability $P(\mathbf{T}, \mathbf{R}, \mathbf{S}|I)$,

$$\hat{\mathbf{T}}, \hat{\mathbf{R}}, \hat{\mathbf{S}} = arg \max_{\mathbf{T}, \mathbf{R}, \mathbf{S}} P(\mathbf{T}, \mathbf{R}, \mathbf{S}|I). \quad (2.22)$$

In machine learning based object detection approaches, the posterior probability $P(\mathbf{T}, \mathbf{R}, \mathbf{S}|I)$ is estimated using a classifier. As shown in [12], if an AdaBoost classifier is trained to distinguish positive and negative pose hypotheses $(\mathbf{T}, \mathbf{R}, \mathbf{S})$, the probability computed from the AdaBoost classifier (refer to Eq. (2.17)) is a good estimate of the posterior probability.

If the posterior probability is complex, as in most real applications, many weak classifiers, often a few hundred, need to be integrated to approximate well the posterior probability. The PBT classifier as used in our implementation approaches the target posterior probability by data augmentation and tree expansion through a divide-and-conquer strategy. Note that other classifiers, such as the random forests [2] or support vector machine [30], can also provide an approximation of the posterior probability.

To search for an optimal pose of the target object, all possible combinations of the three transformations, $\mathbf{T}$, $\mathbf{R}$, and $\mathbf{S}$, need to be tested by the trained classifier.

---

[1]The reduced error of Nonrigid MSL is achieved by combining the technique of Constrained MSL presented in Chap. 4. Using Constrained MSL, we can reduce the mean E_{p2m} error from 7.44 to 7.12 mm. By estimating three more PCA coefficients of the nonrigid deformation, the mean error is further reduced to 6.65 mm.

Due to the exponential increase of the number of pose hypotheses with respect to the dimensionality of the pose parameter space, exhaustive search is impractical for 3D object detection. In MSL, we split the search into multiple steps. The posterior probability $P(\mathbf{T}, \mathbf{R}, \mathbf{S}|I)$ can be factorized as

$$P(\mathbf{T}, \mathbf{R}, \mathbf{S}|I) = P(\mathbf{T}|I)P(\mathbf{R}, \mathbf{S}|\mathbf{T}, I)$$
$$= P(\mathbf{T}|I)P(\mathbf{R}|\mathbf{T}, I)P(\mathbf{S}|\mathbf{T}, \mathbf{R}, I). \tag{2.23}$$

The position classifier of MSL gives an approximation of the posterior probability $P(\mathbf{T}|I)$. However, in the following estimation steps, we do not estimate the conditional probabilities $P(\mathbf{R}|\mathbf{T}, I)$ and $P(\mathbf{S}|\mathbf{T}, \mathbf{R}, I)$ directly. Instead, the position-orientation classifier estimates probability $P(\mathbf{T}, \mathbf{R}|I)$ and the position-orientation-scale classifier estimates $P(\mathbf{T}, \mathbf{R}, \mathbf{S}|I)$. Nevertheless, the conditional probabilities can be derived as

$$P(\mathbf{R}|\mathbf{T}, I) = \frac{P(\mathbf{T}, \mathbf{R}|I)}{P(\mathbf{T}|I)} \tag{2.24}$$

and

$$P(\mathbf{S}|\mathbf{T}, \mathbf{R}, I) = \frac{P(\mathbf{T}, \mathbf{R}, \mathbf{S}|I)}{P(\mathbf{T}, \mathbf{R}|I)}. \tag{2.25}$$

In MSL, when we evaluate position-orientation hypothesis $(\mathbf{T}, \mathbf{R})$ to get an estimate of $P(\mathbf{T}, \mathbf{R}|I)$, the probability $P(\mathbf{T}|I)$ is already estimated by the position classifier. So, the conditional probability $P(\mathbf{R}|\mathbf{T}, I)$ can be derived using Eq. (2.24) without an additional evaluation of $P(\mathbf{T}|I)$. The same is true to the calculation of $P(\mathbf{S}|\mathbf{T}, \mathbf{R}, I)$.

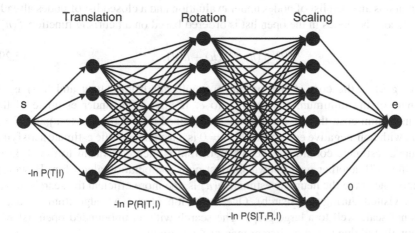

Fig. 2.18 In marginal space learning, object pose estimation can be formulated as searching for the shortest path from the start node s to the end node e in a graph

By factorizing joint probability $P(\mathbf{T},\mathbf{R},\mathbf{S}|I)$, the object detection problem as formulated in Eq. (2.22) is converted to

$$\hat{\mathbf{T}},\hat{\mathbf{R}},\hat{\mathbf{S}} = arg \max_{\mathbf{T},\mathbf{R},\mathbf{S}} P(\mathbf{T}|I)P(\mathbf{R}|\mathbf{T},I)P(\mathbf{S}|\mathbf{T},\mathbf{R},I). \tag{2.26}$$

In the following, we cast it to the classical shortest path computation problem by defining a path cost function $f(\mathbf{T},\mathbf{R},\mathbf{S})$ as

$$
\begin{aligned}
f(\mathbf{T},\mathbf{R},\mathbf{S}) &= -\ln P(\mathbf{T},\mathbf{R},\mathbf{S}|I) \\
&= -\ln P(\mathbf{T}|I) - \ln P(\mathbf{R}|\mathbf{T},I) - \ln P(\mathbf{S}|\mathbf{T},\mathbf{R},I). \tag{2.27}
\end{aligned}
$$

Then, the object pose estimation problem is converted to

$$\hat{\mathbf{T}},\hat{\mathbf{R}},\hat{\mathbf{S}} = arg \min_{\mathbf{T},\mathbf{R},\mathbf{S}} -\ln P(\mathbf{T}|I) - \ln P(\mathbf{R}|\mathbf{T},I) - \ln P(\mathbf{S}|\mathbf{T},\mathbf{R},I). \tag{2.28}$$

Figure 2.18 shows the graph of the shortest path computation problem for object pose estimation. The start node s is connected to all position hypotheses $\mathbf{T}$ with a weight $-\ln P(\mathbf{T}|I)$. Each position hypothesis is connected to all orientation hypotheses $\mathbf{R}$ with a weight $-\ln P(\mathbf{R}|\mathbf{T},I)$. Similarly, each orientation hypothesis is connected to all scale hypotheses $\mathbf{S}$ with a weight $-\ln P(\mathbf{S}|\mathbf{T},\mathbf{R},I)$. Finally, each scale hypothesis is connected to the end node e with zero cost. Under this formulation, object pose estimation is equivalent to searching for an optimal path from s to e with a minimum cost.

Exhaustive search guarantees to find a global optimal path by evaluating all potential paths, but it is too time consuming. The A* algorithm [15] is a more efficient search algorithm that also guarantees to find an optimal path if all edge costs are non-negative as ours. Figure 2.19 shows the pseudo code the A* algorithm. It maintains an open list of nodes under evaluation and a closed list of nodes already processed. The nodes in the open list is ordered based on a heuristic function $f(n)$

$$f(n) = g(n) + h(n), \tag{2.29}$$

where $g(n)$ is the cost of the current optimal path from s to n and $h(n)$ is an estimate of the minimum cost from n to e. If $h(n)$ is an under estimate of the real minimum cost, the A* algorithm is guaranteed to find the shortest path. For a graph with non-negative edge costs, $h(n) = 0$ is a trivial heuristic estimate satisfying the under-estimate condition. The A* algorithm is then equivalent to the Dijkstra algorithm [7], another well-known shortest path computation algorithm. However, the more accurate the heuristic estimate $h(n)$ is, the more efficient the search (fewer nodes visited during the search). One limitation of the A* algorithm is that it does not scale well to a large graph. The search with an unbounded open list will eventually fail due to either time or memory constraint.

Create two empty lists: an open list (for nodes under evaluation) and a closed list (for nodes already processed). For each node n in these lists, we record the cost $g(n)$ of the current optimal path from the start node s to n. For each node n in the open list, we also record a heuristic estimate $f(n)$ of the full path cost from s to the end node e passing through n.

Add the start node s ($g(s) = 0$) to the open list

Repeat the following procedure until the open list is empty
    Remove the first element n from the open list
    If n is the end node e
        A shortest path has been found. Terminate the algorithm.
    Else /* n is not the end node */
        Add n to the closed list
        Expand the path to all successor nodes of n.
        For each successor m
            Update cost $g(m) = g(n) + e(n,m)$, where $e(n,m)$ is edge cost from n to m.
            Estimate the cost $h(m)$ of the remaining path from m to e.
            Calculate the heuristic cost $f(m) = g(m) + h(m)$
            If the successor node m is not in the closed list
                Add m to the open list
            Else /* The successor node is in the closed list */
                If $g(m)$ is smaller than its recorded cost in the closed list
                    Add m to the open list
                    Remove m from the closed list
              End
            End
        End
    End
    Sort the open list in the ascending order using the estimated cost $f(n) = g(n) + h(n)$
End

Fig. 2.19 Pseudo code of the A* search algorithm [15]

In many real applications, searching for the exact global shortest path is not absolutely necessary. An efficient algorithm is more desirable if it can find a near-optimal path much faster than the exact algorithms. Object detection is such an application. First, there are many good pose hypotheses. For 3D object detection, in total, there are at least $2^9 = 512$ pose hypotheses within one searching step distance to the ground truth. Any of them is good enough. Second, the PBT classification score is just an approximation of the posterior probabilities $P(\mathbf{T}|I)$, $P(\mathbf{T},\mathbf{R}|I)$, and $P(\mathbf{T},\mathbf{R},\mathbf{S}|I)$. That means the edge cost is a noisy measurement. Although the pose hypothesis corresponding to the global optimal path is generally a good estimate, it may not be the one closest to the ground truth.

Many greedy search algorithms have been proposed to reduce the searching time and memory footprint of exact search algorithms. Beam search is a greedy search that was first used in the Harpy Speech Recognition System developed at Carnegie Mellon University in mid-1970s [23]. The basic idea of beam search is that instead of maintaining all paths currently under evaluation, it only maintains a limited number of most promising paths [1]. The upper limit of the number of maintained paths is called beam width, which is a critical parameter to control the trade-off between search speed (as well as memory footprint) and optimality of the generated path. If the beam width is infinity, the algorithm is equivalent to an exact search that can generate a global optimal path, but at the cost of longer search time and larger memory footprint. With a small beam width, the algorithm is efficient but often generates a path with a large cost or fails to generate a solution at all since an optimal (or feasible) path may be pruned erroneously during the search. To the extreme, with a beam width of one, the algorithm is equivalent to the hill-climbing algorithm, which often outputs a locally optimal solution of poor quality [32].

Although the idea is simple, beam search works well on a lot of problems, e.g., planning [35], scheduling [6], speech recognition [23], and machine translation [27]. It works especially well on problems with a lot of near-optimal solutions [6] like our object pose estimation problem. A recent comparison [32] on a variety of graph search problems shows that beam search offers a better trade-off between speed and accuracy than other greedy search algorithms. It is well suited for large search problems when other algorithms fail to generate a solution at all. In addition, beam search can be integrated into different exact search algorithms, e.g., the A* algorithm.

Note that a tree can be searched in different orders, e.g., depth-first, breadth-first, or best-first, where the nodes are ordered using a heuristic cost estimate. From this point of view, the MSL uses the classical breadth-first beam search. Our graph is basically a tree if the end node e is removed. (The node e is added to convert the graph search problem to a shortest path computation problem. The tree leaf nodes are connected to e with edges of a zero cost.) In the breadth-first search order, a tree is searched level by level. First, the root node is searched; then, all children of the root node are searched; and next, all grand-children of the root node are searched. This search order is propagated level by level until all leaf nodes have been searched.

In MSL, after each step, a limited number of pose hypotheses are preserved and all other pose hypotheses with a low classification score are discarded. The beam width (i.e., the number of preserved candidates after each step) is tuned to get a good trade-off between the estimation accuracy and speed. As shown in Fig. 2.13 for heart chamber detection, a beam width of one (equivalent to the hill-climbing algorithm) is too restrictive and good pose candidates are likely to be pruned erroneously. When the beam width is increased to 100, the best position hypotheses (which are closest to the ground truth) are almost sure to be preserved for the left ventricle detection, as shown in Fig. 2.13a. For the following position-orientation and position-orientation-scale estimation, with a small beam width, we start to lose some of the best pose candidates. Fortunately, our problem contains a lot of near-optimal solutions, and the MSL successfully preserves many good pose candidates, as shown in Fig. 2.13b and c.

2.7.2 Relation to Particle Filtering

The MSL can also be regarded as a special type of particle filter [9] for which the particles are propagated in the sequence of subspaces (Eq. (2.5)) of increasingly larger dimension, namely, the marginal spaces. A typical particle filter propagates particles in the same space; hence, the MSL contributes to an extended filtering process, by allowing the space dimensions to vary between estimation steps. For a given marginal space, the MSL prunes the particles through classifiers trained in that subspace, while the propagation to the next subspace involves adding more parameters, thus increasing the particle dimensionality, and adding more particles to cover the new subspace. The last space in the estimation is the pose parameter space of the object that needs to be detected.

2.8 Conclusions

In this chapter, we discussed in detail the Marginal Space Learning (MSL) paradigm, demonstrating its efficiency and robustness. By progressively learning in subspaces of increasing dimensions called Marginal Spaces, the MSL achieves early pruning of irrelevant hypotheses. This property makes MSL an ideal tool for fast pose estimation. The chapter also covered the entire framework of an MSL application in 3D with a focus on heart chamber detection in CT volumes, analyzing its 3D image features and a default classifier, the PBT. Finally we presented an extension to Nonrigid MSL and related the MSL concept to prior search and estimation strategies.

References

1. Bisiani, R.: Beam search. In: S.C. Shapiro (ed.) Encyclopedia of Artificial Intelligence, pp. 56–58. John Wiley & Sons (1987)
2. Breiman, L.: Random forests. Machine Learning 45(1), 5–32 (2001)
3. Breiman, L., Friedman, J.H., Olshen, R.A., Stone, C.J.: Classification and regression trees. Chapman and Hall/CRC (1984)
4. Cootes, T.F., Edwards, G.J., Taylor, C.J.: Active appearance models. IEEE Trans. Pattern Anal. Machine Intell. 23(6), 681–685 (2001)
5. Cootes, T.F., Taylor, C.J., Cooper, D.H., Graham, J.: Active shape models—their training and application. Computer Vision and Image Understanding 61(1), 38–59 (1995)
6. Dashti, M.T., Wijs, A.J.: Pruning state spaces with extended beam search. In: Proc. Int'l Conf. Automated Technology for Verification and Analysis, pp. 543–552 (2007)
7. Dijkstra, E.W.: A note on two problems in connexion with graphs. Numerische Mathematik 1(1), 269–271 (1959)
8. Dollár, P., Tu, Z., Belongie, S.: Supervised learning of edges and object boundaries. In: Proc. IEEE Conf. Computer Vision and Pattern Recognition, pp. 1964–1971 (2006)

9. Doucet, A., Johansen, A.: A tutorial on particle filtering and smoothing: Fifteen years later. Technical Report, Department of Statistics, University of British Columbia (2008)
10. Ecabert, O., Peters, J., Weese, J.: Modeling shape variability for full heart segmentation in cardiac computed-tomography images. In: Proc. of SPIE Medical Imaging, pp. 1199–1210 (2006)
11. Freund, Y., Schapire, R.E.: A decision-theoretic generalization of on-line learning and an application to boosting. J. Computer and System Sciences 55(1), 119–139 (1997)
12. Friedman, J., Hastie, T., Tibbshirani, R.: Additive logistic regression: A statistical view of boosting. The Annals of Statistics 28(2), 337–407 (2000)
13. Fritz, D., Rinck, D., Unterhinninghofen, R., Dillmann, R., Scheuring, M.: Automatic segmentation of the left ventricle and computation of diagnostic parameters using regiongrowing and a statistical model. In: Proc. of SPIE Medical Imaging, pp. 1844–1854 (2005)
14. Georgescu, B., Zhou, X.S., Comaniciu, D., Gupta, A.: Database-guided segmentation of anatomical structures with complex appearance. In: Proc. IEEE Conf. Computer Vision and Pattern Recognition, pp. 429–436 (2005)
15. Hart, P.E., Nilsson, N.J., Raphael, B.: A formal basis for the heuristic determination of minimum cost paths. IEEE Trans. Systems Science and Cybernetics 4(2), 100–107 (1968)
16. Heimann, T., Münzing, S., Meinzer, H.P., Wolf, I.: A shape-guided deformable model with evolutionary algorithm initialization for 3D soft tissue segmentation. In: Proc. Information Processing in Medical Imaging, pp. 1–12 (2007)
17. Henry, W.L., DeMaria, A., Gramiak, R., King, D.L., Kisslo, J.A., Popp, R.L., Sahn, D.J., Schiller, N.B., Tajik, A., Teichholz, L.E., Weyman, A.E.: Report of the American Society of Echocardiography Committee on Nomenclature and Standards in two-dimensional echocardiography. Circulation 62(2), 212–215 (1980)
18. Karney, C.F.F.: Quaternions in molecular modeling. Journal of Molecular Graphics and Modeling 25(5), 595–604 (2007)
19. Kelm, B.M., Wels, M., Zhou, S.K., Seifert, S., Suehling, M., Zheng, Y., Comaniciu, D.: Spine detection in CT and MR using iterated marginal space learning. Medical Image Analysis 17(8), 1283–1292 (2013)
20. Kelm, B.M., Zhou, S.K., Suehling, M., Zheng, Y., Wels, M., Comaniciu, D.: Detection of 3D spinal geometry using iterated marginal space learning. In: Proc. MICCAI Workshop Medical Computer Vision — Recognition Techniques and Applications in Medical Imaging, pp. 96–105 (2010)
21. Kusiak, A.: Feature transformation methods in data mining. IEEE Trans. Electronics Packaging Manufacturing 24(3), 214–221 (2001)
22. Lorenz, C., von Berg, J.: A comprehensive shape model of the heart. Medical Image Analysis 10(4), 657–670 (2006)
23. Lowerre, B.: The Harpy speech recognition system. Ph.D. thesis (1976)
24. Oren, M., Papageorgiou, C., Sinha, P., Osuna, E., Poggio, T.: Pedestrian detection using wavelet templates. In: Proc. IEEE Conf. Computer Vision and Pattern Recognition, pp. 193–199 (1997)
25. Quinlan, J.R.: Induction of decision trees. Machine Learning 1(1), 81–106 (1986)
26. Schapire, R.E., Singer, Y.: Improved boosting algorithms using confidence-rated predictions. Machine Learning 37(3), 297–336 (1999)
27. Tillmann, C., Ney, H.: Word reordering and a dynamic programming beam search algorithm for statistical machine translation. Computational Linguistics 29(1), 97–133 (2003)
28. Tu, Z.: Probabilistic boosting-tree: Learning discriminative methods for classification, recognition, and clustering. In: Proc. Int'l Conf. Computer Vision, pp. 1589–1596 (2005)
29. Tu, Z., Zhou, X.S., Barbu, A., Bogoni, L., Comaniciu, D.: Probabilistic 3D polyp detection in CT images: The role of sample alignment. In: Proc. IEEE Conf. Computer Vision and Pattern Recognition, pp. 1544–1551 (2006)
30. Vapnik, V.: The Nature of Statistical Learning Theory. Springer-Verlag (1995)
31. Viola, P., Jones, M.: Rapid object detection using a boosted cascade of simple features. In: Proc. IEEE Conf. Computer Vision and Pattern Recognition, pp. 511–518 (2001)

32. Wilt, C., Thayer, J., Ruml, W.: A comparison of greedy search algorithms. In: Proc. Symposium on Combinatorial Search, pp. 1–8 (2010)
33. Zheng, Y., Barbu, A., Georgescu, B., Scheuering, M., Comaniciu, D.: Fast automatic heart chamber segmentation from 3D CT data using marginal space learning and steerable features. In: Proc. Int'l Conf. Computer Vision, pp. 1–8 (2007)
34. Zheng, Y., Barbu, A., Georgescu, B., Scheuering, M., Comaniciu, D.: Four-chamber heart modeling and automatic segmentation for 3D cardiac CT volumes using marginal space learning and steerable features. IEEE Trans. Medical Imaging 27(11), 1668–1681 (2008)
35. Zhou, R., Hansen, E.A.: Beam-stack search: Integrating backtracking with beam search. In: Int'l Conf. on Automated Planning and Scheduling, pp. 90–98 (2005)

Chapter 3
Comparison of Marginal Space Learning and Full Space Learning in 2D

3.1 Introduction

Discriminative learning based approaches have been shown to be efficient and robust for many 2D object detection problems [3, 4, 9, 13, 16]. In these methods, object detection or localization is formulated as a classification problem: whether an image block contains the target object or not. The object is found by scanning the classifier exhaustively over all possible combinations of location, orientation, and scale. As a result, a classifier only needs to tolerate limited variation in object pose, since the pose variability is covered through exhaustive search. Most of the previous methods [3, 9, 13, 16] under this framework only estimate the position and isotropic scaling of a 2D object (three parameters in total). However, in order increase the accuracy of estimation, especially when the object rotates or has anisotropic scale variations, more pose parameters need to be estimated.

In many 2D applications, the task is to estimate an oriented bounding box of the object, which has five degrees of freedom: two for translation, one for orientation, and two for anisotropic scaling. It is a challenge to extend the learning-based approaches to a high dimensional space since the number of hypotheses increases exponentially with respect to the dimensionality of the parameter space. However, a five dimensional pose parameter searching space is still manageable by using a coarse-to-fine strategy. Since the learning and detection are performed in the full parameter space, we call this approach Full Space Learning (FSL).

The diagram of FSL using the coarse-to-fine strategy is shown in Fig. 3.1. First, a coarse search step is used for each parameter to limit the number of hypotheses to a tractable level. For example, the search step size for position can be set to as large as eight pixels to generate around 1,000 position hypotheses for an image with a size of 300×200 pixels. The orientation search step size is set to 20 degrees to generate 18 hypotheses for the whole orientation range. Similarly, the search step size for scales are also set to a large value. Even with such coarse search steps, the total number of hypotheses can easily exceed one million (see Sect. 3.3). Bootstrapping can be exploited to further improve the robustness of coarse detection. In the fine search

Y. Zheng and D. Comaniciu, *Marginal Space Learning for Medical Image Analysis: Efficient Detection and Segmentation of Anatomical Structures*, DOI 10.1007/978-1-4939-0600-0_3, © Springer Science+Business Media New York 2014

step, we search around each candidate using a smaller step size, typically, reducing the search step size by half. This refinement procedure can be iterated several times until the search step size is small enough. For example, in the diagram shown in Fig. 3.1, we iterate the fine search step twice.

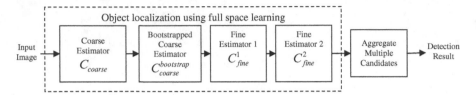

Fig. 3.1 Object localization using full space learning with a coarse-to-fine strategy. ©2009 SPIE. Reprinted, with permission, from Zheng, Y., Lu, X., Georgescu, B., Littmann, A., Mueller, E., Comaniciu, D.: Automatic left ventricle detection in MRI images using marginal space learning and component-based voting. In: *Proc. of SPIE Medical Imaging*, vol. 7259, pp. 1–12 (2009)

In this chapter, we adapt the MSL to the Left Ventricle (LV) detection in 2D Magnetic Resonance Imaging (MRI)—see Fig. 3.2. Furthermore, we compare the performance of the MSL and FSL. A thorough comparison experiment on the LV detection in MRI images shows that the MSL significantly outperforms FSL, on both the training and test sets.

The remainder of this chapter is organized as follows. The adaptation of the MSL for LV detection in 2D long axis cardiac MR images is presented in Sect. 3.2. We then present our implementation of the FSL using a coarse-to-fine strategy for LV detection in Sect. 3.3. The quantitative comparison between the MSL and FSL on a large cardiac MR dataset is performed in Sect. 3.4.

3.2   Marginal Space Learning for 2D Object Detection

In this section, we present a 2D object detection scheme using the computational framework of Marginal Space Learning (MSL). The training procedure of 2D MSL is similar to the 3D variant. In the following, we use the LV detection in 2D MRI images as an example to illustrate the whole training workflow. The training parameters (e.g., criteria for positive/negative samples and the number of hypotheses retained after each step in MSL) are given in this section to facilitate the in-depth understanding of the system by the interested reader. For other 2D object detection tasks, the training parameters can be tuned to further improve the detection accuracy. To cope with different scanning resolutions, the input images are first normalized to the 1 mm resolution.

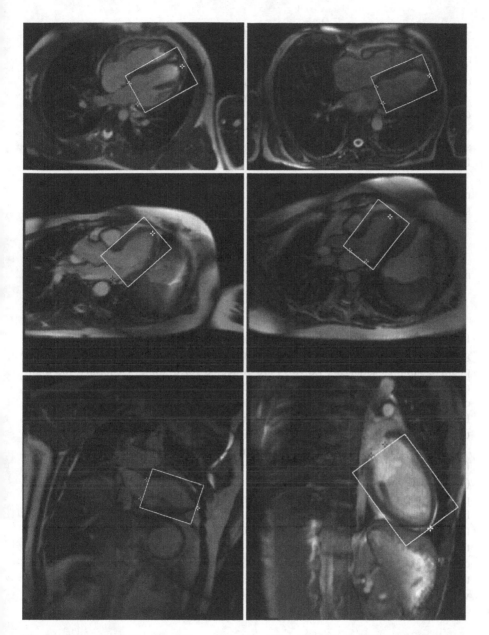

Fig. 3.2 Detection results of the left ventricle (the oriented bounding boxes) and its landmarks (white stars for the left ventricle apex and dark stars for two annulus points on the mitral valve)

3.2.1 Training of Position Estimator

To localize a 2D object, we need to estimate five parameters: two for position, one for orientation, and two for anisotropic scaling. As shown in Fig. 2.3, we first estimate the position of the object in an image. We treat the orientation and scales as the intra-class variations; therefore, learning is constrained in a marginal space with two dimensions. Haar wavelet features are very fast to compute and have been shown to be effective for many applications [13]. We also use Haar wavelet features for learning during this step.

Given a set of position hypotheses, we split them into two groups, positive and negative, based on their distances to the ground truth. A positive sample (X, Y) should satisfy

$$\max\{|X - X_t|, |Y - Y_t|\} \leq 2 \text{ mm}, \tag{3.1}$$

and a negative sample should satisfy

$$\max\{|X - X_t|, |Y - Y_t|\} > 4 \text{ mm}. \tag{3.2}$$

Here, (X_t, Y_t) is the ground truth of the object center. Samples within $(2, 4]$ mm to the ground truth are excluded in training to avoid confusing the learning algorithm. All positive samples satisfying Eq. (3.1) are collected for training. Generally, the total number of negative samples from the whole training set is quite large. Due to the computer memory constraint, we can only train on a limited number of negatives. For this purpose, we randomly sample about three million negatives from the whole training set, which corresponds to a sampling rate of 17.2%.

Given a set of positive and negative training samples, we extract 2D Haar wavelet features for each sample and train a classifier using the Probabilistic Boosting-Tree (PBT) [10]. We use the trained classifier to scan a training image, pixel by pixel, and preserve top N_1 candidates. The number of preserved candidates should be tuned based on the performance of the trained classifier and the target detection speed of the system. Experimentally, we set $N_1 = 1,000$. This number is about 10 times larger than the corresponding parameter for 3D MSL [19, 20] discussed in the previous chapter (3D LV detection application in CT volumes). The reason is perhaps due to more LV shape variability of the slice-based representation and more appearance variability in the case of Cardiac MRI versus Cardiac CT.

3.2.2 Training of Position-Orientation Estimator

For a given image, suppose we have N_1 preserved candidates, (X_i, Y_i), $i = 1, \ldots, N_1$, of the object position. We then estimate both the position and orientation. The parameter space for this stage is three dimensional (two for position and one for orientation), so we need to augment the dimension of candidates. For each candidate of the position, we sample the orientation space uniformly to generate hypotheses for orientation estimation. The orientation search step is set to be five degrees, corresponding to 72 orientation hypotheses. Among all these hypotheses, some are close to the ground truth (positive) and others are far away (negative). The learning goal is to distinguish the positive and negative samples using image features. A hypothesis (X, Y, θ) is regarded as a positive sample if it satisfies both Eq. (3.1) and

$$|\theta - \theta_t| \leq 5 \text{ degrees}, \tag{3.3}$$

and a negative sample satisfies either Eq. (3.2) or

$$|\theta - \theta_t| > 10 \text{ degrees}, \tag{3.4}$$

where θ_t represents the ground truth of the object orientation. Similarly, we random sample three million negatives, corresponding to a sampling rate of 6.6 % on our training set.

Since the alignment of Haar wavelet features to a specific orientation is not efficient, involving image rotations, we employ the steerable features to avoid such image rotations (see Sect. 2.3.2 of Chap. 2). A trained PBT classifier is used to prune the hypotheses to preserve only top $N_2 = 100$ candidates for object position and orientation.

3.2.3   Training of Position-Orientation-Scale Estimator

The full-parameter estimation step is analogous to position-orientation estimation excepting that learning is performed in the full five dimensional similarity transformation space. The dimension of each candidate is augmented by scanning the scale subspace uniformly and exhaustively. The ranges of S_x and S_y of the LV bounding box are [56.6, 131.3] mm and [37.0, 110.8] mm, respectively, deduced from the training set. The search step for scales is set to 6 mm. To cover the whole range, we generate 14 uniformly distributed samples for S_x and 13 for S_y, corresponding to 182 hypotheses for the scale space.

A hypothesis (X, Y, θ, S_x, S_y) is regarded as a positive sample if it satisfies Eqs. (3.1), (3.3), and

$$\max\{|S_x - S_x^t|, |S_y - S_y^t|\} \leq 6 \text{ mm}, \tag{3.5}$$

and a negative sample satisfies any of Eqs. (3.2), (3.4), or

$$\max\{|S_x - S_x^t|, |S_y - S_y^t|\} > 12 \text{ mm}, \tag{3.6}$$

where S_x^t and S_y^t represent the ground truth of the object scales in x and y directions, respectively. Similarly, three million negative samples are randomly selected, corresponding to a sampling rate of 12.0 % on our training set. The steerable features and the PBT are used for training.

3.2.4 Object Detection in Unseen Images

This section provides a summary on running the LV detection procedure on an unseen image. The input image is first normalized to the 1 mm resolution. All pixels are tested using the trained position classifier and the top 1,000 candidates, (X_i, Y_i), $i = 1, \ldots, 1{,}000$, are kept. Next, each candidate is augmented with 72 hypotheses about orientation, (X_i, Y_i, θ_j), $j = 1, \ldots, 72$. The trained position-orientation classifier is used to prune these $1{,}000 \times 72 = 72{,}000$ hypotheses and the top 100 candidates are retained, $(\hat{X}_i, \hat{Y}_i, \hat{\theta}_i)$, $i = 1, \ldots, 100$. Similarly, we augment each candidate with a set of hypotheses about scaling and use the trained position-orientation-scale classifier to rank these hypotheses. For LV bounding box detection, we have 182 scale combinations, resulting in a total of $100 \times 182 = 18{,}200$ hypotheses. For a typical image of 300×200 pixels, in total, we test $300 \times 200 + 1{,}000 \times 72 + 100 \times 182 = 150{,}200$ hypotheses. The final detection result is obtained using cluster analysis on the top 100 candidates after position-orientation-scale estimation.

3.3 Full Space Learning for 2D Object Detection

Table 3.1 Parameters for full space learning. The "H" columns show the number of hypotheses for each parameter. The "S" columns show the search step size for each parameter. The step sizes are measured in millimeters for the translation and scale. The "Total H" column lists the total number of hypotheses tested by each classifier. The "Preserve" column lists the number of candidates preserved after each step

	X		Y		θ		S_x		a			
	H	S	H	S	H	S	H	S	H	S	Total H	Preserve
C_{coarse}	36	8	23	8	18	20°	15	16	6	0.2	1,341,360	10,000
$C_{coarse}^{bootstrap}$	1	8	1	8	1	20°	1	16	1	0.2	$10{,}000 \times 1$	200
C_{fine}^1	3	4	3	4	3	10°	3	8	3	0.1	200×243	100
C_{fine}^2	3	2	3	2	3	5°	3	4	3	0.05	100×243	100

For comparison, we also implemented a Full Space Learning (FSL) system that directly learns classifiers in the original five-dimensional space. The full pose parameter space has five parameters (X, Y, θ, S_x, S_y). Alternatively, we can use the aspect ratio $a = S_y/S_x$ to replace S_y as the last parameter. Due to the high dimension of the search space, a coarse-to-fine strategy is used. The system diagram is shown in Fig. 3.1 and comprising the training and use of four classifiers.

At the coarse level, we use large search steps to reduce the total number of testing hypotheses. To detect the LV bounding box in a typical image (around 300×200 pixels), we search 36 hypotheses for X, 23 hypotheses for Y, 18 hypotheses for θ, 15 hypotheses for S_x, and 6 hypotheses for the aspect ratio a. The corresponding search steps are shown in the row labeled as "C_{coarse}" in Table 3.1. In total, we search $36 \times 23 \times 18 \times 15 \times 6 = 1,341,360$ hypotheses at the coarse level. Due to the constraint of limited computer memory, we randomly sample three million negative samples for training, corresponding to a sampling rate of 0.35 % on the training set.

The Haar wavelet features are computed for classification and since they cannot be efficiently extracted under an arbitrary rotation, the image needs to be rotated according to the hypothesis about the orientation. Each pose hypothesis corresponds to an oriented bounding box. According to [1], the image patch inside a bounding box is cropped and the cropped image is normalized to the same size (e.g., 80×60 pixels), before extracting Haar wavelet features. Such image cropping and size normalization is time consuming if performed for each pose hypothesis (with more than one million hypotheses for one image); therefore, we calculate a set of the rotated images in a preprocessing step. To match the finest orientation search step, 72 rotated images are calculated with an incremental rotation of $5°$ to cover the full orientation space. Given a pose hypothesis, the Haar wavelet features are extracted on the corresponding rotated image.

The PBT is used to train the coarse classifier C_{coarse}. Since the resulting classifier is not robust enough, we keep as many as 10,000 candidates after the coarse classification step to make sure that most training images have some true positives included in the candidates.

Next step we train a bootstrapped classifier, still at the coarse search level. We split the 10,000 top candidates from the previous step into positive and negative sets based on their distances to the ground truth and train a classifier $C_{coarse}^{bootstrap}$ to discriminate them. Using the bootstrapped classifier $C_{coarse}^{bootstrap}$, we prune those 10,000 candidates to preserve the 200 top candidates.

As shown in Fig. 3.1, we use two iterations of fine level search to improve the estimation accuracy. In each iteration, the search step for each parameter is reduced by half. Around each candidate, we search three hypotheses for each parameter, a total of $3^5 = 243$ hypotheses around each candidate. Therefore, for the first fine classifier C_{fine}^1 we test $200 \times 243 = 48,600$ hypotheses. We preserve the top 100 candidates after the first fine-search step; then, we reduce the search step by half again and train another fine classifier C_{fine}^2. Finally, similarly to the MSL pipeline, we derive the detection result by clustering the top 100 candidates.

The number of hypotheses and search step sizes for each classifier are listed in Table 3.1. In total, we test $1,341,360 + 10,000 + 46,800 + 23,400 = 1,424,260$ hypotheses. For comparison, only 150,200 hypotheses are tested in MSL. The speed of the system is roughly proportional to the number of tested hypotheses; therefore, by using MSL we gain a speed-up by a factor of nine.

3.4   Performance Comparison Experiment for MSL and FSL Detection

In this section, we quantitatively evaluate the performance of Marginal Space Learning (MSL) and Full Space Learning (FSL) for LV detection in MRI images.

Automatic LV detection in MRI images is a challenging problem. First, unlike CT, MRI provides physicians the flexibility in selecting the orientation of the imaging plane to capture the best view for diagnosis. On the other hand, this flexibility presents a huge challenge for an automatic detection system since both the position and orientation of the LV are unconstrained in an image. Roughly, the LV is rotation symmetric around its long axis (the axis connecting the LV apex to the center of the mitral valve). The long-axis views are often captured to perform LV measurement. However, the orientation of the LV long axis in the image is unconstrained (as shown in Fig. 3.2). Previous work [2, 15] on LV detection was focused on short-axis views where the LV shape is roughly circular and consistent during the cardiac cycle, thus making the detection problem much easier.

Second, a 2D MRI image used in this application only captures a 2D intersection of a 3D object; therefore, a lot of information is lost. Although the LV and the Right Ventricle (RV) have quite different 3D shapes, in the 2D four-chamber view, the LV is likely to be confused with the RV for an untrained eye (see the top two examples in Fig. 3.2).

Third, the LV shape changes significantly in a cardiac cycle. The heart is a nonrigid organ that keeps beating to pump blood into the body. In order to study the dynamics of the heart, a cardiologist needs to capture images from different cardiac phases. The LV shape changes significantly from the End-Diastolic (ED) phase (when the LV is the largest) to the End-Systolic (ES) phase (when the LV is the smallest).

Last but not least, the images captured by different scanners with different imaging protocols have large variations in intensity (see Fig. 3.2).

We collected and annotated 795 MRI images of the LV long-axis view. As shown in Fig. 3.2, the dataset has large variations in the orientation, size, shape, and image intensity for the LV. We randomly select 400 images for training and reserve the remaining 395 images for testing. Two error measurements are used for quantitative evaluation, the center-center distance and the vertex-vertex distance. Given a box with four vertices V_1, V_2, V_3, V_4, we can consistently sort these four vertices based on the box orientation. The vertex-vertex distance of boxes A and B is defined as the mean Euclidean distance between the corresponding vertices,

$$D_v(A, B) = \frac{1}{4} \sum_{i=1}^{4} \|V_i^A - V_i^B\|. \tag{3.7}$$

The center-center distance only measures the detection accuracy of the box center, while the vertex-vertex distance measures the overall estimation accuracy in all five pose parameters.

Table 3.2 Comparison of Marginal Space Learning (MSL) and Full Space Learning (FSL) for LV bounding box detection on the training set (400 images). The errors are measured in millimeters

	Center-Center Distance			Vertex-Vertex Distance		
	Mean	Std	Median	Mean	Std	Median
FSL	9.73	25.62	1.79	17.31	37.32	5.07
MSL	**1.31**	**0.84**	**1.15**	**3.09**	**1.63**	**2.82**

Table 3.3 Comparison of Marginal Space Learning (MSL) and Full Space Learning (FSL) for LV bounding box detection on the test set (395 images). The errors are measured in millimeters

	Center-Center Distance			Vertex-Vertex Distance		
	Mean	Std	Median	Mean	Std	Median
FSL	43.88	45.01	21.01	63.26	52.09	46.49
MSL	**13.49**	**24.61**	**5.77**	**21.39**	**30.99**	**10.19**

Tables 3.2 and 3.3 show detection errors of the LV bounding box obtained by both methods on the training set and test set, respectively. The MSL clearly outperforms the FSL on both the training and test sets. On the training set, the MSL achieves quite accurate results with 1.31 mm in the center-center error and 3.09 mm in the vertex-vertex error. The FSL does not perform well even on the training set with much larger errors. On the test set, the mean center-center error is 13.49 mm for MSL and 43.88 mm for FSL. The MSL achieves 21.39 mm in the mean vertex-vertex error, compared to 63.26 mm for FSL.

The MSL was originally proposed to accelerate 3D object detection; nevertheless, in this application on 2D object detection it achieves higher detection accuracy than the FSL. The system performance is dominated by the first detector, the MSL position detector and the FSL coarse detector C_{coarse}. If a true hypothesis is missed by the first detector, it cannot be picked up in the following steps. Studying these two detectors can give us hints for the difference in detection accuracy. Since the same feature sets (Haar wavelet features) and learning algorithm (the PBT) are used by both detectors, the MSL superior performance might come from the following two factors: the sampling ratio of the negative training set and the variation of positive samples.

Generally, in a learning-based approach, the number of negative samples is much larger than the number of positive samples. Due to computer memory constraints, however, almost all learning-based systems [4, 13] can only be trained on a limited number of negative samples. In our case, we randomly select three million negatives to train the classifiers for both MSL and FSL. In the FSL case, the sampling ratio for negative samples is about 0.35 % since there are so many hypotheses to test. On the selected training set with three million negatives, the classifier C_{coarse} in FSL was well trained, but did not generalize well on unseen data since it was trained on relatively too few samples. This is an intrinsic limitation of the FSL due to the exponential increase of hypotheses to be tested. On the contrary, the MSL position detector has a search space of only two dimensions, hence a much smaller number of testing hypotheses. With the same number of negative training samples (three million), the sampling ratio is significantly higher (about 17.2 % of the whole negative set). Therefore, the generalization capability of the MSL position detector is much better.

The second reason for the performance difference might be given by the variations in the positive samples. To make the trained system robust, the positive samples should be accurately aligned [11]. On the other hand, to achieve a reasonable speed, we have to set large search steps for the FSL coarse classifier. Therefore, the FSL positive samples have large variations in all five parameters (position, orientation, and scale). For the MSL position detector, the positive samples also have large variations in orientation and scale, actually larger than in the FSL case. However, they are accurately aligned in position. Since position is intuitively the most important pose parameter, with smaller position variations in the MSL positive samples, the MSL classification boundary might be easier to learn.

The MSL is significantly faster than the FSL since much fewer hypotheses need to be tested. As shown in Sect. 3.3, the number of MSL hypotheses tested by is about 10.5 % of FSL hypotheses, and the speed is roughly proportional to the number of testing hypotheses. On a computer with a 3.2 GHz processor and 3 GB memory, the MSL detection speed is about 1.49 s/image, while the FSL takes about 13.12 s to process one image. Both algorithms are well suited for parallel computation to make full use of multiple CPU cores of a computer. The processing speed reported here is obtained without parallel computation.

Although the MSL pipeline outperforms the FSL on both speed and accuracy, the MSL detection robustness still has room for improvement. For this challenging application, in addition to the LV bounding box, we also want to detect a few important LV landmarks (the LV apex and mitral valve annulus); therefore, we train three detectors, one for the LV bounding box, one for the apex, and the other for the mitral valve annulus. During detection, each detector is run independently to generate a list of top candidates (e.g., 100). Based on the geometric relationship of the candidates, we learn a ranking model to select the best LV bounding box among all LV candidates. We then run the apex and base detectors again within a constrained range to refine the landmark detection results. Using the ranking based multi-detector aggregation approach, we can significantly reduce the detection outliers [21, 22]. Please refer to Sect. 5.3 of Chap. 5 for more details on this approach.

3.5 Conclusions

In this chapter we discussed the application of the MSL to detect 2D objects and demonstrated it on LV detection in 2D MRI images. In addition, we performed a thorough comparison between the two computational pipelines: MSL and FSL. Experiments showed that the MSL outperforms the FSL, on both the training and test sets. As it will be shown later on, the MSL superior performance in both detection speed and accuracy, determines its use for many 2D object detection problems, for different medical imaging modalities, e.g., ultrasound transducer [5, 7], balloon marker [6, 14], and various catheters [12, 17] in fluoroscopy; multiple landmarks and organs in topograms [18]; and the left ventricle in 2D ultrasound [8].

References

1. Dollár, P., Tu, Z., Belongie, S.: Supervised learning of edges and object boundaries. In: Proc. IEEE Conf. Computer Vision and Pattern Recognition, pp. 1964–1971 (2006)
2. Duta, N., Jain, A.K., Dubuisson-Jolly, M.P.: Learning-based object detection in cardiac MR images. In: Proc. Int'l Conf. Computer Vision, pp. 1210–1216 (1999)
3. Felzenszwalb, P., McAllester, D., Ramanan, D.: A discriminatively trained, multiscale, deformable part model. In: Proc. IEEE Conf. Computer Vision and Pattern Recognition, pp. 1–8 (2008)
4. Georgescu, B., Zhou, X.S., Comaniciu, D., Gupta, A.: Database-guided segmentation of anatomical structures with complex appearance. In: Proc. IEEE Conf. Computer Vision and Pattern Recognition, pp. 429–436 (2005)
5. Heimann, T., Mountney, P., John, M., Ionasec, R.: Learning without labeling: Domain adaptation for ultrasound transducer localization. In: Proc. Int'l Conf. Medical Image Computing and Computer Assisted Intervention, vol. 3, pp. 49–56 (2013)
6. Lu, X., Chen, T., Comaniciu, D.: Robust discriminative wire structure modeling with applications to stent enhancement in fluoroscopy. In: Proc. IEEE Conf. Computer Vision and Pattern Recognition, pp. 1121–1127 (2011)
7. Mountney, P., Ionasec, R., Kaizer, M., Mamaghani, S., Wu, W., Chen, T., John, M., Boese, J., Comaniciu, D.: Ultrasound and fluoroscopic images fusion by autonomous ultrasound probe detection. In: Proc. Int'l Conf. Medical Image Computing and Computer Assisted Intervention, vol. 2, pp. 544–551 (2012)
8. Park, J., Feng, S., Zhou, K.S.: Automatic computation of 2D cardiac measurements from B-mode echocardiography. In: Proc. of SPIE Medical Imaging, vol. 8315, pp. 1–11 (2012)
9. Shet, V.D., Neumann, J., Remesh, V., Davis, L.S.: Bilattice-based logical reasoning for human detection. In: Proc. IEEE Conf. Computer Vision and Pattern Recognition, pp. 1–8 (2007)
10. Tu, Z.: Probabilistic boosting-tree: Learning discriminative methods for classification, recognition, and clustering. In: Proc. Int'l Conf. Computer Vision, pp. 1589–1596 (2005)
11. Tu, Z., Zhou, X.S., Barbu, A., Bogoni, L., Comaniciu, D.: Probabilistic 3D polyp detection in CT images: The role of sample alignment. In: Proc. IEEE Conf. Computer Vision and Pattern Recognition, pp. 1544–1551 (2006)
12. Tzoumas, S., Wang, P., Zheng, Y., John, M., Comaniciu, D.: Robust pigtail catheter tip detection in fluoroscopy. In: Proc. of SPIE Medical Imaging, vol. 8316, pp. 1–8 (2012)
13. Viola, P., Jones, M.: Rapid object detection using a boosted cascade of simple features. In: Proc. IEEE Conf. Computer Vision and Pattern Recognition, pp. 511–518 (2001)
14. Wang, Y., Chen, T., Wang, P., Rohkohl, C., Comaniciu, D.: Automatic localization of balloon markers and guidewire in rotational fluoroscopy with application to 3D stent reconstruction. In: Proc. European Conf. Computer Vision, pp. 428–441 (2012)
15. Weng, J., Singh, A., Chiu, M.Y.: Learning-based ventricle detection from cardiac MR and CT images. IEEE Trans. Medical Imaging 16(4), 378–391 (1997)
16. Wu, B., Nevatia, R., Li, Y.: Segmentation of multiple, partially occluded objects by grouping, merging, assigning part detection responses. In: Proc. IEEE Conf. Computer Vision and Pattern Recognition, pp. 1–8 (2008)

17. Wu, W., Chen, T., Barbu, A., Wang, P., Strobel, N., Zhou, S.K., Comaniciu, D.: Learning-based hypothesis fusion for robust catheter tracking in 2D X-ray fluoroscopy. In: Proc. IEEE Conf. Computer Vision and Pattern Recognition, pp. 1097–1104 (2011)
18. Zhang, W., Mantlic, F., Zhou, S.K.: Automatic landmark detection and scan range delimitation for topogram images using hierarchical network. In: Proc. of SPIE Medical Imaging, vol. 7623, pp. 1–8 (2010)
19. Zheng, Y., Barbu, A., Georgescu, B., Scheuering, M., Comaniciu, D.: Fast automatic heart chamber segmentation from 3D CT data using marginal space learning and steerable features. In: Proc. Int'l Conf. Computer Vision, pp. 1–8 (2007)
20. Zheng, Y., Barbu, A., Georgescu, B., Scheuering, M., Comaniciu, D.: Four-chamber heart modeling and automatic segmentation for 3D cardiac CT volumes using marginal space learning and steerable features. IEEE Trans. Medical Imaging **27**(11), 1668–1681 (2008)
21. Zheng, Y., Lu, X., Georgescu, B., Littmann, A., Mueller, E., Comaniciu, D.: Automatic left ventricle detection in MRI images using marginal space learning and component-based voting. In: Proc. of SPIE Medical Imaging, pp. 1–12 (2009)
22. Zheng, Y., Lu, X., Georgescu, B., Littmann, A., Mueller, E., Comaniciu, D.: Robust object detection using marginal space learning and ranking-based multi-detector aggregation: Application to automatic left ventricle detection in 2D MRI images. In: Proc. IEEE Conf. Computer Vision and Pattern Recognition, pp. 1343–1350 (2009)

Chapter 4
Constrained Marginal Space Learning

4.1 Introduction

In the previous chapters we showed how the computational framework of Marginal Space Learning (MSL) achieves efficient and robust object detection by selectively focusing on the classification in marginal spaces of increasing dimensionality. The MSL strategy is to start object detection in a lower dimension space, such as the position space, and add more and more parameters in the subsequent detection stages, by also including the object's orientation, scale and non-rigid deformation.

As the title of this chapter suggests, further constraints imposed on marginal spaces can increase the efficiency of the MSL process. First, from the training set we compute the distribution range of each parameter and uniformly sample in that range to generate test hypotheses. Since the location/center of an object cannot be arbitrarily close to the volume border, we can safely skip those hypotheses around volume border during the object pose estimation.

Second, in many applications the pose parameters are not independent. A large organ, for example, is likely to have larger values in all three directions. We can exploit such correlations among pose parameters to reduce the number of testing hypotheses and implicitly increase the MSL efficiency [14, 15]. We rely on the joint distribution of parameters in the training set to drive the hypothesis generation and sample only the regions with high probabilities. The estimation of the joint distribution is, however difficult, due to the limited number of positive samples, typically hundreds. Therefore, to generate testing hypotheses, we use uniform kernels in the joint parameter space, centered on the training samples, a process called *example-based sampling* [2, 16]. We start by uniformly sampling the marginal space to get a large set, S_u. For each training sample, we add its neighboring hypotheses in S_u to the test set S_t. Repeating the above process for all training samples and consolidating redundant hypotheses in S_t, we derive a much smaller test set than S_u.

Y. Zheng and D. Comaniciu, *Marginal Space Learning for Medical Image Analysis:* 79
Efficient Detection and Segmentation of Anatomical Structures,
DOI 10.1007/978-1-4939-0600-0_4, © Springer Science+Business Media New York 2014

The constrained marginal space learning defined as above improves the detection speed by an order of magnitude when compared to the standard MSL. Besides the speed-up, constraining the search to a small valid region can reduce the likelihood of detection outliers, therefore improving the detection accuracy.

Let us now discuss the representations and sampling in the orientation space. As discussed in Chap. 2, for the original MSL we used three Euler angles to represent the 3D orientation space, an approach that has several limitations: (1) There are multiple sets of values that can yield the same orientation, leading to a fundamental ambiguity. (2) The Euclidean distance in the Euler angle space is used in the original MSL as the distance measurement between two orientations. However, since the mapping from Euler angles to orientation space is not distance-preserving, uniform sampling in the Euler angle space is not uniform in the orientation space [4, 7], this effect introducing degradations in the results.

In this chapter we introduce the use of *quaternions* [4] to overcome all the above limitations. Quaternions provide a straightforward orientation representation that can effectively handle the rotation problem and help calculating the correct distance between two orientations.

In summary, we make two major improvements to the original MSL.

1. After analyzing the challenges of Euler angles for 3D orientation representation, we employ quaternions to overcome the limitations of Euler angles.
2. We develop efficient ways to further constrain the search spaces in the MSL and improve the detection speed by an order of magnitude. As a result, it takes less than half a second to detect a 3D anatomical structure in a typical data volume.

The remainder of this chapter is organized as follows. In Sect. 4.2, we compare Euler angles and quaternions for 3D orientation representation and discuss the limitations of Euler angles as used in the original MSL. We also show how to uniformly sample an orientation space to generate orientation hypotheses and calculate the mean orientation to aggregate multiple top candidates into a single estimate. Section 4.3 presents our approach to constraining the search space in the MSL. Extensive comparison experiments on large medical datasets in Sect. 4.4 demonstrate the efficiency of the constrained MSL. This chapter concludes with Sect. 4.5.

4.2   3D Orientation

In this section, we first analyze the drawbacks of Euler angles for 3D orientation representation in the original MSL and then propose to use quaternions to solve all the limitations of Euler angles.

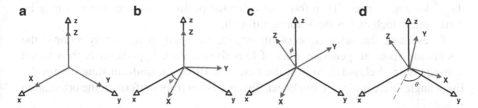

Fig. 4.1 Euler angles in the ZXZ convention. (**a**) Initial orientation with x-y-z representing a reference coordinate system and X-Y-Z representing the rotating coordinate system. (**b**) After rotation around the Z axis with an amount ψ. (**c**) After rotation around the X axis with an amount ϕ. (**d**) Final orientation after rotation around the Z axis with an amount θ

4.2.1   Representation with Euler Angles

It is well known that 3D orientation has three degrees of freedom and can be represented as three Euler angles. An advantage of Euler angles is that they have an intuitive physical meaning. For example, an orientation with Euler angles of ψ, ϕ, and θ in the ZXZ convention is achieved by rotating the original coordinate system around the Z axis with an amount ψ, followed by a rotation around the X axis with an amount ϕ, and lastly a rotation around the Z axis again with an amount θ. Figure 4.1 shows each rotation step of the above example. The rotation operation is not commutable. That means we cannot change the order of rotations. The rotations can either occur about the axes of the fixed coordinate system (extrinsic rotations) or about the axes of a rotating coordinate system, which is initially aligned with the fixed one and modifies its orientation after each elemental rotation (intrinsic rotations). From now on, we will focus on intrinsic rotations, as shown in Fig. 4.1.

To train a classifier to distinguish correct orientation estimates from wrong ones, we need to provide both positive and negative training samples. The Euclidean distance[1] in the Euler angle space can be used to measure the distance of a hypothesis $O^h = (\psi^h, \phi^h, \theta^h)$ to the ground truth $O^t = (\psi^t, \phi^t, \theta^t)$

$$D_e(O^h, O^t) = \sqrt{\|\psi^h - \psi^t\|^2 + \|\phi^h - \phi^t\|^2 + \|\theta^h - \theta^t\|^2}. \qquad (4.1)$$

If the distance is less than a threshold, it corresponds to a positive sample, otherwise to a negative one. Though convenient, the Euclidean distance is not a good distance measurement of orientations. There are multiple sets of Euler angles that yield the same orientation, leading to a fundamental ambiguity. For example, Euler angles $(\alpha, 0, \beta)$ and $(\gamma, 0, \theta)$ in the ZXZ convention represent the same orientation when $\alpha + \beta = \gamma + \theta$. That means two close orientations may have a large distance in

---

[1]In Chap. 2, a special city-block distance is actually used to split the orientation hypotheses into the positive and negative sets. The city-block distance is less accurate than the Euclidean distance and can be taken as an approximation of the latter.

the Euler angle space. Therefore, the collected positive and negative sets may be confusing, which makes the learning difficult.

To estimate the orientation of an object, we need to uniformly sample the orientation space to generate a set of hypotheses. Each hypothesis is then tested with the trained classifier to pick the best one. However, uniform sampling of the Euler angle space under the Euclidean distance is not truly uniform in the orientation space [7].

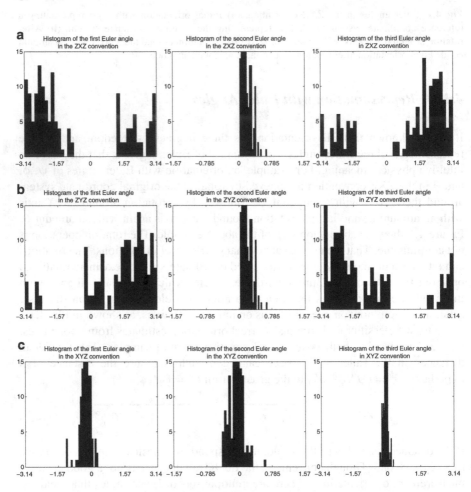

Fig. 4.2 Histograms of three Euler angles of the left ventricle orientation in ultrasound volumes in (**a**) the ZXZ convention, (**b**) the ZYZ convention, and (**c**) the XYZ convention

Another drawback of using Euler angles is that there are 12 possible conventions and a handful are widely used [7]. In the original MSL as presented in Chap. 2, the range of Euler angles is computed from a training set. Each Euler angle is then uniformly sampled within that range to generate hypotheses. Different conventions may give quite different search ranges. For example, if the rotation is only around the y axis, the XYZ convention (where two Euler angles are zero) is more compact than the ZXZ conventions since the latter needs three rotations to generate a pure rotation around the y axis. Figure 4.2 shows the histograms of the Euler angles with the ZXZ, ZYZ, and XYZ conventions for the left ventricle orientation in ultrasound volumes (see Sect. 4.4.3). In this case, the representation with the XYZ convention is more compact. However, for the application of heart chamber detection in cardiac CT volumes (see Sect. 4.4.2), we find that the ZXZ convention is more efficient than the XYZ convention to represent the Euler angle distribution range. In practice, for a new application, we need to try different conventions to select the most compact one.

In summary, previous use of Euler angles for orientation representation in Chap. 2 presents the following challenges:

1. Due to the inherent ambiguity in Euler angle representation, the same orientation can be represented with multiple value sets.
2. The Euclidean distance in the Euler angle space is not a good distance measurement of orientations.
3. Uniform sampling of the Euler angle space is not uniform in the orientation space due to the use of a wrong distance measurement.
4. Among many Euler angle conventions, we need to manually select the convention that represents the search range most compactly.
5. Each Euler angle is uniformly sampled independently to generate orientation hypotheses, without exploiting the correlation among them. Therefore, many more hypotheses are tested than necessary during object detection.

4.2.2 Representation with Quaternions

In this work, we use quaternions to overcome the drawbacks of the Euler angles as used in the original MSL. Introduced in mid-1800s by Hamilton, quaternions provide an elegant conceptual framework, which can solve many problems involving rotations [4]. A quaternion is represented by four numbers

$$\mathbf{q} = [w, x, y, z], \tag{4.2}$$

or as a scalar and a vector

$$\mathbf{q} = [s, \mathbf{v}]. \tag{4.3}$$

In the scalar-vector representation, multiplication of two quaternions becomes

$$\mathbf{q_1 q_2} = [s_1 s_2 - \mathbf{v_1}.\mathbf{v_2}, \quad s_1 \mathbf{v_2} + s_2 \mathbf{v_1} + \mathbf{v_1} \times \mathbf{v_2}], \tag{4.4}$$

where $\mathbf{v_1}.\mathbf{v_2}$ is the vector inner-product and $\mathbf{v_1} \times \mathbf{v_2}$ is the vector cross-product. The multiplication of two quaternions is also a quaternion.

To represent an orientation, we use unit quaternions,

$$|\mathbf{q}| = w^2 + x^2 + y^2 + z^2 = 1. \tag{4.5}$$

A unit quaternion also has three degrees of freedom, the same as the Euler angles. The rotation matrix, $\mathbf{R}$, can be represented by unit quaternions as

$$\mathbf{R} = \begin{vmatrix} 1 - 2y^2 - 2z^2 & 2xy - 2wz & 2xz + 2wy \\ 2xy + 2wz & 1 - 2x^2 - 2z^2 & 2yz - 2wx \\ 2xz - 2wy & 2yz + 2wx & 1 - 2x^2 - 2y^2 \end{vmatrix}. \tag{4.6}$$

A unit quaternion can also be represented in the scalar-vector form as

$$\mathbf{q} = [\cos(\theta/2), \mathbf{v}\sin(\theta/2)], \tag{4.7}$$

where $\mathbf{v}$ is a three-dimensional unit vector. Given a quaternion $\mathbf{p}$, if we left-multiply it with $\mathbf{q} = [\cos(\theta/2), \mathbf{v}\sin(\theta/2)]$, we get a new quaternion $\mathbf{qp}$. The physical meaning of this operation is that $\mathbf{qp}$ represents the orientation after we rotate $\mathbf{p}$ around axis $\mathbf{v}$ with the amount of rotation θ [4]. The conjugate of a quaternion is defined as

$$\bar{\mathbf{q}} = [w, -x, -y, -z] = [\cos(-\theta/2), \mathbf{v}\sin(-\theta/2)]. \tag{4.8}$$

Here, $\bar{\mathbf{q}}$ represents a rotation around axis $\mathbf{v}$ with an amount $-\theta$.

Given two orientations, we can rotate one around an axis to align it to the other [11]. The amount of rotation provides a natural definition of the distance between two orientations. Using quaternions, we can calculate the amount of rotation between two orientations easily. The rotation, $\mathbf{q} = \mathbf{q_1}\bar{\mathbf{q_2}}$, moves $\mathbf{q_2}$ to $\mathbf{q_1}$. Therefore, the amount of rotation between quaternions $\mathbf{q_1}$ and $\mathbf{q_2}$ using the scalar-vector representation in Eq. (4.3) is

$$D_q(q_1, q_2) = \arccos(|s_1 s_2 - \mathbf{v_1}.\mathbf{v_2}|). \tag{4.9}$$

For comparison, the measurement using the Euclidean distance in the Euler angle space D_e (Eq. (4.1)) is often larger than the quaternion-based distance D_q. However, for some cases, $D_e(O_1, O_2) = D_q(O_1, O_2)$. Suppose the XYZ convention is used and the only rotation is around the x axis in an amount less than 180 degrees. In this case, the last two Euler angles are zero. The Euclidean distance in the Euler angle space measures the rotation around the x axis, which is the same to the quaternion distance defined in Eq. (4.9).

4.2.3 Uniform Sampling of 3D Orientation Space

In MSL, we need to generate a set of discrete orientation samples, which are uniformly distributed, as test hypotheses. The problem of uniform sampling can be formulated as, given N sample orientations, we want to distribute them as uniformly as possible. We can define "a covering radius, α, as the maximum rotation needed to align an arbitrary orientation with one of the sample orientations" [4]. For uniform sampling, we want to find an optimal configuration of N sample orientations that gives the smallest α. The optimization procedure is difficult in practice, an interested reader is referred to [4] for more details. A few near-optimal configurations for some N's are listed in Table 4.1 and they are available for download from website http://charles.karney.info/orientation/.

Table 4.1 A few near-optimal uniformly sampled 3D orientation sets. Row N lists the number of orientations in each set and row α lists the covering radius. All the orientation sets are available for download from http://charles.karney.info/orientation/

Name	c48u1	c600v	c48n9	c600vc	c48u27	c48u83	c48u181
N	24	60	216	360	648	1992	4344
α (°)	62.80	44.48	33.48	36.47	20.83	16.29	12.29
Name	c48n309	c48n527	c48u815	c48u1153	c48u1201	c48u1641	c48u2219
N	7416	12648	19560	27672	28824	39384	53256
α (°)	9.72	8.17	7.40	6.60	6.48	5.75	5.27
Name	48u2947	c48u3733	c48u4749	c48u5879	c48u7111	c48u8649	
N	70728	89592	113976	141096	170664	207576	
α (°)	4.71	4.37	4.00	3.74	3.53	3.26	

Since the orientation space has three dimensions, reducing the covering radius α by a half increases the number of samples roughly by a factor of eight. To achieve a reasonable trade-off between speed and accuracy, orientation set c48n309 with $\alpha = 9.72°$ is used for most of our 3D object detection problems. Orientation sets with more dense resolutions up to $\alpha = 0.646°$ are also available from website http://charles.karney.info/orientation/. However, the smallest orientation difference our machine learning based estimator can distinguish cannot approach zero. The actual lower bound is determined by not only the power of the classifier, but also other factors, e.g., the voxel resolution and the ambiguity of orientation definition (which is often affected by the amount of nonrigid deformation of the target object across patients or different scans of the same patients). For rigid objects with less variation across patients, a more densely sampled orientation set may be used if the requirement of orientation estimation accuracy is high. For example, in [5, 6], the orientation of the intervertebral disk needs to be estimated accurately from a low resolution scout scan to set acquisition slice orientation for a high resolution scan. In that application, we used orientation set c48u8649 with $\alpha = 3.26°$ and the actual mean orientation estimation error from automatic detection was 3.9°, only slightly higher than the sampling resolution.

4.2.4 Mean Orientation

After the detection with MSL classifiers, we arrive at a set of top pose candidates. In most applications, it is required to aggregate these top candidates into a single pose estimate. Picking the best candidate with the largest detection score is not robust. In practice, we find that an average (weighted or un-weighted) of the top pose candidates (e.g., 100) gives a superior result. Calculating the average of position and scale hypotheses is simple since these two marginal spaces are an Euclidean space and a simple arithmetic mean can be used. However, it is not trivial to calculate the mean orientation. Suppose there are n orientations represented as rotation matrices $\mathbf{R}_1, \mathbf{R}_2, \ldots, \mathbf{R}_n$ and each orientation $\mathbf{R}_i$ is assigned a weight w_i (which can be the detection score generated by the MSL classifiers). Given a 3D point $\mathbf{X}$, it can be rotated to a new position $\mathbf{R}_i \mathbf{X}$ using rotation $\mathbf{R}_i$. We define the mean orientation R_m as the one that after applying the rotation, point $\mathbf{R}_m \mathbf{X}$ has the smallest sum of weighted residual errors to the other rotated positions $\mathbf{R}_i \mathbf{X}$ [1],

$$\mathbf{R}_m = arg\min_{\mathbf{R}} \sum_{i=1}^{n} w_i \|\mathbf{R}_i \mathbf{X} - \mathbf{R}\mathbf{X}\|, \quad \text{for any 3D point } \mathbf{X}. \tag{4.10}$$

Let $\bar{\mathbf{R}}$ be the weighted average of rotation matrices $\mathbf{R}_i$,

$$\bar{\mathbf{R}} = \frac{\sum_{i=1}^{n} w_i \mathbf{R}_i}{\sum_{i=1}^{n} w_i}. \tag{4.11}$$

It is shown that the optimal solution of Eq. (4.10) is equivalent to [1, 10]

$$\mathbf{R}_m = arg\min_{\mathbf{R}} \text{Trace}(\mathbf{R}^T \bar{\mathbf{R}}), \tag{4.12}$$

where function $\text{Trace}(\mathbf{A})$ is the summation of the diagonal elements of matrix $\mathbf{A}$. Let the singular value decomposition of $\bar{\mathbf{R}}$ be

$$\bar{\mathbf{R}} = \mathbf{U}\Lambda\mathbf{V}^T, \tag{4.13}$$

where Λ is a diagonal matrix; $\mathbf{U}$ and $\mathbf{V}$ are orthogonal matrices. The optimal mean orientation can be represented as [1, 10]

$$\mathbf{R}_m = \mathbf{U}\mathbf{V}^T. \tag{4.14}$$

If the orientation is represented in quaternions, it is not necessary to convert them to rotation matrix to calculate the mean orientation. Suppose $\mathbf{q}_i$ is a quaternion representation of rotation $\mathbf{R}_i$ and

$$\mathbf{Q} = \frac{\sum_{i=1}^{n} w_i \mathbf{q}_i \mathbf{q}_i^T}{\sum_{i=1}^{n} w_i}. \tag{4.15}$$

Let $\mathbf{p}$ be a quaternion representation of $\mathbf{R}$, it can be shown that [10]

$$\text{Trace}(\mathbf{R}^T \bar{\mathbf{R}}) = 4\mathbf{p}^T \mathbf{Q}\mathbf{p} - 1. \tag{4.16}$$

Thus, the optimal mean orientation $\mathbf{p}_m$ is given by the eigenvector corresponding to the largest eigenvalue of $\mathbf{Q}$. Note, in [4], the optimal solution is represented as the eigenvector corresponding to the smallest eigenvalue of $\mathbf{I} - \mathbf{Q}$. Since for each eigenvalue λ of $\mathbf{Q}$, $1 - \lambda$ is the corresponding eigenvalue of $\mathbf{I} - \mathbf{Q}$, these two solutions are equivalent.

4.3 Constrained Search Space for MSL

In this section, we present two methods to effectively constrain the search space in MSL.

4.3.1 Constrained Space for Object Position

Due to the heterogeneity in scanning protocols, the position of an object-of-interest may vary significantly in a volume. Figure 4.3 shows three CT scans (two cardiac scans and one full-torso scan) with various capture ranges, although all contain the heart in the field of view and are used to evaluate our left ventricle detection method (see Sect. 4.4.2). The difference of the capture range between the cardiac and full-torso scans is large and considerable variation is also observed in the two cardiac scans. Similar variation is observed in the liver datasets too (see Figs. 4.8 and 4.9). A learning based object detection system normally tests all voxels as hypotheses of the object center. Therefore, for a big volume, the number of hypotheses is quite large. It is preferable to constrain the search to a smaller region. The challenge is that the scheme should be generic and works for different application scenarios.

In the following, we discuss a generic way to constrain the search space. Our basic assumption is that, to study an organ, we need normally to capture the whole organ in the volume; therefore, the center of the organ cannot be arbitrarily close to the volume border. As shown in Fig. 4.4a and b, for each training volume, we can measure the distance of the object center (e.g., the left ventricle in this case) to the volume border in all six directions (e.g., X^l for the distance to the left volume border, X^r for right, Y^t for top, Y^b for bottom, Z^f for front, and Z^b for back). All the distances should be measured in physical units (e.g., millimeters) to handle different resolution settings in different volumes. The minimum value (e.g., X^l_{min} for the left margin) along each direction can be easily calculated from a training set. These minimum margins define a region (the white box in Fig. 4.4c and d) and we only need to test voxels inside the region as possible position hypotheses. The constraint

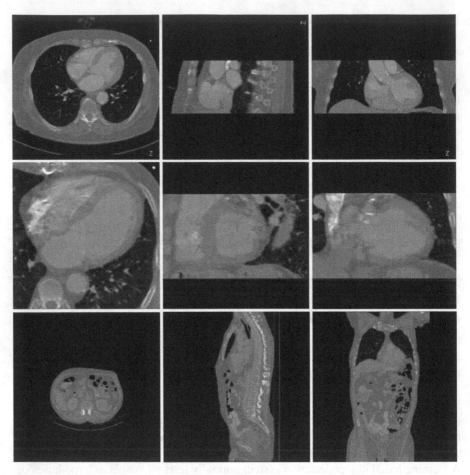

Fig. 4.3 3D CT scans for the heart with various capture ranges. Each row represents three orthogonal views of a volume. The first two are cardiac scans and the last one is a full-torso scan

is more effective for a volume with a small field of view (Fig. 4.4d) than one with a large field of view (Fig. 4.4c).

Using the proposed method, we can reduce the number of test hypotheses quite significantly. On average, we achieve a reduction of 91 % for liver detection (Sect. 4.4.1), 89 % for left ventricle detection in CT (Sect. 4.4.2), and 84 % for left ventricle detection in ultrasound (Sect. 4.4.3). That means we can speed up the position estimation about 10 times. Our strategy is generic and the statistics of the searching range can be easily calculated from the annotated training set. If there is any application-specific prior knowledge available, it can be combined with our strategy to further constrain the position search space.

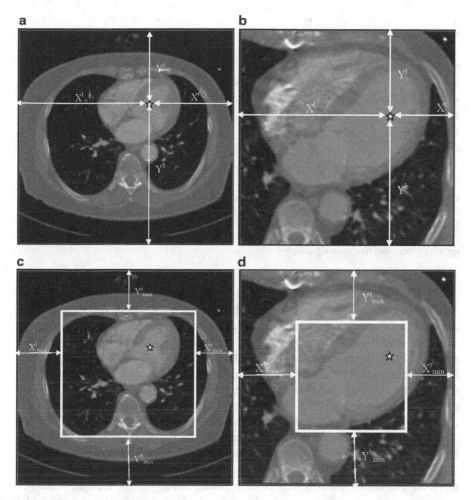

Fig. 4.4 Constraining the search for object center in a volume, illustrated for the left ventricle detection in a CT volume. (**a**) and (**b**) show two training samples on which the distances of the object center to the volume borders are measured. (**c**) and (**d**) show the constrained search space (the region enclosed by the white box) during object center estimation. The constraint is more effective for a volume with a small field of view as shown in (**d**) than one with a large field of view as shown in (**c**)

4.3.2 Constrained Space for Orientation

In this section, we present our example-based sampling strategy to effectively constrain the orientation search space. We use left ventricle detection in CT volumes (Sect. 4.4.2) to illustrate the efficiency of the proposed method. Similar analysis can also be performed for the other two applications presented in Sect. 4.4.

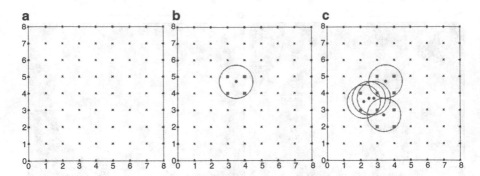

Fig. 4.5 Example-based selection of test hypotheses. (**a**) Uniformly sampled hypotheses, shown as black 'x's. (**b**) After processing the first training sample. The *circular dot* (center of the circle) shows the ground truth and the circle shows the neighborhood range. All hypotheses inside the circle (indicated with *rectangular dots*) are added to the test hypothesis set. (**c**) The test hypothesis set after processing five training samples

For many problems, the orientation of an object is well constrained in a small region. It is not necessary to test the whole orientation space. For example, on the cardiac CT dataset the ranges of Euler angles for the left ventricle using the ZXZ convention are $[-0.9, 39.1]$, $[-60.0, 88.7]$, and $[-68.8, -21.9]$ degrees, respectively. In the original MSL, each Euler angle is sampled independently within its own range and all possible combinations of three Euler angle samples are tested for orientation estimation. However, since three Euler angles should be combined to define an orientation, they are not independent. Sampling each Euler angle independently will generate far more hypotheses than necessary.

To constrain the search space, we can estimate the joint distribution of pose parameters using a training set. We then sample only the region with large probabilities to generate test hypotheses. However, it is not trivial to estimate the joint probability distributions reliably since, usually, only a limited number of positive training samples (a couple of hundred or even fewer) are available. Therefore, we use an example-based sampling strategy to generate test hypotheses (as shown in Fig. 4.5). The procedure is as follows.

1. Uniformly sample the parameter space with a certain resolution r to generate S_u (as shown in Fig. 4.5a).
2. Set the selected hypothesis set S_t to empty.
3. For each training sample, we add its neighboring samples in S_u (which have a distance no more than d) into S_t (as shown by the big rectangular dots in Fig. 4.5b). Here, $d \geq r/2$; otherwise, there may be no sample satisfying the condition. In our experiments, we set $d = r$.
4. Consolidate redundant elements in S_t to get the final test hypothesis set.

To generate the constrained test hypothesis set for orientation, we first need to uniformly sample the whole orientation space to generate the set S_u as discussed in

Sect. 4.2.3. For most 3D object detection problems, we start from a uniform set of 7416 samples distributed in the whole orientation space with $\alpha = 9.72$ degrees as S_u (set c48n309 in Table 4.1). On a dataset of 457 cardiac CT volumes, S_t of the left ventricle orientation has only 66 unique orientations, which is much smaller than S_u (7416) and also smaller than the number of the training volumes (457).

In the original MSL, each Euler angle was uniformly sampled with a step size β to generate hypotheses. The maximum distance for an arbitrary orientation to the closest hypothesis is $\frac{\sqrt{3}}{2}\beta$ using the Euclidean distance measurement. (The maximum distance occurs at the center of neighboring grid nodes. In 3D, it is at the center of a cube formed by eight neighboring grid nodes and it has a distance of $\frac{\sqrt{3}}{2}\beta$ to any node of the cube.) Since different distance measurements are used in constrained MSL (the quaternion distance) and the original MSL (the Euclidean distance), we cannot compare them directly. The Euclidean distance measurement tends to over-estimate the true distance. However, for some special cases, these two distance measurements have the same value. To achieve a nominally equivalent sampling resolution, the search step size β should be $\beta = \frac{2}{\sqrt{3}}\alpha$, that is 11.2 degrees. Suppose the range of a parameter is within $[V_{min}, V_{max}]$. We sample N points, $P_{min}, P_{min} + r, \ldots, P_{max} = P_{min} + (N-1)r$, under resolution r. To fully cover the whole range, we must have $P_{min} \leq V_{min}$ and $P_{max} \geq V_{max}$. Therefore, the number of samples should be

$$N_o = \left\lceil \frac{V_{max} - V_{min}}{r} \right\rceil + 1, \tag{4.17}$$

where $\lceil x \rceil$ returns the smallest integer that is no less than x. On the cardiac CT dataset, sampling Euler angles under the resolution of 11.2 degrees, we need $5 \times 15 \times 6 = 450$ samples to cover the orientation space. Using the quaternion representation and exploiting the correlation among orientation parameters, we reduce the number of hypotheses by 85 % to 66 samples.

4.3.3 Constrained Space for Scale

In the MSL framework, we estimate three scales of an anisotropic similarity transformation. The three scale parameters are often highly correlated. Figure 4.6 shows the distribution of scales of the left ventricle calculated from a dataset with 457 CT scans. The left ventricle has a roughly rotation symmetric shape: Two scales (we denote them as S_x and S_y) perpendicular to the left ventricle long axis (represented as the z axis) are roughly the same. Therefore, the correlation of these two scales is higher (with a correlation coefficient of 0.88 as shown in Fig. 4.6a) than the correlation to scale S_z along the long axis (with correlation coefficients of 0.81 as shown in Fig. 4.6b and 0.79 as shown in Fig. 4.6c, respectively). The distribution of the scales is clearly clustered. In the original MSL, such correlation is totally ignored. The whole region inside the box in Fig. 4.6d (which constrains the range for each scale dimension) is uniformly sampled and tested, resulting in far more scale hypotheses than necessary. On the other extreme, if only a single isotropic scale parameter is estimated, the dispersion of the distribution is ignored since it is equivalent to fit a straight line to the distribution. The object cannot be localized accurately, resulting in poor shape initialization.

No matter how complicated the distribution may be, the same example-based sampling technique can be applied to the scale space to generate scale hypotheses. The range of the scales of the left ventricle calculated from the 457 training volumes are [53.0, 91.1] mm for S_x, [49.9, 94.0] mm for S_y, and [72.3, 128.4] mm for S_z, respectively. If we uniformly sample each scale independently using a resolution of 6 mm, we need $8 \times 9 \times 11 = 792$ samples. Using our example-based sampling strategy, we only need 240 samples to cover the whole training set under the same sampling resolution of 6 mm.

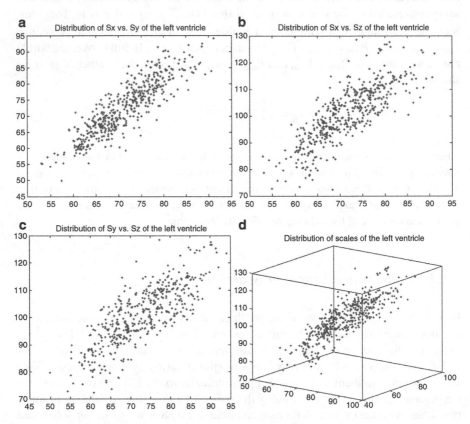

Fig. 4.6 Distribution of the scales of the left ventricle calculated from a dataset with 457 CT scans. Two scales (S_x and S_y) are defined perpendicular to its long axis and the other (S_z) is defined along the long axis. (**a**) Distribution of S_x vs. S_y, which has a high correlation coefficient of 0.88. (**b**) Distribution of S_x vs. S_z with a correlation coefficient of 0.81. (**c**) Distribution of S_y vs. S_z with a correlation coefficient of 0.79. (**d**) Distribution of scales in 3D

4.4 Experiments on Constrained Marginal Space Learning

In this section, we present three experiments to demonstrate the improved efficiency of constrained MSL, compared to the original MSL.

4.4.1 Liver Detection in CT Volumes

Our database contains 226 challenging 3D CT volumes, coming from largely diverse sources. In particular, the volumes come from patients whose disease affects various anatomies (Table 4.2) and therefore are often scanned under different protocols. This heterogeneity causes a large variation in both shape deformation and texture patterns of livers. Moreover, diagnosis of different diseases often requests different contrast agent injection protocols, or no contrast at all. For example, in our database, only about half of the volumes are contrast enhanced around the liver region, while previous studies usually use enhanced volumes only. Due to the different scanning protocols, the volumes have various dimensionality: the inter-slice resolution varies from 1.0 to 8.0 mm; the number of slices varies from 40 to 524; the actual volume height (the scan range along the patient's toe to head direction) varies from 122 to 766 mm. Moreover, the position of livers changes a lot, which presents significant challenges to atlas based approaches such as [9,17]. The statistics of volume heights, inter-slice resolution, and liver center positions are shown in Fig. 4.7.

The MSL detection speed is roughly proportional to the number of test hypotheses. The analysis presented in Sect. 4.3 shows that constrained MSL significantly reduces the number of test hypotheses. Table 4.3 shows the break-down computation time for all three steps in MSL. The detection speed is measured on a desktop computer with a 3.2 GHz dual-core processor and 3 GB memory. Overall, constrained MSL uses only 470.3 ms to process one volume, while unconstrained MSL uses 6590.8 ms. Using constrained MSL, we achieve a speed-up by a factor of 14.

In the following, we compare the accuracy of constrained MSL and the original MSL. After object localization, we align a mean shape (a surface mesh calculated from a training set) to the estimated transformation. The accuracy of initial shape estimate is measured with the symmetric point-to-mesh distance, E_{p2m}. For each point on a mesh, we search for the closest point on the other mesh to calculate the minimum distance. We calculate the point-to-mesh distance from the detected

Table 4.2 Disease distribution of the dataset used for liver detection evaluation. The items in the first row indicate the anatomies under diagnosis

Organ	Liver	Colon	Lymph Node	Thorax	Pancreas	Kidney	Other	Unknown
#Volume	60	32	20	19	6	3	2	84
Percentage (%)	26.6	15.6	8.9	8.4	2.7	1.3	0.9	37.2

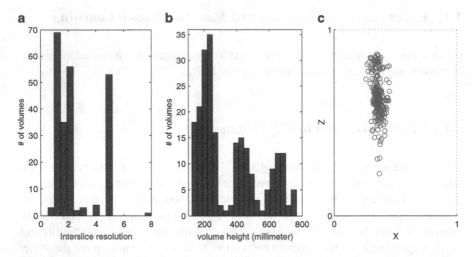

Fig. 4.7 Heterogeneity of the liver dataset. (**a**) The distribution of inter-slice resolution. (**b**) The distribution of volume heights along the z axis (pointing from patient's toe to head). (**c**) The distribution of liver locations. Each circle indicates the normalized x (pointing from patient's right shoulder to left shoulder) and z coordinates of a liver centroid (i.e., a volume dimension is normalized to $1 \times 1 \times 1$)

Table 4.3 Comparison of unconstrained and constrained MSL on the number of test hypotheses and computation time for liver detection in CT volumes

	Unconstrained MSL		Constrained MSL	
	Hypotheses	Speed (ms)	Hypotheses	Speed (ms)
Position	~403,000	2088.7	~38,000	167.1
Orientation	2686	2090.0	42	59.5
Scale	1664	1082.8	303	243.7
Overall		6590.8		470.3

mesh to the ground truth and vice verse to make the measurement symmetric. After initialization, we can deform the mesh to fit the image boundary to further reduce the error. In this work, we focus on object localization. Therefore, in the following we only measure the error of the initialized shapes for comparison purpose.

Constrained MSL also slightly improves detection accuracy. As shown in Table 4.4, constrained MSL reduces the mean E_{p2m} error from 7.44 to 7.12 mm, and

Table 4.4 Comparison of unconstrained and constrained MSL on liver detection accuracy in CT volumes. Average point-to-mesh error E_{p2m} (in millimeters) of the initialized shape is used for evaluation

	Mean	Standard Deviation	Median	Mean of Worst 10 %
Unconstrained MSL	7.44	2.26	6.99	12.32
Constrained MSL	7.12	2.15	6.73	11.88

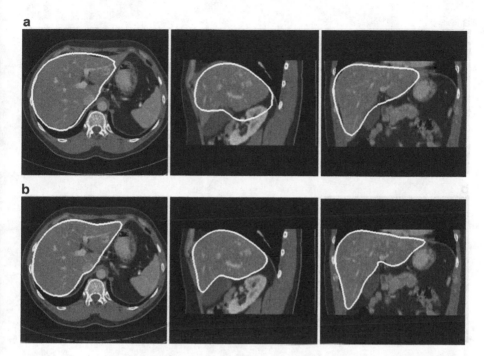

Fig. 4.8 Liver segmentation results of a CT volume with a small field of view. (**a**) Initialization by constrained MSL. (**b**) Final segmentation result. From left to right: transaxial, sagittal, and coronal views

the median E_{p2m} error from 6.99 to 6.73 mm, in a threefold cross-validation. The accuracy improvement arises from two parts. First, as we constrain the search to a smaller but more meaningful region, the likelihood of detection outliers is reduced. Second, quaternions are used for orientation distance measurement, which reduces the confusion caused by the wrong distance measurement used in the original MSL.

Figures 4.8 and 4.9 show typical liver segmentation results on two CT volumes. Accurate boundary delineation is achieved starting from the good initial estimate of the shape generated by constrained MSL. After applying our learning-based nonrigid deformation estimation method [8], the final E_{p2m} error is 1.45 mm, which is comparable or better than the state-of-the-art [3].

4.4.2 Left Ventricle Detection in CT Volumes

In this experiment, we compare unconstrained and constrained MSL on left ventricle detection in cardiac CT angiography data. We collected and annotated 457 CT volumes from 186 patients with various cardiovascular diseases. The imaging protocols are heterogeneous with different capture ranges and resolutions. A volume

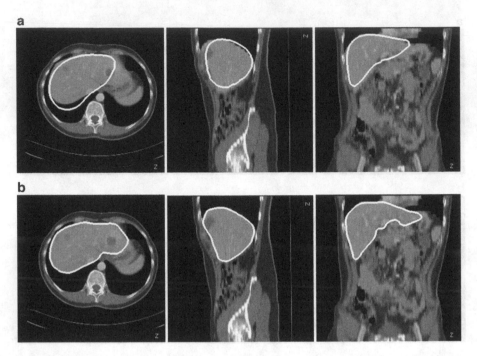

Fig. 4.9 Liver segmentation result of a another CT volume with a large field of view. (**a**) Initialization by constrained MSL. (**b**) Final segmentation result. From left to right: transaxial, sagittal, and coronal views

Table 4.5 Comparison of unconstrained and constrained MSL on the number of test hypotheses and computation time for left ventricle detection in CT volumes

	Unconstrained MSL		Constrained MSL	
	Hypotheses	Speed (ms)	Hypotheses	Speed (ms)
Position	~158,000	784.3	~18,000	75.9
Orientation	450	351.5	66	52.6
Scale	792	193.3	240	60.4
Overall		1329.3		188.9

Table 4.6 Comparison of unconstrained and constrained MSL on left ventricle detection accuracy in CT volumes. Average point-to-mesh error E_{p2m} (in millimeters) of the initialized shape is used for evaluation

	Mean	Standard Deviation	Median	Mean of Worst 10 %
Unconstrained MSL	2.66	1.00	2.45	4.73
Constrained MSL	2.62	0.84	2.45	4.43

contains 80–350 slices and the size of each slice is 512×512 pixels. The resolution inside a slice is isotropic and varies from 0.28 to 0.74 mm, while the distance between neighboring slices varies from 0.4 to 2.0 mm.

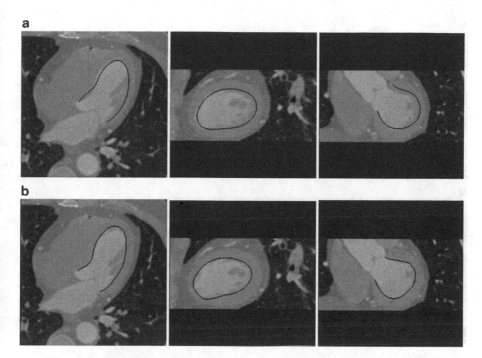

Fig. 4.10 Left ventricle segmentation results of a cardiac CT volume. (**a**) Initialization by constrained MSL. (**b**) Final segmentation result. From left to right: transaxial, sagittal, and coronal views

Similar to the previous experiments, constrained MSL also significantly reduces the number of test hypotheses and speeds up the detection consequently. Table 4.5 shows the break-down computation time for all three steps in MSL. Overall, constrained MSL uses only 188.9 ms to process one volume, while unconstrained MSL uses 1329.3 ms. (Note that the heart chamber detection speed of 0.5 s reported in [12, 13] already used constrained search space for position estimation, while the orientation and scale hypotheses are generated using exhaustive search. The overall detection speed will be slower (1.3 s) if the position space is not constrained either.) Using constrained MSL, we achieve a speed-up by a factor of seven.

Table 4.6 shows the quantitative evaluation based on a fourfold cross-validation for both unconstrained and constrained MSL. Constrained MSL achieves a slightly smaller mean error than unconstrained MSL (2.62 mm vs. 2.66 mm). We also check the worst 10 % cases (46 cases). The mean error for the worst 10 % cases is 4.43 mm of constrained MSL, about 6.3 % less than 4.73 mm of unconstrained MSL. It is clear that constraining the search space, we can reduce the likelihood of detection outliers. Please note that the mean initialization error of 2.66 mm achieved by unconstrained MSL is better than 3.17 mm reported in Chap. 2 for the left ventricle endocardium, although the same algorithm is used. In Chap. 2, we treat the whole left ventricle (including both the endocardium and epicardium) as

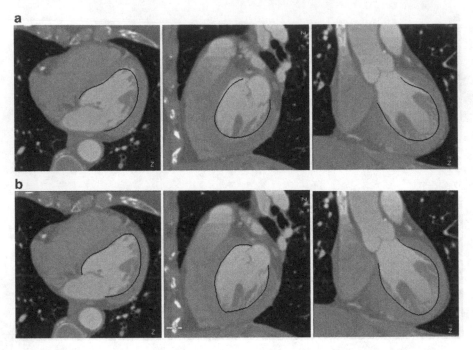

Fig. 4.11 Left ventricle segmentation results of another cardiac CT volume. (**a**) Initialization by constrained MSL. (**b**) Final segmentation result. From left to right: transaxial, sagittal, and coronal views

a single object and use MSL to estimate its pose. The size of the left ventricle is determined by its outer surface (which is the epicardium), not the endocardium. Therefore, the initialized shape is more accurate for the epicardium (2.51 mm) than the endocardium (3.17 mm). In this experiment, we focus on the endocardium detection only. Therefore, the mean shape calculated from the training set and the detected left ventricle pose are more accurate to approximate the endocardium surface.

Figures 4.10 and 4.11 show typical segmentation results of the left ventricle on two CT volumes. Constrained MSL can provide a quite good initial estimate of the shape. After nonrigid deformation estimation (refer to Chap. 7), we can achieve accurate boundary delineation results.

4.4.3 Left Ventricle Detection in Ultrasound Volumes

In this experiment, we compare unconstrained and constrained MSL on left ventricle detection in 3D ultrasound data. We collected 505 expert-annotated 3D ultrasound volumes. A typical volume size is about $160 \times 144 \times 208$ voxels and the resolution

Table 4.7 Comparison of unconstrained and constrained MSL on the number of test hypotheses and computation time for left ventricle detection in ultrasound volumes

	Unconstrained MSL		Constrained MSL	
	Hypotheses	Speed (ms)	Hypotheses	Speed (ms)
Position	~233,000	1487.3	~37,000	163.6
Orientation	882	696.3	99	12.7
Scale	2340	769.7	296	219.3
Overall		2953.3		395.6

Table 4.8 Comparison of unconstrained and constrained MSL on left ventricle detection accuracy in ultrasound volumes. Average point-to-mesh error E_{p2m} (in millimeters) of the initialized shape is used for evaluation

	Mean	Standard Deviation	Median	Mean of Worst 10 %
Unconstrained MSL	3.28	2.50	2.76	7.89
Constrained MSL	3.25	2.09	2.74	7.46

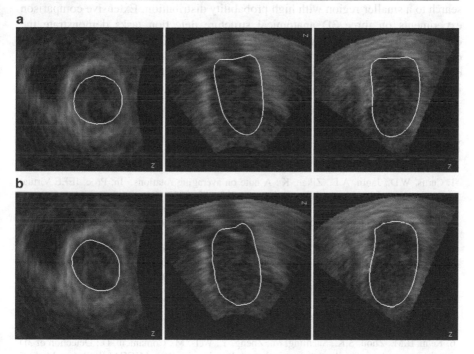

Fig. 4.12 Left ventricle segmentation results of an ultrasound volume. (**a**) Initialization by constrained MSL. (**b**) Final segmentation result. Three standard cardiac views are shown in each row

ranges are [1.24, 1.42], [1.34, 1.42], and [0.85, 0.90] mm along different directions. A fourfold cross-validation is performed to evaluate our algorithm. Similar to the previous experiments, using constrained MSL we can speed up the detection by a factor of seven (Table 4.7), while achieving a comparable detection accuracy (Table 4.8). Figure 4.12 shows the segmentation result for one example volume.

4.5 Conclusions

In this chapter, we described two major improvements to the original Marginal Space Learning (MSL). First, quaternions are used for 3D orientation representation to overcome the limitations of Euler angles. Second, a constrained MSL technique is introduced to reduce the search space. Based on the statistics of the minimum distance from the object center to volume border, the object position space is constrained to a region of interest and the volume margin can be safely skipped during position estimation. Instead of quantizing each orientation and scale parameter independently, an example-based sampling strategy is exploited to constrain the search to a smaller region with high probability distribution. Extensive comparison experiments on three 3D anatomical structure detection tasks demonstrate the efficiency of the method. It significantly accelerates the detection speed by an order of magnitude, resulting in a system that can process one volume in 0.2–0.5 s, depending on the application. At the same time, constrained MSL can also slightly improve the detection accuracy by reducing the likelihood of detection outliers.

References

1. Curtis, W.D., Janin, A.L., Zikan, K.: A note on averaging rotations. In: Proc. IEEE Virtual Reality Annual International Symposium, pp. 377–385 (1993)
2. Georgescu, B., Zhou, X.S., Comaniciu, D., Gupta, A.: Database-guided segmentation of anatomical structures with complex appearance. In: Proc. IEEE Conf. Computer Vision and Pattern Recognition, pp. 429–436 (2005)
3. van Ginneken, B., Heimann, T., Styner, M.: 3D segmentation in the clinic: A grand challenge. In: MICCAI Workshop on 3D Segmentation in the Clinic: A Grand Challenge (2007)
4. Karney, C.F.F.: Quaternions in molecular modeling. Journal of Molecular Graphics and Modeling **25**(5), 595–604 (2007)
5. Kelm, B.M., Wels, M., Zhou, S.K., Seifert, S., Suehling, M., Zheng, Y., Comaniciu, D.: Spine detection in CT and MR using iterated marginal space learning. Medical Image Analysis **17**(8), 1283–1292 (2013)
6. Kelm, B.M., Zhou, S.K., Suehling, M., Zheng, Y., Wels, M., Comaniciu, D.: Detection of 3D spinal geometry using iterated marginal space learning. In: Proc. MICCAI Workshop Medical Computer Vision — Recognition Techniques and Applications in Medical Imaging, pp. 96–105 (2010)
7. Kuffner, J.J.: Effective sampling and distance metrics for 3D rigid body path planning. In: Proc. IEEE Int'l Conf. Robotics and Automation, pp. 3993–3998 (2004)
8. Ling, H., Zhou, S.K., Zheng, Y., Georgescu, B., Suehling, M., Comaniciu, D.: Hierarchical, learning-based automatic liver segmentation. In: Proc. IEEE Conf. Computer Vision and Pattern Recognition, pp. 1–8 (2008)

9. Okada, T., Shimada, R., Sato, Y., Hori, M., Yokota, K., Nakamoto, M., Chen, Y.W., Nakamura, H., Tamura, S.: Automated segmentation of the liver from 3D CT images using probabilistic atlas and multi-level statistical shape model. In: Proc. Int'l Conf. Medical Image Computing and Computer Assisted Intervention, vol. 1, p. 86–93 (2007)

10. Rancourt, D., Rivest, L.P., Asselin, J.: Using orientation statistics to investigate variations in human kinematics. Applied Statistics **49**(1), 81–94 (2000)

11. Shoemake, K.: Animating rotation with quaternion curves. In: Proc. SIGGRAPH, pp. 245–254 (1985)

12. Zheng, Y., Barbu, A., Georgescu, B., Scheuering, M., Comaniciu, D.: Fast automatic heart chamber segmentation from 3D CT data using marginal space learning and steerable features. In: Proc. Int'l Conf. Computer Vision, pp. 1–8 (2007)

13. Zheng, Y., Barbu, A., Georgescu, B., Scheuering, M., Comaniciu, D.: Four-chamber heart modeling and automatic segmentation for 3D cardiac CT volumes using marginal space learning and steerable features. IEEE Trans. Medical Imaging **27**(11), 1668–1681 (2008)

14. Zheng, Y., Georgescu, B., Comaniciu, D.: Marginal space learning for efficient detection of 2D/3D anatomical structures in medical images. In: Proc. Information Processing in Medical Imaging, pp. 411–422 (2009)

15. Zheng, Y., Georgescu, B., Ling, H., Zhou, S.K., Scheuering, M., Comaniciu, D.: Constrained marginal space learning for efficient 3D anatomical structure detection in medical images. In: Proc. IEEE Conf. Computer Vision and Pattern Recognition, pp. 194–201 (2009)

16. Zheng, Y., Zhou, X.S., Georgescu, B., Zhou, S.K., Comaniciu, D.: Example based non-rigid shape detection. In: Proc. European Conf. Computer Vision, pp. 423–436 (2006)

17. Zhou, X., Kitagawa, T., Hara, T., Fujita, H., Zhang, X., Yokoyama, R., Kondo, H., Kanematsu, M., Hoshi, H.: Constructing a probabilistic model for automated liver region segmentation using non-contrast X-ray torso CT images. In: Proc. Int'l Conf. Medical Image Computing and Computer Assisted Intervention, vol. 2, pp. 856–863 (2006)

Chapter 5
Part-Based Object Detection and Segmentation

5.1 Introduction

The computational framework of Marginal Space Learning (MSL) formulates the detection of an anatomical structure as a whole object. Nevertheless, an object might exhibit different degrees of variations due to many factors, e.g., nonrigid deformation, anatomical variations, or diversity in scanning protocols. When variations are too large for the object to maintain a globally consistent shape or appearance, the MSL cannot be applied directly or the detection robustness may be degraded. To deal with this problem we observe that complex anatomical structures can be naturally split into different parts. For example, the aorta can be decomposed into the aortic root, ascending aorta, aortic arch, and descending aorta. Although the global object might exhibit large variations, an object part is subject to less distortion due to its smaller size and better specification, therefore it can be detected more reliably [50, 51].

In some cases, in spite of the fact that the global object can still be detected, the shape initialization accuracy for the subsequent boundary delineation may be degraded due to a large shape variation. The MSL based detection and segmentation uses a mean shape aligned to the estimated pose to provide initial segmentation. If the shape variation is too big, the mean shape cannot represent the whole shape population well; therefore, the shape initialization accuracy may be poor. If the object partitioning is properly implemented, the object parts have a more consistent shape and the MSL can be applied to achieve accurate segmentation of the parts. The part segmentation can then be consolidated into a complete segmentation of the global object. For objects with a large shape variation, a part-based segmentation approach may be more accurate than the holistic approach that treats the anatomical structure as a single object [52, 53].

The anatomical variations are one major challenge in many automatic detection/segmentation problems and these are typical in the case of Left Atrium (LA) and Pulmonary Veins (PVs). Accurate segmentation of the whole LA, including the chamber, appendage, and PVs, has important applications in planning and visual

Y. Zheng and D. Comaniciu, *Marginal Space Learning for Medical Image Analysis:*   103
Efficient Detection and Segmentation of Anatomical Structures,
DOI 10.1007/978-1-4939-0600-0__5, © Springer Science+Business Media New York 2014

guidance for catheter based ablation to treat atrial fibrillation. An automatic segmentation algorithm has to handle all the common anatomical variations. To achieve this, we note that each LA part has a more consistent shape and the anatomical variation is mainly on the connections among the parts. Therefore we developed a part-based detection method to achieve robust and accurate segmentation of the LA. The whole LA structure is split into six parts, namely, the LA chamber, Left Atrial Appendage (LAA), and four major PVs. We train an MSL pose detector for each part. However, if each part is detected independently, detection outliers may happen. For example, due to the similar shape and proximity of neighboring PVs, one PV may be detected as another PV. The solution is to enforce statistical shape constraints among different parts during the detection process, to reduce outliers.

The automatic and precise detection of the Left Ventricle (LV) in Magnetic Resonance Imaging (MRI) is important not only for the analysis of the LV function, but also during the image acquisition process. In the following, we consider the problem of detecting the LV in a long axis view, when the image plane passes through the LV axis, defined by the apex and two basal points on the mitral valve annulus. As a result of the weak constraint, the LV shape variations and changes in the background surrounding the LV are large. In addition, when the four chambers of the heart are visible in the image plane the LV and Right Ventricle (RV) have a similar appearance. A physician needs to rely on more subtle difference to distinguish the LV and RV (e.g., myocardium thickness). The cardiac motion is another cause of large shape changes for this application. A normal LV pumps at least 50 % of blood out of its cavity; therefore, the size and shape of the LV change significantly from the end-diastolic phase (when the LV size is the largest) to the end-systolic phase (when the LV is the smallest).

Due to all these variations, our approach to the LV detection problem is to use multiple part detectors and an intelligent aggregation scheme that exploits the redundancy among detectors and improves the overall robustness. We call this method ranking based multi-detector aggregation for LV detection in 2D MRI. In addition to the LV detector of the whole chamber, we train two part detectors, one for the LV apex and the other for the base around the mitral valve. During detection, first, each detector is independently run on an input image to generate a few top candidate detections. A ranking based approach is developed to aggregate all information to pick the best detection result.

Another source of variability comes from an object being imaged with different field-of-views across scans. For example, in a C-arm Computed Tomography (C-arm CT) scan for Transcatheter Aortic Valve Implantation (TAVI), the aortic arch and descending aorta may be captured in some volumes, but missing in others. To address this challenge, we developed a part-based aorta model. The whole aorta is represented with four parts: aortic root, ascending aorta, aortic arch, and descending aorta. Since the aortic root and aortic arch are more consistent, we train two MSL pose detectors, one for each part. The length of the ascending aorta and descending aorta varies quite a lot; hence, it is difficult to treat them as a consistent object. Instead, they are detected through a tracking approach, by noting that their 2D transaxial view has a shape close to a circle. Starting from the detected aortic root or arch, we track the intersection circle using a trained circle detector. As a result, using a part-based approach, we achieve superior performance even for cases when aorta is not fully captured by the acquisition. Depending on the parts that are detected, different workflows can be exploited; therefore, a large structural variation can be elegantly handled.

The remainder of this chapter is organized as follows. In Sect. 5.2, we present a part-based detection scheme to handle anatomical variations of the PVs. The ranking based multi-detector aggregation approach is presented in Sect. 5.3 to improve the detection robustness of the LV in 2D MRI. In Sect. 5.4, we describe a part-based aorta detection method to handle variations in the scanning field of view. Conclusions are presented in Sect. 5.5.

5.2   Part-Based Left Atrium Detection and Segmentation in C-arm CT

Affecting more than three million people in the USA [28], Atrial Fibrillation (AF) is the most common cardiac arrhythmia, involving irregular heart beats. AF is associated with an increased risk of stroke, heart failure, cognitive dysfunction, and reduced quality of life. For example, AF patients have a fivefold increased risk of stroke compared to those without AF and about 15–20 % of strokes can be attributed to AF [41]. A widely used minimally invasive surgery to treat AF, the catheter based ablation procedure uses high radio-frequency energy to eliminate the sources of ectopic foci. With the improvement in the ablation technology, this procedure was adopted quickly with 15 % annual increase rate from 1990 to 2005 [22] and the latest estimate of the number of ablations is approximately 50,000/year in the USA and 60,000/year in Europe [9]. The ablation is mainly performed inside the Left Atrium (LA), especially around the ostia of the Pulmonary Veins (PV). Sometimes, other regions may also be ablated, e.g., the roof of the LA chamber, mitral isthmus, and the Left Atrial Appendage (LAA), to treat persistent AF.

Automatic segmentation of the LA has important applications in pre-operative assessment and intra-operative guidance for the ablation procedure [19, 21, 26]. However, there are large variations in the PV drainage patterns [27]. Majority of the population have two separate PVs on each side of the LA chamber, namely the Left Inferior PV (LIPV) and Left Superior PV (LSPV) on the left side, and the Right Inferior PV (RIPV) and Right Superior PV (RSPV) on the right side (Fig. 5.1). A significant proportion (about 20–30 %) of the population have anatomical variations and the most common variations are extra right PVs, where, besides the RIPV and RSPV, one or more extra PVs emerge separately from the right side of the LA chamber, and the left common PV, where the LIPV and LSPV merge into one before joining the chamber. A personalized LA model can help to translate a generic ablation strategy to the patient's specific anatomy, thus making the ablation strategy more effective for the patient. Fusing the patient-specific LA model together with

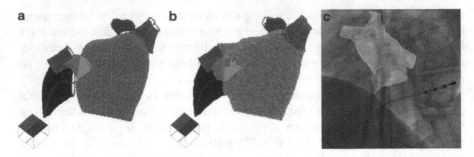

Fig. 5.1 The part-based Left Atrium (LA) mesh model. (**a**) Meshes of the separate LA parts. (**b**) Final consolidated mesh model. (**c**) Overlay of the model onto a fluoroscopic image to provide visual guidance during catheter based ablation

electro-anatomical maps or overlaying the result onto 2D real-time fluoroscopic images also provides valuable visual guidance during the intervention (Fig. 5.1c).

Most of the existing LA segmentation methods work on Computed Tomography (CT) or MRI data with electrocardiography-gated (i.e., ECG-gated or gated for short) acquisitions, where the boundary between the LA and the surrounding tissues is sufficiently clear to facilitate the segmentation. There is one reported work on LA segmentation on non-gated C-arm Computed Tomography (C-arm CT) [26], which is the most closely related work to ours. To handle the severe imaging artifacts of C-arm CT (e.g., cardiac motion blur), it uses model-based approaches to exploit the prior shape constraints to improve the segmentation robustness. However, using a single holistic shape model to initialize the LA segmentation, Manzke et al.'s method [26] has difficulty to handle anatomical variations of the PVs, e.g., the left common PV and extra right middle PVs. The right middle PVs are missing in their LA model. Furthermore, their model does not include the LA appendage. Although the LA appendage itself is less important than the PVs in the catheter based ablations, the ridge between the LA appendage and the LSPV is an important ablation region. Including the LA appendage into the shape model provides better visual guidance for physicians to ablate the ridge. Furthermore, the LA appendage is important for other catheter based interventions, e.g., the occlusion of the LA appendage in AF patients to reduce the risk of stroke [17].

In the following we present a fully automatic LA segmentation system on C-arm CT data. Compared to conventional CT or MRI, one advantage of C-arm CT is that the overlay of the 3D patient-specific LA model onto a 2D fluoroscopic image is straightforward since both the 3D and 2D images are captured on the same device within a short time interval. Normally, a non-gated acquisition is performed for C-arm CT; therefore, it may contain cardiac motion artifacts. On a C-arm system with a small X-ray detector panel (20×20 cm^2), part of the body may be missing in some 2D X-ray projections due to the limited field of view, resulting in significant artifacts around the margin of a reconstructed volume. In addition, there may be streak artifacts caused by various catheters inserted in the heart, which are less common in CT/MRI. All these present challenges to non-model based segmentation approaches [19,21,24], which assume no or little prior knowledge of the LA shape, although they may work well on highly-contrasted CT/MRI data. In our work, these challenges are addressed using a model based approach, that also takes advantage of the machine learning based object pose detector and boundary detector.

Instead of using one mean shape model as in [26], the PV anatomical variations are addressed using a part-based model, where the whole LA is split into the chamber, appendage, and four major PVs. Each part is a much simpler anatomical structure compared to the holistic one, therefore can be detected and segmented using a model based approach. In order to increase robustness, we detect the most reliable structure (the LA chamber in this case) first and use it to constrain the detection of other parts (the appendage and PVs). Experiments show that it is better to treat the LA chamber and appendage as a single object to improve the detection robustness of the appendage. Due to the anatomical variations (e.g., the presence of the left common PV), the relative position of the major PVs to the LA chamber varies. A statistical shape model is used to enforce a proper constraint during the detection of the PVs, i.e., estimating their pose parameters, including position, orientation, and size.

After segmenting the LA parts, a consolidated mesh is generated by resolving the gaps and overlaps among the parts [49]. Extra right middle PVs are then extracted using a graph cuts based approach [4,5]. To avoid segmentation leakage, the right middle PV extraction is constrained in a region of interest defined by the already segmented RIPV and RSPV [43].

Our segmentation accuracy of the LA chamber and major PVs is comparable to [26], although our validation involves hundreds of datasets, versus the only 33 datasets in [26]. In addition to [26], we also extract the LA appendage and right middle PVs. Taking about 2.6 s to process a volume with $256 \times 256 \times 250$ voxels, the proposed method is much faster than [26]. Our method also compares favorably with the other methods in computation speed, e.g., 5 s in [20] and 5–45 s in [19]. Although the atlas-based methods have the potential to handle anatomical variations by using multiple atlases, their computational efficiency is low, since it may take more than two hours to process one dataset [8].

5.2.1   Part-Based Left Atrium Model

As shown in Fig. 5.1a, our part-based LA model includes the LA chamber body, appendage, and four major PVs. We reuse the LA chamber model from our four-chamber heart model [45,47]. The LA chamber surface mesh is composed of 545 mesh points and 1,056 triangles with an opening at the mitral valve.

For AF ablation, physicians only care about a short PV trunk connected to the LA chamber; therefore, we only detect a trunk of 20 mm in length, originating from its ostium. In the case of left common PV, the PVs after the bifurcation at the distal end of the common PV are modeled, as shown in Fig. 5.2c and d. Each PV is represented as an open-ended tubular structure with a proximal opening on the LA chamber side

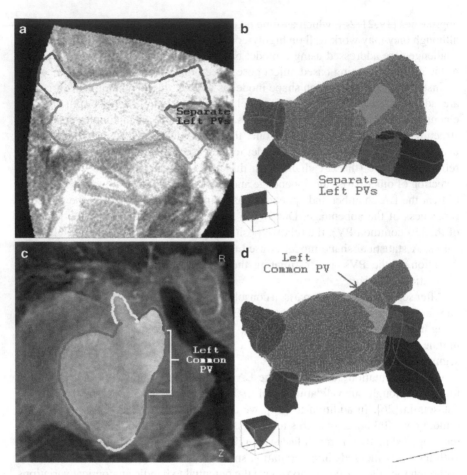

Fig. 5.2 Pulmonary Vein (PV) segmentation results on two datasets. (**a**) and (**b**) show a patient with separate left inferior and superior PVs. (**c**) and (**d**) show a patient with a left common PV

and a distal opening away from the LA chamber. On the PV mesh, the two openings are represented as two closed contours, namely the proximal ring and the distal ring, respectively. The PV mesh is uniformly resampled to nine rings (including the proximal and distal rings) perpendicular to its centerline and each ring is uniformly resampled to 24 points; therefore, the PV mesh is composed of a total of 216 points and 384 triangles.

The LA appendage has a complicated shape, which is composed of a lot of small cavities. On C-arm CT, the boundary between cavities is often blurred due to the cardiac motion artifacts. In our application, it is accurate enough to use a smooth mesh tightly enclosing all the appendage cavities. The shape of the appendage mesh is close to a tilted cone with an opening (called a proximal ring) at the connection to the LA chamber. The centerline from the proximal ring center to the appendage tip defines the orientation of the tilted cone. Similar to the PVs, the appendage mesh is also represented as a set of uniformly distributed circular rings perpendicular to its centerline. Since the appendage is larger and has a more complicated shape than the PVs, it is represented as a denser mesh with 18 rings and each ring with 33 points. The most distal ring is represented as a single point to close the mesh at the appendage tip.

The right middle PVs are an optional component of our part-based LA model as they are only present in a relatively small proportion of patients. The right middle PVs originate on the LA chamber around the area between two major right PVs. Majority of the population (70–80 %) have no middle PVs. However, some patients may have up to three middle PVs [27]. If the origin of a PV is too close to a major PV, it is often difficult to identify if this PV is an independent middle PV or just a side branch of a major PV. Due to these difficulties, we do not have a consistent mesh presentation of the right middle PVs. They are extracted using a non-model based graph cuts approach [5].

Our LA model does not include the side branches of a PV since the AF ablation is normally performed around the PV ostia on the LA chamber surface. A side branch may improve the aesthetic effect of the 3D visualization, but is not clinically relevant. The variation of the left PVs is dominated by the left common PV (Fig. 5.2) and it is extremely rare to have extra middle PVs on the left side [27]; therefore, the left middle PVs are not included in our model. Note that the part-based LA model is an internal representation to facilitate the segmentation process in handling anatomical variations. The final LA model presented to physicians is a consolidated mesh with different parts labeled with different colors, as shown in Fig. 5.1b.

5.2.2 Constrained Detection of Left Atrium Parts

Compared to the holistic approach [26], the part-based approach can handle large anatomical variations. The MSL based detection/segmentation method works well for the LA chamber. However, independent detection of other parts is not robust, either due to low contrast at the appendage or small size of PVs. In C-arm CT, the appendage is particularly difficult to detect since the appendage is a pouch without outlet and the blood flow is slow inside the appendage, preventing complete filling of contrast agent. In many datasets, the appendage is only barely visible. The MSL detector may pick the neighboring LSPV, which often touches the appendage and has higher contrast. However, the relative position of the appendage to the chamber is quite consistent. Experiments show that the best performance is achieved by treating the appendage and chamber as a consolidated object. One MSL based pose detector is trained to detect the combined object.

Through comparison experiments, we found that neither a holistic approach nor independent detection worked well for the PVs (refer to Sect. 5.2.3.2). Therefore, we selected a method to enforce a statistical shape constraint in PV detection. The Point Distribution Model (PDM) [7] is often used to enforce the statistical shape constraint among a set of landmarks in an Active Shape Model (ASM) based segmentation. The shape variation is decomposed into orthogonal deformation modes through Principal Component Analysis (PCA). A deformed shape is projected into a low dimensional deformation subspace to enforce a statistical shape constraint. For each PV, an MSL pose detector can estimate nine pose parameters, i.e., three position parameters (T_x, T_y, T_z), three orientation Euler angles (O_x, O_y, O_z), and three anisotropic scaling parameters (S_x, S_y, S_z). Different to the conventional PDM, we also want to enforce constraint among the estimated orientation and size of PVs. One solution is to stack all PV pose parameters into a long vector to perform PCA. However, the position and orientation parameters are measured in different units. If not weighted properly, the extracted deformation modes may be dominated by one part of the transformation. Furthermore, the Euler angles are periodic (with a period of 2π), which prevents the application of PCA. Boisvert et al. [3] proposed to build a shape model on a Riemannian manifold that has an intrinsic measurement of the orientation distance. However, they still need to heuristically assign proper weights to the distances in the translation and orientation spaces.

In our solution we use a new representation of the pose parameters to avoid the above problems. The object pose can be fully represented by the object center $\mathbf{T}$ together with three scaled orthogonal axes. Alternative to the Euler angles, the object orientation can be represented as a rotation matrix $\mathbf{R} = (\mathbf{R_x}, \mathbf{R_y}, \mathbf{R_z})$ where each column of $\mathbf{R}$ defines an axis. The object pose parameters are then given by a four-point set $(\mathbf{T}, \mathbf{V_x}, \mathbf{V_y}, \mathbf{V_z})$, where

$$\mathbf{V_x} = \mathbf{T} + S_x \mathbf{R_x},$$

$$\mathbf{V_y} = \mathbf{T} + S_y \mathbf{R_y},$$

$$\mathbf{V_z} = \mathbf{T} + S_z \mathbf{R_z}. \tag{5.1}$$

The pose of each PV is represented by four points. Besides the constraint among the PVs, we also add the already detected LA chamber center and appendage center to stabilize the detection. In total, we get a set of 18 points and the point distribution shape subspace is learned on the training set.

After independent detection of the position, orientation, size of the PVs, we project their poses into a subspace with eight dimensions, which explains about 75 % of the total variation, to enforce a statistical shape constraint. Note that the percentage of preserved variations in the sub-space is lower than the typical 95 % used for object segmentation [7]. In a typical setting, the ASM is used for object boundary segmentation; therefore, the sub-space needs to be large enough to achieve a flexible and precise segmentation. In our case, the ASM is used to constrain the PV pose estimation. Since the robustness is more important than precision, we found a subspace with a lower dimension is better. The additional variations can be compensated by the following boundary segmentation process.

After enforcing a statistical shape constraint, the new PV center is given by the point $\hat{\mathbf{T}}$. We can recover the orientation ($\hat{\mathbf{R}}$) and scale ($\hat{\mathbf{S}}$) from points $\mathbf{V_x}$, $\mathbf{V_y}$, and

V_z by simple inversion of Eq. (5.1). However, the estimate $\hat{R}$ is generally not a true rotation matrix ($\hat{R}^T \hat{R} \neq I$). We want to find the nearest rotation matrix R_0 to minimize the sum of squares of elements in the difference matrix $R_0 - \hat{R}$, which is equivalent to

$$R_0 = arg\min_{R} \text{Trace}((R - \hat{R})^T (R - \hat{R})), \qquad (5.2)$$

subject to $R_0{}^T R_0 = I$. Here, Trace(.) is sum of the diagonal elements. The optimal solution [18] is given by

$$R_0 = \hat{R}(\hat{R}^T \hat{R})^{-1/2}. \qquad (5.3)$$

Using the statistical shape constraint, a proper configuration of the different LA parts is preserved by the segmentation results. As mentioned before, for image data acquired with a C-arm system equipped with a small X-ray detector panel, a significant portion of a PV may be outside of the field of view. Using the proposed method, the partially missing PV can still be detected correctly.

After segmenting the LA parts, a consolidated mesh is generated by resolving the gaps and overlaps among the parts. Please refer to [49, 53] for more details.

5.2.3 Experiments on Left Atrium Segmentation in C-arm CT

5.2.3.1 Data Sets

We collected 687 C-arm CT datasets, scanned by Siemens Axiom Artis zee C-arm systems at 18 clinical sites in Europe and the USA from June 2006 to April 2011. Among them 253 datasets were scanned with large X-ray detector panels (30×40 cm^2) and reconstructed to volumes composed of 85–254 slices, each slice containing 256×256 pixels. The resolution varies from 0.61 to 1.00 mm. A typical large volume has $256 \times 256 \times 190$ voxels with an isotropic resolution of 0.90 mm. The other 434 datasets were scanned with small X-ray detectors (20×20 cm^2). Each volume contains 164–251 slices and each slice has 256×256 pixels. The resulting volume resolution also varies. A typical small volume has $256 \times 256 \times 245$ voxels with an isotropic resolution of 0.44 mm. Because of the limited field of view of small X-ray detectors, the reconstructed volumes may contain artifacts, especially around the volume margin.

The contrast agent is injected via a pigtail catheter inside the pulmonary artery trunk. A single sweep of the C-arm involving a rotation of 200° in 5 s is performed to capture 2D projections and a 3D volume is reconstructed from all 2D projections belonging to various cardiac phases (the so-called non-gated reconstruction). Such non-gated acquisition often results in significant amount of motion blur, especially around the septum wall of the LA. In most cases, the LA has sufficient contrast, but inhomogeneous contrast filling is often observed, especially between the left and right PVs because of the different transition time of the contrast agent from the pulmonary artery trunk to the PVs. The LA appendage often lacks contrast because of the slow blood flow inside the appendage. Different to [26, 35], our imaging protocol uses a single scan to reduce the amount of contrast agent and radiation dose, even for a C-arm system with a small X-ray detector.

To train the proposed segmentation system and perform quantitative evaluation, the LA needs to be annotated on all datasets. The annotation is generated sequentially. First, the LA chamber, appendage, and four major PVs are annotated using the part model presented in Sect. 5.2.1 and are then used to train the part detectors (Sect. 5.2.2). A consolidated mesh is generated from the LA parts using the methods presented in [49]. The mesh is then double checked and segmentation errors are manually corrected if necessary.

5.2.3.2   Quantitative Evaluation of Left Atrium Segmentation

Table 5.1 Left atrium segmentation errors (based on a fourfold cross-validation) on 253 large C-arm CT volumes. The symmetric point-to-mesh errors, measured in millimeters (mm), are reported

	Holistic		Independent		Proposed	
	Mean	Median	Mean	Median	Mean	Median
LA Chamber	1.52	1.38	1.45	1.26	**1.41**	1.26
Appendage	3.16	2.51	3.39	2.52	**2.87**	2.20
Left Inf. PV	2.68	2.10	1.67	1.32	**1.60**	1.30
Left Sup. PV	2.45	1.74	1.72	1.38	**1.55**	1.15
Right Inf. PV	3.24	2.39	1.85	1.30	**1.67**	1.34
Right Sup. PV	2.31	1.86	1.42	1.15	**1.36**	1.21
Whole Mesh Average	2.08	1.94	1.85	1.59	**1.70**	1.50
Whole Mesh (No Part Label)	1.72	1.61	1.51	1.37	**1.47**	1.30
Whole Mesh (No Part Label + No LAA)	1.55	1.45	1.30	1.15	**1.27**	1.14

A fourfold cross-validation is performed to evaluate the LA segmentation accuracy. The whole dataset is randomly split into four roughly equal sets. Three sets are used to train the system and the remaining set is reserved for testing. The configuration is rotated, until each set has been tested once. Due to the heterogeneity of the datasets, we train two separate systems, one for the large volumes and one for the small ones, respectively. The evaluation is performed separately for each system.

The LA segmentation accuracy is measured using the symmetric point-to-mesh distance [46]. For each point on a mesh, we search for the closest point on the other mesh to calculate the minimum distance. Different anatomical parts are labeled differently on our consolidated mesh. To include the mesh part labeling errors in the evaluation, when we search for the closest corresponding point, the search is constrained to the region with the same part label. The minimum distances of all mesh points are averaged to calculate the mesh-level error. We calculate the distance from the detected mesh to the ground truth and vice versa to make the measurement symmetric. Our consolidated mesh has an opening around the mitral valve so that the physicians can have an endocardium view inside the LA. The mesh is closed around the distal PVs, although there is no image boundary around that region. Similar to [26], the artificial closing around the distal PVs are excluded from the evaluation (which corresponds to about 5.5 % mesh triangles excluded).

Table 5.2 Left atrium segmentation errors (based on a fourfold cross-validation) on 434 small C-arm CT volumes. The symmetric point-to-mesh errors, measured in millimeters (mm), are reported

	Holistic		Independent		Proposed	
	Mean	Median	Mean	Median	Mean	Median
LA Chamber	1.45	1.26	1.42	1.22	**1.34**	1.16
Appendage	2.41	1.98	3.11	2.32	**2.40**	1.95
Left Inf. PV	2.71	1.97	1.94	1.22	**1.66**	1.18
Left Sup. PV	2.73	1.72	2.23	1.33	**1.60**	1.03
Right Inf. PV	2.80	2.19	1.83	1.30	**1.58**	1.31
Right Sup. PV	2.21	1.71	1.63	1.07	**1.36**	1.05
Whole Mesh Average	1.90	1.68	1.84	1.56	**1.57**	1.39
Whole Mesh (No Part Label)	1.60	1.45	1.47	1.29	**1.35**	1.22
Whole Mesh (No Part Label + No LAA)	1.51	1.36	1.31	1.14	**1.23**	1.09

In the following experiment, to evaluate how constrained detection of LA parts improves the segmentation accuracy, the right middle PVs are excluded (not detected at all). Please refer to [43] for a quantitative evaluation of our method on detecting and segmenting the right middle PVs.

Tables 5.1 and 5.2 show segmentation errors of the consolidated mesh using various approaches on the large and small volumes, respectively. The comparison is limited to the variations in the LA part detection approaches to provide an initial shape. After that, we use the same procedure for boundary delineation and consolidated mesh generation [49]. The break-down error of each mesh part is shown and the row *"Whole Mesh Average"* shows the average error of the whole mesh. If we treat the whole LA as a holistic object, the segmentation errors are large, especially for the PVs due to the anatomical variations. Independent detection of the parts can significantly improve the PV segmentation accuracy. However, the LA appendage segmentation accuracy is deteriorated. Using the proposed method, we achieve consistent improvement for all LA parts on both the large and small volumes. On average, we achieve an error of 1.70 mm for the large volumes, which corresponding to 18 % reduction compared to the holistic approach and 8 % reduction to the independent detection. A slightly smaller average error of 1.57 mm is achieved for the small volumes, partially due to the higher voxel resolution and stronger contrast inside the LA. In addition, we have more small volumes for training and cross-validation (434 vs. 253). This error corresponds to 17 % reduction

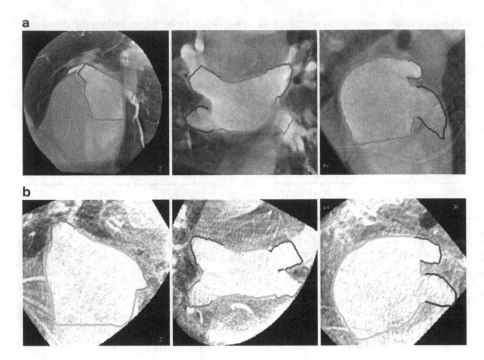

Fig. 5.3 The left atrium segmentation results on (**a**) a large volume and (**b**) a small volume. Three orthogonal views are shown for each volume

to the holistic approach and 15 % reduction to the independent detection. Figure 5.3 shows the segmentation results on a large volume and a small volume using the proposed method.

In our approach, the inferior PVs have larger errors than the superior PVs since they are more likely to be cut by the volume borders. However, for the independent detection method, the LSPV has the largest error (2.23 mm) among all PVs on the small volumes. If the LSPV is partially out of the volume, the appendage is often detected as the LSPV, resulting in a large segmentation error.

We cannot directly compare our segmentation accuracy with those reported in the literature due to the difference in imaging modalities, datasets, and LA models, etc. There is no quantitative evaluation available in [19, 21]. To our knowledge, there is one previous work [26] on LA segmentation in C-arm CT, which was validated on a small database (33 patients) from a single clinical site. A mean error of 1.31 mm was reported in [26] without including the challenging LA appendage in their model. Their point-to-mesh error does not include the part labeling error. In our case, for a mesh part, we measure the distance to the corresponding part in the ground truth, therefore both the segmentation and mesh part labeling errors are penalized. To make a more direct comparison, the row "*Whole Mesh (No Part Label)*" in Tables 5.1 and 5.2 reports the similar error without considering the part label. That means the closest point is searched on the whole mesh when we calculate the mesh error, not restricted to the part with the same label. The LA appendage can be further excluded as reported in row "*Whole Mesh (No Part Label + No LAA)*" of Tables 5.1 and 5.2. Under this condition, we achieve a mean error of 1.27 mm and 1.23 mm for the large and small volumes, respectively. These errors are comparable with the 1.31 mm mean error reported in [26]. Their segmentation is initialized with a holistic mean shape. It is not clear if patients with a left common PV are included in their test set, since a holistic approach has difficulty to handle such anatomical variations.

5.3 Ranking Based Multi-Detector Aggregation for Left Ventricle Detection in 2D MRI

When an object is subject to large variations and is surrounded by cluttered background, it is hard to be detected reliably. In such scenarios, besides the global detector, we can train multiple part detectors and use an intelligent aggregation scheme to exploit the redundancy among the results of multi-detectors to improve robustness.

Part-based detection approaches have been previously proposed to detect the human body (under occlusion, in surveillance video) [32, 42] or other generic nonrigid objects [11]. In [42], the hierarchical human body model has a fixed geometry, e.g., the foot box is exactly the lower half of the whole-body box. With this rigid geometric model, for each detected part box candidate, a whole-body box can be inferred. After that, all following reasoning is performed at the whole-body level. Shet et al. [32] proposed a logic-based method to detect humans, exploiting a more flexible part model. However, domain specific knowledge needs to be manually coded in the logic rule templates. To the other extremity, a loosely coupled star model was used in [11] to model the nonrigid deformation of an object. The detection always starts from the whole-object detector and a whole-object candidate is confirmed if we can detect a part in the expected position. Such a manually defined aggregation scheme cannot fully exploit the rich information embedded in the detected candidates.

In the following we present a ranking based multi-detector aggregation algorithm for Left Ventricle (LV) detection in 2D Magnetic Resonance Imaging (MRI). We assume that the 2D MRI data contains a long axis view of the LV, the imaging plane passing through the LV axis, defined by the apex and two basal points on the mitral valve annulus. Note however, that with this definition the LV appearance can vary substantially, since the rotation along the long axis is not constrained. As a result, the datasets may contain two, three, or four chamber views, thus making the LV detection problem challenging, not only due to the LV shape and appearance variations, but also due to varying background tissue and sometimes similar appearance of the right ventricle.

In Chap. 3, we extended Marginal Space Learning (MSL) to detect the bounding box of the LV on 2D MRI and demonstrated its superior performance compared to Full Space Learning (FSL). However, due to the large variations in the appearance and shape of the LV, the performance of MSL still has room for improvement. We will present a learning-based aggregation scheme to further increase the detection robustness. Besides the LV body, we also want to detect a few important LV landmarks (i.e., apex and mitral valve annulus); therefore, we train three detectors, one for the LV bounding box, one for the apex, and the other for the base (for the mitral valve annulus), as shown in Fig. 5.4. During detection, each detector is run independently to generate a list of top candidates. A detector tends to fire up around the true position multiple times, while the fire-ups at wrong positions may be sporadic. This property has been exploited in the cluster analysis based aggregation scheme [37]. According to this observation, a correct LV bounding box should have many surrounding LV candidates. Furthermore, around the apex of a correct LV box, there should be many detected apex candidates. This is also true for the base candidates. Based on the geometric relationship of the candidates, we learn a ranking model [12] to select the best LV bounding box among all LV candidates. After detecting the LV, we run the apex and base detectors again within a constrained range to refine the detection results of landmarks. After that, it is straightforward to recover the landmarks (the apex and two annulus points) from the detected apex and base boxes.

5.3.1 Part-Based Left Ventricle Model

In this section, we present a part model of the LV. Besides the LV bounding box (the white box in Fig. 5.4), we also detect the LV apex (point A in Fig. 5.4) and two annulus points (points C and D in Fig. 5.4) on the mitral valve. Instead of defining these landmarks as points and training a position detector for each, we define them as boxes. A base box (the black box in Fig. 5.4) is defined as a square that tightly bounds two annulus points. The base box is aligned with the axis connecting the annulus points. The apex box is defined as a square centered at the apex and aligned with the LV long axis. We define the LV long axis as the axis connecting the apex and the basal center (point B in Fig. 5.4), which is the center of two annulus points. There is no obvious way to define the box size for the apex; hence, we set it to half of the distance from the apex to the basal center. Detecting these landmark points as boxes, we can exploit the orientation and implicit size information of the region around the landmarks. The detection results are more robust than using a position detector only. The LV box is defined as a bounding box of the myocardium and aligned with the LV long axis. There are some constraints or geometric relationships encoded in our part model. For example, the LV box and the apex box have the same orientation, while the base box has a similar orientation to the LV box. From the LV bounding box, we can get a rough estimate of the position of the apex and basal

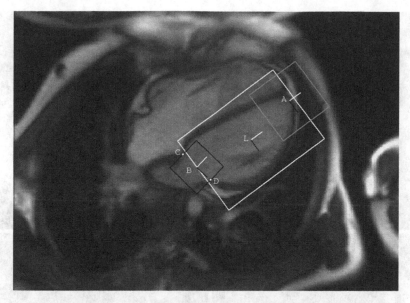

Fig. 5.4 A part-based Left Ventricle (LV) model with white for the LV bounding box, black for the bounding box of two annulus points (points C and D), and gray for the LV apex (point A). ©2009 IEEE. Reprinted, with permission, from Zheng, Y., Lu, X., Georgescu, B., Littmann, A., Mueller, E., Comaniciu, D.: Robust object detection using marginal space learning and ranking-based multi-detector aggregation: Application to automatic left ventricle detection in 2D MRI images. In: *Proc. IEEE Conf. Computer Vision and Pattern Recognition*, pp. 1343–1350 (2009)

center. These geometric relationships are exploited to select the best detection box for the LV using a ranking-based approach.

The independent detection of each LV part may lack robustness due to other similar anatomies. Figure 5.5 shows one example image of the canonical four-chamber view, on which the LV and RV are similar in both shape and appearance. The LV whole-body detector picks the RV as the final detection result. We previously proposed a simple voting based scheme [48] to exploit the geometric constraints among the LV parts. Figure 5.6 shows the final detection after voting, which generates correct detection for all three LV parts. The voting based scheme is based on a few manually crafted rules, which may not be optimal in exploiting the geometric constraints embedded in the part model. Here, we present a machine learning based approach for aggregating multi-part detectors, which is more power-ful and robust.

5.3.2 Ranking Features

We define a RankBoost model [12] to select the best LV bounding box among all LV detection candidates. The features used to train the RankBoost model are

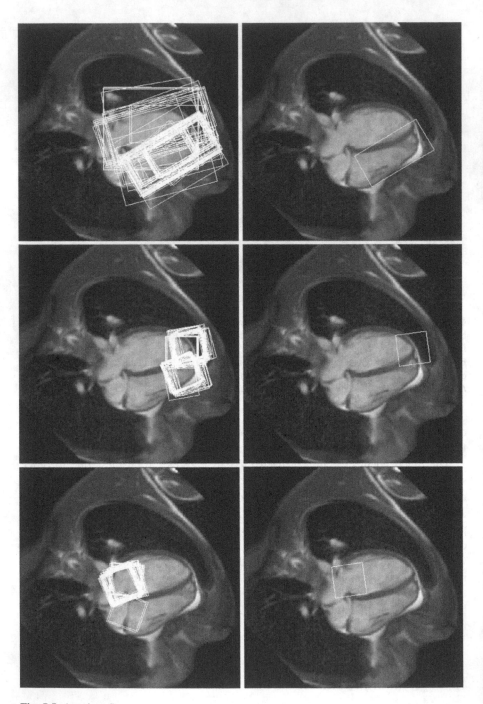

Fig. 5.5 (continued)

based on the geometric relationship between the box under study and the other candidate boxes. A box can be presented as five parameters (X, Y, θ, S_x, S_y), where (X, Y) is the box center; θ represents the box orientation; and S_x and S_y are the length and width of the box, respectively. Given boxes $\mathbf{A}$ $(X^A, Y^A, \theta^A, S_x^A, S_y^A)$ and $\mathbf{B}$ $(X^B, Y^B, \theta^B, S_x^B, S_y^B)$, we can calculate the following four geometric relationships.

1. The center-center distance, defined as

$$D_c(\mathbf{A}, \mathbf{B}) = \sqrt{(X^A - X^B)^2 + (Y^B - Y^B)^2}. \quad (5.4)$$

2. The orientation distance, defined as

$$D_o(\mathbf{A}, \mathbf{B}) = \|\theta^A - \theta^B\|. \quad (5.5)$$

3. The overlapping ratio, defined as the intersection area of $\mathbf{A}$ and $\mathbf{B}$ divided by the area of the union,

$$O(\mathbf{A}, \mathbf{B}) = \frac{\mathbf{A} \cap \mathbf{B}}{\mathbf{A} \cup \mathbf{B}}. \quad (5.6)$$

4. The vertex-vertex distance, $D_v(\mathbf{A}, \mathbf{B})$. A box is fully represented by its four vertices $\mathbf{V}_1, \mathbf{V}_2, \mathbf{V}_3, \mathbf{V}_4$. Given a box, we can consistently sort its vertices based on the box orientation. The vertex-vertex distance is defined as the mean Euclidean distance between the corresponding vertices,

$$D_v(\mathbf{A}, \mathbf{B}) = \frac{1}{4} \sum_{i=1}^{4} \|\mathbf{V}_i^A - \mathbf{V}_i^B\|. \quad (5.7)$$

Among all these features, the center-center and orientation distances only partially measure the difference between two boxes. The overlapping ratio has an ambiguity w.r.t. orientation: rotating box $\mathbf{A}$ around its center by 180 degrees does not change its overlapping ratio to any other boxes. The vertex-vertex distance is the most comprehensive distance measure: $D_v(\mathbf{A}, \mathbf{B}) = 0$ if and only if boxes $\mathbf{A}$ and $\mathbf{B}$ are the same.

Fig. 5.5 Independent detection of the Left Ventricle (LV) parts: the LV whole body (*top row*), apex (*middle row*), and base (*bottom row*). The left column shows the top 100 detected candidates and the right column shows the aggregated final detection for each anatomy after cluster analysis. The LV body detector picks the Right Ventricle (RV) as the final detection result and the apex detector is lucky to pick the correct one. The appearance around the base region is more distinctive; therefore the LV base is detected correctly. ©2009 SPIE. Reprinted, with permission, from Zheng, Y., Lu, X., Georgescu, B., Littmann, A., Mueller, E., Comaniciu, D.: Automatic left ventricle detection in MRI images using marginal space learning and component-based voting. In: *Proc. of SPIE Medical Imaging*, vol. 7259, pp. 1–12 (2009)

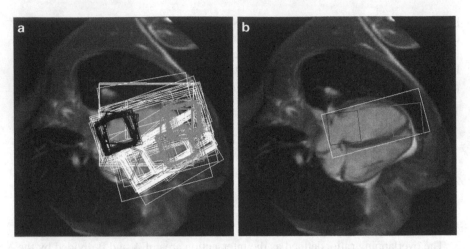

Fig. 5.6 Left Ventricle (LV) detection result of the example shown in Fig. 5.5 after aggregating part detection candidates. (**a**) Top 100 candidates for each LV part: the LV whole body (*white*), apex (*gray*), and base (*black*). (**b**) Final result after aggregation using part-based voting [48]. ©2009 SPIE. Reprinted, with permission, from Zheng, Y., Lu, X., Georgescu, B., Littmann, A., Mueller, E., Comaniciu, D.: Automatic left ventricle detection in MRI images using marginal space learning and component-based voting. In: *Proc. of SPIE Medical Imaging*, vol. 7259, pp. 1–12 (2009)

Assume that for each detector we retain 100 bounding box candidates. Given an LV bounding box **A**, three groups of features are extracted and used to learn the ranking model. The first group of features is extracted from the other 99 LV candidate boxes. First, all the other LV boxes are sorted using the vertex-vertex distance to box **A**. Therefore, we can assign a consistent ordering to the extracted feature set, across different boxes. Suppose box **B** is another LV box, we extract five features from it, including its detection score (which is assigned by the PBT classifier [36]) and all the above four geometric features between boxes **A** and **B**. In total, we extract $99 \times 5 = 495$ features in this group. The second group of features is based on the geometric relationship of box **A** to all 100 LV apex candidates. From box **A**, we can predict the position of its apex, $\mathbf{C}_p^A$. (We assign $\mathbf{C}_p^A$ as the center of the box edge on the apex side.) To assign a consistent ordering to the extracted feature set, the LV apex candidates are sorted w.r.t. the distance to the predicted apex position, $\mathbf{C}_p^A$. Given an apex box **C**, three features are extracted: (1) detection score of box **C**, (2) distance to the predicted position, and (3) orientation distance, $D_o(\mathbf{A}, \mathbf{C})$. In total, we extract $100 \times 3 = 300$ features in this group. The third group of features is extracted from the base candidate boxes. Similar to the features from the apex candidates, 300 features are extracted based on the geometric relationship of box **A** and the top 100 candidates of the LV base. Including the detection score of box **A** itself, we have $1 + 495 + 300 + 300 = 1,096$ features.

5.3.3 Ranking-Based Aggregation

In this section, we present the RankBoost [12] learning algorithm, used to select the best LV box from a set of candidates. The goal of RankBoost learning is minimizing the (weighted) number of pairs of boxes that are mis-ordered by the final ranking, relative to the given ground truth. The learner is provided with ground truth about the relative ranking of an individual pair of boxes x_0 and x_1 based on the vertex-vertex distance to the ground truth. Suppose box x_1 should be ranked above box x_0; otherwise, a penalty $D(x_0, x_1)$ is imposed. An equally weighted penalty $D(x_0, x_1) = 1$ normalized to a probability distribution is selected at the beginning. The learning goal is searching for the final ranking function H that minimizes the ranking loss

$$rloss_D(H) = \sum_{x_0, x_1} D(x_0, x_1)\delta[H(x_1) \leq H(x_0)]. \tag{5.8}$$

Here, $\delta[.]$ is 1 if the predicate holds and 0 otherwise. Note that the instances are sorted in the descending order with respect to H.

Given: Initial distribution D over $\mathscr{X} \times \mathscr{X}$.
Initialize: $D_1 = D$.
For $t = 1, 2, ..., T$

- Train weak learner using distribution D_t to get weak ranking $h_t : \mathscr{X} \to R$.
- Choose optimal $\alpha_t \in R$.
- Update:
$$D_{t+1}(x_0, x_1) = \frac{D_t(x_0, x_1)\exp[\alpha_t(h_t(x_0) - h_t(x_1))]}{Z_t}$$
Here, Z_t is a normalization factor (chosen so that D_{t+1} will be a distribution).

Output the final ranking: $H(x) = \sum_{t=1}^T \alpha_t h_t(x)$.

Fig. 5.7 The RankBoost algorithm. ©2009 IEEE. Reprinted, with permission, from Zheng, Y., Lu, X., Georgescu, B., Littmann, A., Mueller, E., Comaniciu, D.: Robust object detection using marginal space learning and ranking-based multi-detector aggregation: Application to automatic left ventricle detection in 2D MRI images. In: *Proc. IEEE Conf. Computer Vision and Pattern Recognition*, pp. 1343–1350 (2009)

The RankBoost algorithm (as shown in Fig. 5.7) exploits the boosting technique [31] to minimize the ranking loss (Eq. (5.8)). In Fig. 5.7, h_t is a weak ranking function, which corresponds to each individual feature presented in Sect. 5.3.2. The final learned ranking function H is an optimal linear combination of T ($T = 25$ in our experiments) features,

$$H(x) = \sum_{t=1}^T \alpha_t h_t(x). \tag{5.9}$$

The general RankBoost algorithm listed in Fig. 5.7 does not specify how to select the best weak feature h_t and the corresponding weight α_t in each iteration. It is difficult to search for a global optimal solution to minimize the ranking loss of Eq. (5.8). However, there is an upper-bound of the ranking loss $rloss_D(H)$ on the training set. At time t, let

$$Z_t = \sum_{x_0,x_1} D_t(x_0,x_1) \exp\left[\alpha_t(h_t(x_0) - h_t(x_1))\right]. \tag{5.10}$$

It can be shown that the ranking loss of H on the training set is upper-bounded as [12]

$$rloss_D(H) \leq \Pi_{t=1}^T Z_t. \tag{5.11}$$

Instead of minimizing the ranking loss directly, the RankBoost algorithm minimizes the ranking loss Z_t of each iteration. For any given weak ranking function h_t, it can be shown that Z_t is a convex function of α_t and has a unique minimum [31]. The optimal α_t can be found numerically using the Newton-Raphson method. In our approach, each weaker learner uses only one feature. For each feature, we search for an optimal α_t to minimize Z_t. The feature with the smallest Z_t value is selected as the weaker learner. So, the weaker learner training and optimal α_t searching are finished in one step.

The training process of the RankBoost algorithm is expensive in terms of space and computation if we want to preserve the ordering of all pairs of LV candidate boxes. There is a more efficient implementation of RankBoost for a special form of ground truth [12]. We say that the ranking ground truth is bipartite if there exists disjoint subsets X_0 and X_1 of $\mathscr{X}$ such that the ground truth ranks all instances in X_1 above all instances in X_0 and says nothing about any other pairs. In our application, for each training sample, we want to use the RankBoost model to pick a single LV candidate box that has the smallest distance to the ground truth box. We do not care about the relative ranking of non-optimal boxes. Therefore, for each training sample, X_0 is composed of the best candidate box and the remaining boxes are assigned to X_1. Although our ground truth is bipartite for each training sample, the overall ground truth is not bipartite but a union of bipartite subsets. Note that we do not care about the relative ranking of boxes from different training samples. The efficient implementation of RankBoost is still applicable for this case (see [12] for details).

5.3.4   Experiments on Ranking-Based Aggregation

In this experiment, we evaluate the performance of our ranking-based multi-detector aggregation method. We train three detectors (one for the LV bounding box, apex, and base, respectively) on the randomly selected 400 MRI images and tested on the remaining 395 unseen images. The left half of Table 5.3 shows the detection

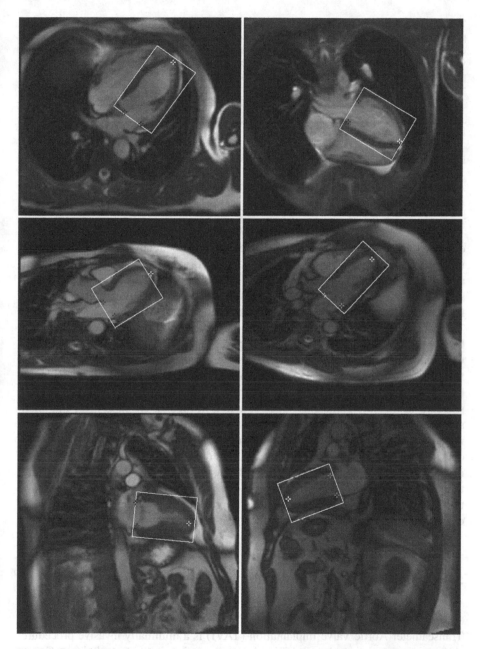

Fig. 5.8 Detection results of the left ventricle (the oriented bounding boxes) and its landmarks (*white stars* for the apex and *dark stars* for two annulus points on the mitral valve)

Table 5.3 Quantitative evaluation for Left Ventricle (LV) bounding box, apex, and mitral annulus point detection accuracy with/without ranking-based multi-detector aggregation on an unseen dataset with 395 MRI images. The errors are measured in millimeters. For the LV bounding box, we list both the center-center and vertex-vertex errors. For the landmarks (the apex and annulus points), we list the Euclidean distance to the ground truth

	Independent Detection				Ranking-Based Aggregation			
	Mean	Std	Median	Worst 10%	Mean	Std	Median	Worst 10%
LV Bounding Box (Center-Center)	13.49	24.61	5.77	74.71	9.86	16.44	5.24	48.66
LV Bounding Box (Vertex-Vertex)	21.39	30.99	10.19	106.74	17.51	24.71	9.79	82.58
Apex	22.81	45.16	6.09	148.09	14.56	28.33	5.76	86.18
Annulus Points	15.77	21.30	7.35	72.00	12.72	16.35	7.02	54.62

errors on unseen data if we run three detectors independently (see also the results in Chap. 3). A fourfold cross-validation is performed to test our ranking-based aggregation scheme. We randomly split 395 unseen images to four roughly equal sets. Three sets are used to train the RankBoost model, and the remaining set is used for testing. The configuration is rotated until each set has been used for testing once. The detection errors for the LV bounding box after multi-detector aggregation are listed on the right half of Table 5.3. Using our ranking-based aggregation scheme, we significantly reduce the detection error. The mean center-center error is reduced from 13.49 to 9.86 mm, a 26.9 % reduction. The mean vertex-vertex error is reduced by 18.1 % (from 21.39 to 17.51 mm). Ranking-based aggregation also reduces the standard deviation significantly. The reduction in median errors is more marginal since most improvement comes from the images with large detection errors. That means the ranking-based aggregation scheme improves the system robustness to detection outliers. Using the detected LV bounding box to constrain the searching range for the apex and base, we also achieve much better results than detecting them independently. The mean error of the apex is reduced by 36.1 %, from 22.81 to 14.56 mm. We also see considerable improvement for annulus points. A few examples of the detection results are shown in Fig. 5.8.

5.4 Part-Based Aorta Detection and Segmentation from C-arm CT

Transcatheter Aortic Valve Implantation (TAVI) is a minimally invasive procedure to treat severe aortic valve stenosis. As an emerging imaging technique, C-arm CT plays a more and more important role in TAVI on both pre-operative surgical planning (e.g., providing 3D valve measurements) and intra-operative guidance (e.g., determining a proper C-arm angulation). Automatic aorta segmentation together with aortic valve landmark detection in a C-arm CT volume facilitates the seamless integration of C-arm CT into the TAVI workflow and improve the patient care.

Several methods have been proposed to segment the aorta. However, most of them work on well established imaging modalities, such as CT or MRI. Automatic segmentation of the aorta in a C-arm CT volume is far more challenging. First, the image quality from different clinical sites is variable since C-arm CT is too new to have a well accepted scanning protocol. We also observed significant variations coming from the same clinical site since physicians were testing different scanning parameters such as the amount of contrast agent and the timing of the image acquisition. Conventional image processing techniques, e.g., intensity-based thresholding, region growing, and the watershed method, are usually not robust under such large variations. The solution is to use machine learning techniques to exploit the rich information embedded in an expert-annotated dataset.

Second, the field of view varies quite a lot for C-arm CT. For example, the aortic arch and descending aorta may be captured in some volumes, but missing in others. To address this challenge, we design a part-based aorta model. The whole aorta is split into four parts: aortic root, ascending aorta, aortic arch, and descending aorta. Using the part-based model, the whole aorta does not need to be fully present in the image data. Depending on the parts that can be detected, different workflows are exploited; therefore, a large structural variation can be elegantly handled.

5.4.1 Part-Based Aorta Segmentation

5.4.1.1 System Diagram

Due to the variation in the field of view, the aorta in a C-arm CT volume has no consistent structure; therefore, the MSL based approach cannot be applied directly. To address this challenge, we present a part-based aorta model (as shown in Fig. 5.9) by splitting the whole aorta into: aortic root, ascending aorta, aortic arch, and descending aorta. The aortic root and aortic arch are consistent in anatomy; therefore, we can apply the MSL to train two separate detectors with one for each part. The length of the ascending and descending aorta parts varies; therefore, we use a tracking-based method to handle this variation.

Figure 5.10 shows the system diagram of the part-based aorta segmentation method. We first detect the aortic root since it should always be present in the volume. The aortic arch detector is then applied. If the aortic arch is not present, therefore, not detected, the descending aorta is often also missing in the volume.[1]

---

[1] Volumes with missing aortic arch are reconstructed with slice size of 256×256 pixels, instead of 512×512 pixels. The slice resolution is roughly the same, resulting in a much smaller transaxial field of view. Therefore, the descending aorta is also outside the volume.

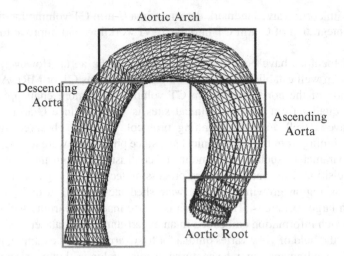

Fig. 5.9 A part-based aorta model. The whole aorta is split into four parts, namely aortic root, ascending aorta, aortic arch, and descending aorta

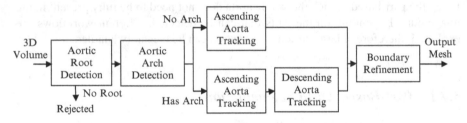

Fig. 5.10 System diagram for part-based aorta segmentation

We track the ascending aorta starting from the aortic root until the top volume border. If the aortic arch is detected, we track the ascending aorta starting from the aortic root until the arch. We also track the descending aorta downward from the arch if the arch is detected. After tracking, we get the centerline of the whole aorta and a tube is synthesized as an initial rough estimate of the shape. We then adjust each mesh point along the surface normal to an optimal position, which has the largest response from a learning-based boundary detector. Generic mesh smoothing [33] is applied to enforce the smoothness constraint. Mesh point adjustment and mesh smoothing can be iterated a few times to improve the boundary delineation accuracy.

5.4.1.2   Aortic Root Segmentation

The aortic root refers to the aorta segment between the aortic hinges and the sinotubular junction. Previous non-model-based approaches [16, 39, 40] have difficulty to exactly delineate the boundary between the aortic root and the Left

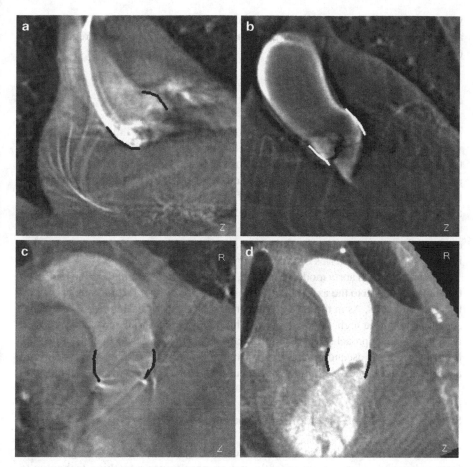

Fig. 5.11 Aortic root segmentation results under the variations of contrast agent and aortic valve regurgitation

Ventricular Outflow Tract (LVOT) since they are fully connected and both contrasted in Computed Tomography Angiography (CTA). In C-arm CT, the contrast agent is directly applied to the aortic root; therefore, the boundary is clear if the aortic valve is fully closed. However, due to the aortic valve regurgitation, the contrast agent may leak into the LVOT in about 20–30 % of cases. The amount of leakage varies depending on the severity of the regurgitation, which creates an extra challenge to an automatic segmentation method. As a consistent anatomy, the aortic root is segmented using the MSL in our system by fitting a surface mesh model into the data. Figure 5.11 shows the aortic root segmentation results on a few data sets, demonstrating the robustness of the MSL under variations of contrast agent and presence of aortic valve regurgitation. The contrast of the first three volumes is weak, while the last volume has quite strong contrast. The amount of regurgitation also varies quite a lot from no regurgitation (Fig. 5.11a and b) to severe regurgitation (Fig. 5.11c and d).

5.4.1.3 Aortic Arch Segmentation

The aortic arch is missing in about half of our dataset due to the limited field of view of the C-arm CT; therefore, the missing or presence of the aortic arch needs to be detected automatically. Since the aorta has a tubular shape, the intersection perpendicular to its centerline is close to a circle. A tracking based approach is often used to trace the circular shape, which works well on the ascending and descending aorta parts. However, the aorta centerline orientation needs to be estimated and updated robustly during the tracking of the bending arch [29]. Otherwise, a tracking error may be propagated to the following slices, resulting in a failure (e.g., tracing into the supra-aortic arteries or the nearby pulmonary artery).

In our part-based aorta model (Fig. 5.9), the aortic arch is defined as the part from the top of the aorta to the axial slice where the intersection of the aorta diverges into two separate parts. As in the case of the aortic root, the MSL is applied to detect and segment the aortic arch. By segmenting the bending the aortic root and arch with a model based approach, the remaining parts are much easier to handle. Since the intersection of the ascending and descending aorta parts to an axial slice is close to a circle, it can be tracked efficiently without estimating the centerline orientation.

5.4.1.4 Tracking of Ascending and Descending Aorta Parts

The length of the visible ascending and descending aorta parts varies significantly from volume to volume. Consequently, we propose to use a tracking technique to deal with this variation. Instead of using a time-consuming Hough transform based circle detector [39, 40], we use machine learning technique to train a 2D circle detector on an axial image slice using 2D Haar wavelet features [37]. The tracking of the ascending aorta starts from the top of the aortic root and is performed slice by slice, moving toward the patient's head. The detected circle on a slice is propagated to the next slice and the circle detector is applied in a neighborhood of 6×6 mm^2 around the initial estimate. For an image slice containing the ascending aorta, it is normal for the detector to find multiple circle candidates around the true position. We pick the one closest to the circle on the previous slice. If the aortic arch is detected in the volume, the tracking procedure stops on the slice touching the aortic arch; otherwise, it stops when no aortic circles are detected or it reaches the top volume border. Tracking of the descending aorta is similar. It starts from the aortic arch, moves toward the patient's abdomen, and stops on the slice with no aortic circles detected.

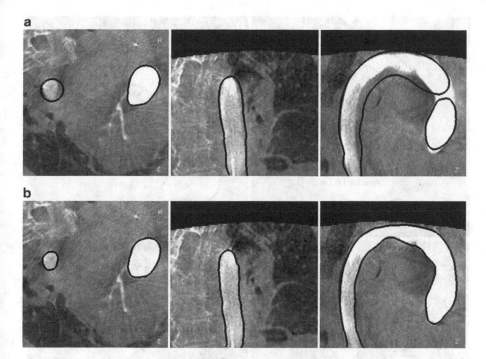

Fig. 5.12 Aorta boundary refinement. (**a**) Initial synthesized tubular mesh after tracking the ascending and descending aorta parts. (**b**) Final segmentation after boundary refinement. Three orthogonal cuts of the volume are shown

5.4.1.5   Aorta Boundary Refinement

After tracking the ascending and descending aorta parts, we get the centerline of the whole aorta. A generalized-cylinder model is synthesized as an initial estimate of the aorta shape and the radius at each centerline point is set to the radius of the detected circle. Figure 5.12a shows the synthesized tube after tracking. The initialization is close to the true aorta boundary; however, a circle does not fit the boundary exactly. A learning based boundary detector is exploited for final boundary delineation. Interested readers are referred to [46] for more details of the learning based boundary detector. One difference to the boundary delineation of the aortic root or arch is that we cannot use the Active Shape Model (ASM) [7] to enforce prior shape constraint since the aorta is not consistent in structure due to the variation in the field of view. Instead, a generic mesh smoothing technique [33] is used to achieve a smooth surface for the segmented aorta. To be specific, a two-step iterative approach is used.

1. Use the learning-based boundary detector to adjust each mesh point along the surface normal to the optimal position where the response of the boundary detector is the largest.

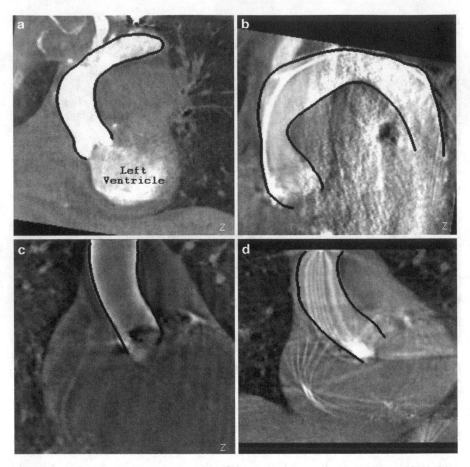

Fig. 5.13 Automatic aorta segmentation on a few example volumes. (**a**) Good contrast, however, with severe valve regurgitation. (**b**) Fair image quality. (**c**) Contrast agent is almost washed out due to bad timing. (**d**) Streak artifacts caused by the catheters. Please note, the aortic arch and descending aorta are missing in the last two volumes

2. Apply generic mesh smoothing.

The above two steps are iterated a couple of times to improve the boundary delineation accuracy. Figure 5.12b shows the result after boundary refinement. More examples of the aorta segmentation results are shown in Fig. 5.13.

Note that, almost all previous work uses bottom-up approaches [2, 6, 29, 30, 44] to track the aorta centerline to handle variations. They are neither automatic nor robust on noisy images. In comparison, we use the top-down MSL to detect the aortic root and arch, and use bottom-up tracking to detect ascending and descending aorta parts, which have large variations in length. Our system exploits the benefits of both approaches.

5.4.2 Evaluation of Aorta Segmentation

We collected a dataset of 319 C-arm CT volumes from 276 patients from 11 clinical sites, mainly from Germany, Australia, Japan, Canada, and USA. The size of each slice in a volume is 256×256 or 512×512 pixels. A volume contains around 200–300 slices. The image resolution is isotropic and varies from volume to volume in the range of [0.70, 0.84] mm.

Aorta segmentation accuracy is measured using the symmetric point-to-mesh distance [46]. The contrast agent gradually fades out along the descending aorta; therefore, the length of the segmented aorta may differ from the manual annotation since it is difficult to determine consistently where the segmentation should stop. When we calculate the error between the segmented mesh and the ground truth, we exclude the extra distal part of the descending aorta from evaluation. On average, the length of the excluded part is about 35 mm, which corresponds to about 15 % of the descending aorta. Based on a fourfold cross-validation, the mean segmentation error of the remaining aorta is 1.08 mm, with a standard deviation of 0.56 mm. Figure 5.13 shows aorta segmentation results on a few volumes. Our method is robust under variations of the field of view, contrast agent, scan timing, and valve regurgitation.

Regarding the segmentation accuracy, we cannot compare our error with those reported in the literature directly because they used different datasets captured from different imaging modalities. Most of the previous aorta segmentation methods did not present a quantitative evaluation of the segmentation accuracy [14,15,23,25,30, 40] or reported in different error criteria [1, 10, 13, 29]. Table 5.4 lists the reported aorta mesh errors available in the literature. Roughly, our accuracy is comparable with the state-of-the-art, e.g., 1.55 mm reported in [44] on 104 MRI datasets, and 1.4 mm reported in [6] on 23 CT datasets. In [38], Waechter et al. reported a mean error of 0.5 mm in aorta segmentation, which is smaller than ours. The errors are evaluated on a small cardiac CT dataset with 20 volumes. Normally, cardiac CT has a higher resolution (often around 0.3–0.4 mm for in-slice resolution) than our C-arm CT (0.70–0.84 mm). Unfortunately, Waechter et al. did not report the volume resolution of their dataset. If standard high-resolution cardiac CT is used in [38] and the errors are measured in voxels, our accuracy in aorta segmentation is comparable with [38].

Our approach is computationally efficient, taking about 0.8 s to segment the aorta in a volume on a computer with 2.33 GHz quad-core processors and 3 GB memory. It is at least 10 times faster than the previous methods [34,44].

5.5 Conclusions

In this chapter, we demonstrated the robustness and accuracy of part-based object detection and segmentation on several applications. A part-based approach may improve the detection robustness if the detection results of multiple part detectors

Table 5.4 Comparison with previous aorta segmentation methods with reported quantitative mesh errors

	Modality	Patients/Subjects	Resolution (mm)	Automatic	Speed	Mesh Error
Zhao et al. [44]	MRI	104	$1.5 \times 1.5 \times 1.5$ to $2.0 \times 2.0 \times 2.0$	No	5 min/subject	1.55 mm
Bruijne et al. [6]	CT	23	$0.448 \times 0.448 \times 2.0$	No	450 s/volume	1.4 mm[a]
Waechter et al. [38]	CT	20	N/A	Yes	N/A	0.5 mm[b]
Our Method	C-arm CT	276	0.70–0.84 isotropic	Yes	0.8 s/volume	1.08 mm

[a] If an aortic aneurysm is present, the outer wall of the aneurysm is segmented, which is more difficult than lumen segmentation
[b] The mesh error includes the aortic root and the valve leaflets

can be aggregated intelligently to exploit the redundancy. For other applications, a part-based approach may provide more accurate shape initialization for each part. After merging the part segmentation into a consolidated mesh, more accurate segmentation can be achieved. Different applications may require different methods to split the object into parts, enforce constraint during part detection, and aggregate the results of part detectors.

References

1. Al-Agamy, A.O., Osman, N.F., Fahmy, A.S.: Segmentation of ascending and descending aorta from magnetic resonance flow images. In: Cairo International Biomedical Engineering Conference, pp. 41–44 (2010)
2. Behrens, T., Rohr, K., Stiehl, H.H.: Robust segmentation of tubular structures in 3-D medical images by parametric object detection and tracking. IEEE Trans. Syst., Man, Cybern. B 33(14), 554–561 (2003)
3. Boisvert, J., Pennec, X., Labelle, H., Cheriet, F., Ayache, N.: Principal spine shape deformation modes using Riemannian geometry and articulated models. In: Proc. Conf. Articulated Motion and Deformable Objects, pp. 346–355 (2006)
4. Boykov, Y., Funka-Lea, G.: Graph cuts and efficient N-D image segmentation. Int. J. Computer Vision 70(2), 109–131 (2006)
5. Boykov, Y.Y., Jolly, M.P.: Interactive graph cuts for optimal boundary and region segmentation of objects in N-D images. In: Proc. Int'l Conf. Computer Vision, pp. 105–112 (2001)
6. de Bruijne, M., van Ginneken, B., Viergever, M.A., Niessen, W.J.: Adapting active shape models for 3D segmentation of tubular structures in medical images. In: Proc. Information Processing in Medical Imaging, pp. 136–147 (2003)
7. Cootes, T.F., Taylor, C.J., Cooper, D.H., Graham, J.: Active shape models—their training and application. Computer Vision and Image Understanding 61(1), 38–59 (1995)
8. Depa, M., Sabuncu, M.R., Holmvang, G., Nezafat, R., Schmidt, E.J., Golland, P.: Robust atlas-based segmentation of highly variable anatomy: Left atrium segmentation. In: MICCAI Workshop on Statistical Atlases and Computational Models of the Heart: Mapping Structure and Function (STACOM), pp. 85–94 (2010)
9. D'Silva, A., Wright, M.: Advances in imaging for atrial fibrillation ablation. Radiology Research and Practice 2011, 1–10 (2011)
10. Egger, J., Freisleben, B., Setser, R., Renapuraar, R., Biermann, C., O'Donnel, T.: Aorta segmentation for stent simulation. In: Proc. MICCAI Workshop on Cardiovascular Interventional Imaging and Biophysical Modeling, pp. 1–7 (2009)
11. Felzenszwalb, P., McAllester, D., Ramanan, D.: A discriminatively trained, multiscale, deformable part model. In: Proc. IEEE Conf. Computer Vision and Pattern Recognition, pp. 1–8 (2008)
12. Freund, Y., Iyer, R., Schapire, R.E., Singer, Y.: An efficient boosting algorithm for combining preferences. J. Machine Learning Research 4(6), 933–970 (2004)
13. Galante, V., Corsi, C., Veronesi, F., Russo, V., Fattori, R., Lamberti, C.: Dynamic characterization of aorta morphology and function in presence of an aneurysm. In: Proc. Computers in Cardiology, vol. 34, pp. 765–678 (2007)
14. Gessat, M., Merk, D.R., Falk, V., Walther, T., Jacobs, S., Nöttling, A., Burgert, O.: A planning system for transapical aortic valve implantation. In: Proc. of SPIE Medical Imaging, vol. 7261, pp. 1–12 (2009)
15. Giri, S.S., Ding, Y., Nishijima, Y., Pedraza-Toscano, A., Burns, P.M., Hamlin, R.L., Simonetti, O.P.: Automated and accurate measurement of aortic pulse wave velocity using magnetic resonance imaging. In: Proc. Computers in Cardiology, vol. 34, pp. 661–664 (2007)

16. Hennemuth, A., Boskamp, T., Fritz, D., Kühnel, C., Bock, S., Rinck, D., Scheuering, M., Peitgen, H.O.: One-click coronary tree segmentation in CT angiographic images. In: Proc. Computer Assisted Radiology and Surgery, pp. 317–321 (2005)

17. Holmes, D.R., Reddy, V.Y., Turi, Z.G., Doshi, S.K., Sievert, H., Buchbinder, M., Mullin, C.M., Sick, P., PROTECT AF Investigators: Percutaneous closure of the left atrial appendage versus warfarin therapy for prevention of stroke in patients with atrial fibrillation: A randomized non-inferiority trial. Lancet **374**(9689), 534–542 (2009)

18. Horn, B.K.P.: Closed-form solution of absolute orientation using orthonormal matrices. Journal of Optical Society of American **5**(7), 1127–1135 (1987)

19. John, M., Rahn, N.: Automatic left atrium segmentation by cutting the blood pool at narrowings. In: Proc. Int'l Conf. Medical Image Computing and Computer Assisted Intervention, vol. 2, pp. 798–805 (2005)

20. Karim, R., Juli, C., Lawes, L.M., Kanangaratnam, P., Davies, D.W., Peters, N.S., Rueckert, D.: Automatic segmentation of left atrial geometry from contrast-enhanced magnetic resonance images using a probabilistic atlas. In: MICCAI Workshop on Statistical Atlases and Computational Models of the Heart: Mapping Structure and Function (STACOM), pp. 134–143 (2010)

21. Karim, R., Mohiaddin, R., Rueckert, D.: Left atrium segmentation for atrial fibrillation ablation. In: Proc. of SPIE Medical Imaging, vol. 6918, pp. 1–8 (2008)

22. Kneeland, P.P., Fang, M.C.: Trends in catheter ablation for atrial fibrillation in the United States. Journal of Hospital Medicine **4**(7), E1–E5 (2009)

23. Krissian, K., Ellsmere, J., Vosburgh, K., Kikinis, R., Westin, C.F.: Multiscale segmentation of the aorta in 3D ultrasound images. In: Proc. Annual Int'l Conf. of the IEEE Engineering in Medicine and Biology Society, pp. 638–641 (2003)

24. Lombaert, H., Sun, Y., Grady, L., Xu, C.: A multilevel banded graph cuts method for fast image segmentation. In: Proc. Int'l Conf. Computer Vision, pp. 259–265 (2005)

25. Loncaric, S., Subasic, M., Sorantin, E.: 3-D deformable model for aortic aneurysm segmentation from CT images. In: Proc. Annual Int'l Conf. of the IEEE Engineering in Medicine and Biology Society, pp. 398–401 (2000)

26. Manzke, R., Meyer, C., Ecabert, O., Peters, J., Noordhoek, N.J., Thiagalingam, A., Reddy, V.Y., Chan, R.C., Weese, J.: Automatic segmentation of rotational X-ray images for anatomic intra-procedural surface generation in atrial fibrillation ablation procedures. IEEE Trans. Medical Imaging **29**(2), 260–272 (2010)

27. Marom, E.M., Herndon, J.E., Kim, Y.K., McAdams, H.P.: Variations in pulmonary venous drainage to the left atrium: Implications for radiofrequency ablation. Radiology **230**, 824–829 (2004)

28. Naccarelli, G.V., Varker, H., Lin, J., Schulman, K.L.: Increasing prevalence of atrial fibrillation and flutter in the United States. American Journal of Cardiology **104**(11), 1534–1539 (2009)

29. Rueckert, D., Burger, P., Forbat, S.M., Mohiaddin, R.D., Yang, G.Z.: Automatic tracking of the aorta in cardiovascular MR images using deformable models. IEEE Trans. Medical Imaging **16**(5), 581–590 (1997)

30. Saur, S.C., Kühnel, C., Boskamp, T., Székely, G., Cattin, P.: Automatic ascending aorta detection in CTA datasets. In: Proc. Workshop Bildverarbeitung für der Medizin, pp. 323–327 (2008)

31. Schapire, R.E., Singer, Y.: Improved boosting algorithms using confidence-rated predictions. Machine Learning **37**(3), 297–336 (1999)

32. Shet, V.D., Neumann, J., Remesh, V., Davis, L.S.: Bilattice-based logical reasoning for human detection. In: Proc. IEEE Conf. Computer Vision and Pattern Recognition, pp. 1–8 (2007)

33. Taubin, G.: Optimal surface smoothing as filter design. In: Proc. European Conf. Computer Vision, pp. 283–292 (1996)

34. Tek, H., Gulsun, M.A., Laguitton, S., Grady, L., Lesage, D., Funka-Lea, G.: Automatic coronary tree modeling. The Insight Journal pp. 1–8 (2008)

35. Thiagalingam, A., Manzke, R., D'avila, A., Ho, I., Locke, A.H., Ruskin, J.N., Chan, R.C., Reddy, V.Y.: Intraprocedural volume imaging of the left atrium and pulmonary veins with

rotational X-ray angiography: Implications for catheter ablation of atrial fibrillation. Journal of Cardiovascular Electrophysiology **19**(3), 293–300 (2008)

36. Tu, Z.: Probabilistic boosting-tree: Learning discriminative methods for classification, recognition, and clustering. In: Proc. Int'l Conf. Computer Vision, pp. 1589–1596 (2005)

37. Viola, P., Jones, M.: Rapid object detection using a boosted cascade of simple features. In: Proc. IEEE Conf. Computer Vision and Pattern Recognition, pp. 511–518 (2001)

38. Waechter, I., Kneser, R., Korosoglou, G., Peters, J., Bakker, N.H., v. d. Boomen, R., Weese, J.: Patient specific models for planning and guidance of minimally invasive aortic valve implantation. In: Proc. Int'l Conf. Medical Image Computing and Computer Assisted Intervention, vol. 1, pp. 526–533 (2010)

39. Wang, C., Smedby, O.: An automatic seeding method for coronary artery segmentation and skeletonization in CTA. The Insight Journal pp. 1–8 (2008)

40. Wang, S., Fu, L., Yue, Y., Kang, Y., Liu, J.: Fast and automatic segmentation of ascending aorta in MSCT volume data. In: Proc. Int'l Conf. Image and Signal Processing, pp. 1–5 (2009)

41. Wolf, P.A., Abbott, R.D., Kannel, W.B.: Atrial fibrillation as an independent risk factor for stroke: The Framingham study. Stroke **22**(8), 983–988 (1991)

42. Wu, B., Nevatia, R., Li, Y.: Segmentation of multiple, partially occluded objects by grouping, merging, assigning part detection responses. In: Proc. IEEE Conf. Computer Vision and Pattern Recognition, pp. 1–8 (2008)

43. Yang, D., Zheng, Y., John, M.: Graph cuts based left atrium segmentation refinement and right middle pulmonary vein extraction in C-arm CT. In: Proc. of SPIE Medical Imaging, pp. 1–9 (2013)

44. Zhao, F., Zhang, H., Wahle, A., Thomas, M.T., Stolpen, A.H., Scholz, T.D., Sonka, M.: Congenital aortic disease: 4D magnetic resonance segmentation and quantitative analysis. Medical Image Analysis **13**(3), 483–493 (2009)

45. Zheng, Y., Barbu, A., Georgescu, B., Scheuering, M., Comaniciu, D.: Fast automatic heart chamber segmentation from 3D CT data using marginal space learning and steerable features. In: Proc. Int'l Conf. Computer Vision, pp. 1–8 (2007)

46. Zheng, Y., Barbu, A., Georgescu, B., Scheuering, M., Comaniciu, D.: Four-chamber heart modeling and automatic segmentation for 3D cardiac CT volumes using marginal space learning and steerable features. IEEE Trans. Medical Imaging **27**(11), 1668–1681 (2008)

47. Zheng, Y., Georgescu, B., Barbu, A., Scheuering, M., Comaniciu, D.: Four-chamber heart modeling and automatic segmentation for 3D cardiac CT volumes. In: Proc. of SPIE Medical Imaging, vol. 6914, pp. 1–12 (2008)

48. Zheng, Y., Georgescu, B., Vega-Higuera, F., Comaniciu, D.: Left ventricle endocardium segmentation for cardiac CT volumes using an optimal smooth surface. In: Proc. of SPIE Medical Imaging, vol. 7259, pp. 1–11 (2009)

49. Zheng, Y., John, M., Boese, J., Comaniciu, D.: Precise segmentation of the left atrium in C-arm CT volumes with applications to atrial fibrillation ablation. In: Proc. IEEE Int'l Sym. Biomedical Imaging, pp. 1421–1424 (2012)

50. Zheng, Y., Lu, X., Georgescu, B., Littmann, A., Mueller, E., Comaniciu, D.: Automatic left ventricle detection in MRI images using marginal space learning and component-based voting. In: Proc. of SPIE Medical Imaging, pp. 1–12 (2009)

51. Zheng, Y., Lu, X., Georgescu, B., Littmann, A., Mueller, E., Comaniciu, D.: Robust object detection using marginal space learning and ranking-based multi-detector aggregation: Application to automatic left ventricle detection in 2D MRI images. In: Proc. IEEE Conf. Computer Vision and Pattern Recognition, pp. 1343–1350 (2009)

52. Zheng, Y., Wang, T., John, M., Zhou, S.K., Boese, J., Comaniciu, D.: Multi-part left atrium modeling and segmentation in C-arm CT volumes for atrial fibrillation ablation. In: Proc. Int'l Conf. Medical Image Computing and Computer Assisted Intervention, vol. 3, pp. 487–495 (2011)

53. Zheng, Y., Yang, D., John, M., Comaniciu, D.: Multi-part modeling and segmentation of left atrium in C-arm CT for image-guided ablation of atrial fibrillation. IEEE Trans. Medical Imaging (2014). In Press

Chapter 6
Optimal Mean Shape for Nonrigid Object Detection and Segmentation

6.1 Introduction

In Marginal Space Learning (MSL) based nonrigid object segmentation, the segmentation process contains two stages: pose estimation and boundary delineation. After estimating the pose of the target object, a pre-calculated mean shape is aligned to the estimated pose to provide an initial shape for the final boundary delineation. Nonrigid deformation is present in almost all anatomical structures across different patients or even for the same patient under different physiological states (e.g., a beating heart at different cardiac phases). How to define the pose of a nonrigid shape is still a problem being researched, although heuristic solutions may exist for specific applications.

In the original MSL, the ground truth of the object pose parameters (position, orientation, and scale) of a training sample is determined by using a bounding box of the annotated mesh. The mean shape is calculated as the average of the normalized shapes in the training set in an object-oriented coordinate system. Such solution does not provide optimality. Since the goal of automatic pose estimation is often to provide an accurate shape initialization for the following segmentation or boundary delineation, in this chapter, we present a method to calculate the optimal mean shape, together with the corresponding optimal pose parameters from a training set to minimize the initialization error. An optimization based approach is defined to generate an optimal mean shape from the training set and the corresponding pose parameters for each training shape. Different to the bounding box based approach that determines the object pose for each training sample independently, the proposed method is based on the optimization on the whole training set.

With the optimally determined pose parameters, the MSL is then applied to learn the intrinsic relationship of the image data and the corresponding target object pose. Such relationship is embedded into the MSL classifiers, which are then applied to unseen data for automatic object detection. Experiments show that the proposed method reduces the shape initialization error not only on the training set, but also on the unseen test set. The final segmentation error can be reduced as well due to

Y. Zheng and D. Comaniciu, *Marginal Space Learning for Medical Image Analysis:* 137
Efficient Detection and Segmentation of Anatomical Structures,
DOI 10.1007/978-1-4939-0600-0_6, © Springer Science+Business Media New York 2014

the more accurate shape initialization. Note that we only change the training step in calculating the optimal mean shape and extracting the pose ground truth of the annotated training samples. There is no computation overhead during the object detection on unseen data.

The remainder of this chapter is organized as follows. We first review the initial bounding box based approach in Sect. 6.2. The optimal mean shape for nonrigid shape initialization is presented in Sect. 6.3. The process is formulated as a generalized Procrustes analysis problem and we then discuss how to align shapes under the similarity transformation and anisotropic similarity transformation. The accuracy of the optimal mean shape is demonstrated on the experiments on aortic valve landmark detection in C-arm Computed Tomography (CT) (Sect. 6.4) and whole-heart segmentation in cardiac CT data (Sect. 6.5). This chapter concludes with Sect. 6.6.

6.2 Heuristic Mean Shape Using a Bounding Box Based Approach

The heuristic approach for calculating a mean shape based on oriented bounding boxes [24, 25] is implemented as follows. For each object, we define an object-orientated coordinate system and calculate the aligned bounding box of the object boundary points, often presented as a surface mesh. Different methods may be used to define the object-oriented coordinate system for different applications. For example, for whole-heart segmentation, the heart coordinate system can be defined based on three landmarks, namely, the aortic valve center, the mitral valve center, and the Left Ventricle (LV) endocardium apex. This local coordinate system actually defines a rotation matrix $\mathbf{R}$ for the transformation between the heart-oriented coordinate system and the world coordinate system. We then calculate a bounding box of the mesh points, aligned with the local coordinate system. The bounding box center gives us the position ground truth X^t, Y^t, and Z^t, and the box size along each side defines the ground truth of scaling S_x^t, S_y^t, and S_z^t.

For each training shape, using the above method, we can calculate its position ($\mathbf{T} = [X,Y,Z]'$), orientation (represented as a rotation matrix $\mathbf{R}$), and anisotropic scaling ($\mathbf{S} = [S_x,S_y,S_z]'$). The transformation from the world coordinate system, $\mathbf{M}_{world}$, to the object-oriented coordinate system, $\mathbf{m}_{object}$ is

$$\mathbf{M}_{world} = \mathbf{R} \begin{bmatrix} S_x & 0 & 0 \\ 0 & S_y & 0 \\ 0 & 0 & S_z \end{bmatrix} \mathbf{m}_{object} + \mathbf{T}. \tag{6.1}$$

Reversing the transformation, we can calculate the position in the object-oriented coordinate system as

$$\mathbf{m}_{object} = \begin{bmatrix} \frac{1}{S_x} & 0 & 0 \\ 0 & \frac{1}{S_y} & 0 \\ 0 & 0 & \frac{1}{S_z} \end{bmatrix} \mathbf{R}^{-1} (\mathbf{M}_{world} - \mathbf{T}). \tag{6.2}$$

After normalizing the similarity transformation (with anisotropic scaling), the mean shape is the average over the whole training set

$$\bar{\mathbf{m}} = \frac{1}{N} \sum_{i=1}^{N} \mathbf{m}_{object}^{i}, \tag{6.3}$$

where N is the number of training samples.

As we can see, the mean shape and the corresponding transformation calculated in this heuristic approach is quite intuitive, however, not optimal from the point of view of how well the mean shape represents the training set.

6.3 Optimal Mean Shape for Nonrigid Shape Initialization

After the MSL based object pose estimation, we align the mean shape to the estimated translation, rotation, and scales as an initial shape for the segmentation process. This initialization needs to be accurate; otherwise, the final boundary evolution may end in a local minimum, due to the clutter of the surrounding tissue around the target object. In this section, we present an optimization based approach to determine the optimal pose parameters and the corresponding mean shape from a training set, thus minimizing the shape initialization error.

6.3.1 Procrustes Optimization for Mean Shape and Pose Parameters

N is the total number of shapes.
$\mathbf{M}_i$, $i = 1, 2, \ldots, N$, represents each shape in the set.
J is the number of points in each shape $\mathbf{M}_i$. Here, we assume all shapes have the same number of points.
$\mathbf{M}_i^j$, $j = 1, 2, \ldots, J$, represents point j in shape i.
$\mathbf{M}_i^j(x), \mathbf{M}_i^j(y), \mathbf{M}_i^j(z)$ are the x, y, z coordinates of point j in shape i, respectively.
$\mathbf{m}$ is a mean shape of the set $\mathbf{M}_i, i = 1, 2, \ldots, N$.
$\bar{\mathbf{m}}$ is an optimal mean shape.

Fig. 6.1 Description of the mathematical symbols used in this chapter

Before going into details, refer to Fig. 6.1 for a description of the mathematic symbols to be used. A group of training shapes, $\mathbf{M}_1, \mathbf{M}_2, \ldots, \mathbf{M}_N$, are supposed to be given, each shape $\mathbf{M}_i$ being represented by J points $\mathbf{M}_i^j, j = 1, \ldots, J$. Point $\mathbf{M}_i^j$ is assumed to have correspondence across volumes. That means it represents the same anatomical position in different volumes. Refer to Chap. 7 for a resampling based approach to establishing mesh point correspondence. To achieve accurate shape initialization, the optimal mean shape $\bar{\mathbf{m}}$ should minimize the residual errors expressed as the Euclidean distance after alignment,

$$\bar{\mathbf{m}} = arg \min_{\mathbf{m}} \sum_{i=1}^{N} \| \mathscr{T}_i(\mathbf{m}) - \mathbf{M}_i \|^2 . \tag{6.4}$$

Here, $\mathscr{T}_i$ is the corresponding transformation from the mean shape $\mathbf{m}$ to each individual shape $\mathbf{M}_i$.

This procedure is called Generalized Procrustes Analysis (GPA) [5] in the shape analysis literature. An iterative approach can be used to search for the locally optimal solution. First, we randomly pick an example shape as a mean shape. We then align each shape to the current mean shape under transformation $\mathscr{T}$. This step of aligning two shapes is called Procrustes analysis. The average of the aligned shapes (the simple average of the corresponding points) is calculated as a new mean shape. The iterative procedure converges to a locally optimal solution after a few iterations. Note that more involved global optimizations exist for the GPA [16].

The similarity transformation with isotropic scaling is often used as the transformation $\mathscr{T}$. A few closed-form solutions have been proposed in the literature to align two shapes under the similarity transformation, as discussed in Sect. 6.3.2. However, the MSL can estimate anisotropic scales of an object efficiently. By covering more deformations, the shape space after alignment is more compact and the mean shape can represent the whole shape population more accurately. Therefore, we use the anisotropic similarity transformation to represent the transformation between two shapes. To our knowledge, there are no closed-form solutions for estimating the anisotropic similarity transformation between two shapes. In Sect. 6.3.3 we present a two-step iterative approach to search for the optimal anisotropic transformation.

6.3.2 Procrustes Analysis Under Isotropic Similarity Transformation

Procrustes analysis is a means to remove the translation, rotation, and scaling between two shapes $\mathbf{M}_1$ and $\mathbf{M}_2$,

$$\hat{\mathscr{T}} = arg \min_{\mathscr{T}} \| \mathscr{T}(\mathbf{M}_1) - \mathbf{M}_2 \|^2 . \tag{6.5}$$

Here, $\mathcal{T}$ is the transformation between two shapes. The similarity transformation is the most widely used transformation in Procrustes analysis,

$$
\hat{\mathbf{T}}, \hat{\mathbf{R}}, \hat{s} = arg \min_{\mathbf{T}, \mathbf{R}, s} \| (s\mathbf{R}\mathbf{M}_1 + \mathbf{T}) - \mathbf{M}_2 \|^2
$$

$$
= arg \min_{\mathbf{T}, \mathbf{R}, s} \sum_{j=1}^{J} \left\| \mathbf{R} \begin{bmatrix} s\mathbf{M}_1^j(x) \\ s\mathbf{M}_1^j(y) \\ s\mathbf{M}_1^j(z) \end{bmatrix} + \mathbf{T} - \begin{bmatrix} \mathbf{M}_2^j(x) \\ \mathbf{M}_2^j(y) \\ \mathbf{M}_2^j(z) \end{bmatrix} \right\|^2 , \tag{6.6}
$$

where $\mathbf{T}$ is translation; $\mathbf{R}$ is a rotation matrix; and s is a scalar for the isotropic scaling. Various methods have been proposed to estimate the similarity transformation between two point sets (2D or 3D). The closed-form solution based on the singular value decomposition of a covariance matrix of the data is the most elegant [2,10,21].

Suppose mean (μ) and variance (σ) of the point sets for shapes $\mathbf{M}_1$ and $\mathbf{M}_2$ are

$$
\mu_1 = \frac{1}{J} \sum_{j=1}^{J} \mathbf{M}_1^j, \tag{6.7}
$$

$$
\sigma_1 = \frac{1}{J} \sum_{j=1}^{J} \| \mathbf{M}_1^j - \mu_1 \|^2, \tag{6.8}
$$

$$
\mu_2 = \frac{1}{J} \sum_{j=1}^{J} \mathbf{M}_2^j, \tag{6.9}
$$

$$
\sigma_2 = \frac{1}{J} \sum_{j=1}^{J} \| \mathbf{M}_2^j - \mu_2 \|^2. \tag{6.10}
$$

Let Σ (a 3×3 matrix) be the covariance matrix of shapes $\mathbf{M}_1$ and $\mathbf{M}_2$,

$$
\Sigma = \frac{1}{J} \sum_{j=1}^{J} (\mathbf{M}_1^j - \mu_1)(\mathbf{M}_2^j - \mu_2)^T. \tag{6.11}
$$

Suppose the singular value decomposition of Σ is

$$
\Sigma = \mathbf{U}\mathbf{D}\mathbf{V}^T, \tag{6.12}
$$

where $\mathbf{D}$ is a diagonal matrix; $\mathbf{U}$ and $\mathbf{V}$ are unitary matrices (i.e., $\mathbf{U}\mathbf{U}^T = \mathbf{I}$ and $\mathbf{V}\mathbf{V}^T = \mathbf{I}$, where $\mathbf{I}$ is an identity matrix). Then, the optimal estimate of the similarity transformation [21] is

$$
\hat{\mathbf{R}} = \mathbf{U}\mathbf{V}^T,
$$

$$
\hat{s} = \frac{1}{\sigma_1^2} Trace(\mathbf{D}),
$$

$$\hat{\mathbf{T}} = \mu_2 - \hat{s}\hat{\mathbf{R}}\mu_1, \tag{6.13}$$

where $Trace(\mathbf{D})$ is the summation of the diagonal elements of matrix $\mathbf{D}$.

The above closed-form solution works well for most cases. However, under some rare conditions, the estimated transformation may include a reflection (i.e., the determinant of $\mathbf{R}$ equals -1, instead of 1). Umeyama [21] provided a simple fix. The reflection happens when the determinant of the shape covariance matrix Σ is negative, $\|\Sigma\| < 0$. In singular value decomposition of Σ, we can re-organize the elements of matrices $\mathbf{D}$, $\mathbf{U}$, and $\mathbf{V}$ so that $\mathbf{D} = diag(d_i)$, where $d_1 \geq d_2 \geq d_3$. Let Λ be

$$\Lambda = \begin{cases} \mathbf{I} & \text{if } \|\Sigma\| \geq 0 \\ diag(1,1,-1) & \text{if } \|\Sigma\| < 0 \end{cases} \tag{6.14}$$

Then, the optimal similarity transformation is

$$\hat{\mathbf{R}} = \mathbf{U}\Lambda\mathbf{V}^T,$$

$$\hat{s} = \frac{1}{\sigma_1^2} Trace(\mathbf{D}\Lambda),$$

$$\hat{\mathbf{T}} = \mu_2 - \hat{s}\hat{\mathbf{R}}\mu_1. \tag{6.15}$$

Refer to [21] for a proof of the optimality of this modified solution.

6.3.3   Procrustes Analysis Under Anisotropic Similarity Transformation

The MSL computational framework estimates efficiently the anisotropic scale of an object. The advantage of covering more deformations is that the shape space after alignment is more compact and the mean shape represents the whole shape population more accurately. This is very helpful for many applications, such as the left ventricle detection and segmentation. The deformation of the left ventricle is dominated by contraction and expansion, and the amount of deformation along different directions is quite different. The deformation along the long axis of the left ventricle is usually smaller than the deformation orthogonal to the long axis. Using three scales to represent the size of the ventricle is more accurate than using a single scale. The capability of estimating anisotropic scales is thus important to build a segmentation system working for all cardiac phases.

In this scenario, the anisotropic scaling needs to be compensated during alignment,

$$\hat{\mathbf{T}}, \hat{\mathbf{R}}, \hat{\mathbf{S}} = arg \min_{\mathbf{T,R,S}} \sum_{j=1}^{J} \left\| \left(\mathbf{R} \begin{bmatrix} S_x & 0 & 0 \\ 0 & S_y & 0 \\ 0 & 0 & S_z \end{bmatrix} \mathbf{M}_1^j + \mathbf{T} \right) - \mathbf{M}_2^j \right\|^2. \tag{6.16}$$

Since there are no closed-form solutions for the alignment under anisotropic scaling [3], we present a two-step iterative approach to search for an optimal solution. Suppose there is a common scale $s = (S_x + S_y + S_z)/3$. Let $S_x' = S_x/s$, $S_y' = S_y/s$, and $S_z' = S_z/s$. Equation (6.16) can be re-written as

$$\hat{\mathbf{T}}, \hat{\mathbf{R}}, \hat{\mathbf{S}} = arg \min_{\mathbf{T,R,S}} \sum_{j=1}^{J} \left\| \left(\mathbf{R}s \begin{bmatrix} S_x' & 0 & 0 \\ 0 & S_y' & 0 \\ 0 & 0 & S_z' \end{bmatrix} \mathbf{M}_1^j + \mathbf{T} \right) - \mathbf{M}_2^j \right\|^2. \tag{6.17}$$

In the first step, suppose we known the anisotropic scaling factors S_x', S_y', and S_z'. (At the beginning, we initialize with isotropic scaling, $S_x' = 1$, $S_y' = 1$, and $S_z' = 1$.) We can apply the anisotropic scaling to each point in shape $\mathbf{M}_1$,

$$\mathbf{P}_1^j(x) = S_x' \mathbf{M}_1^j(x),$$
$$\mathbf{P}_1^j(y) = S_y' \mathbf{M}_1^j(y),$$
$$\mathbf{P}_1^j(z) = S_z' \mathbf{M}_1^j(z), \tag{6.18}$$

for $j = 1, 2, \ldots, J$. Equation (6.17) becomes

$$\hat{\mathbf{T}}, \hat{\mathbf{R}}, \hat{s} = arg \min_{\mathbf{T,R},s} \sum_{j=1}^{J} \left\| \left(\mathbf{R}s \mathbf{P}_1^j + \mathbf{T} \right) - \mathbf{M}_2^j \right\|^2. \tag{6.19}$$

This is the normal similarity transformation estimation as Eq. (6.6) and a closed-form solution is given in Eq. (6.15).

In the second step, assuming the similarity transformation $(\mathbf{T}, \mathbf{R}, s)$ is given, we estimate the optimal anisotropic scaling factors S_x', S_y', and S_z'. The optimization solution to Eq. (6.17) does not change if we left multiply the objective function by $s^{-1}\mathbf{R}^{-1}$, since now $\mathbf{R}$ and s are fixed,

$$\hat{\mathbf{T}}, \hat{\mathbf{R}}, \hat{\mathbf{S}} = arg \min_{\mathbf{T,R,S}} \sum_{j=1}^{J} \left\| s^{-1}\mathbf{R}^{-1} \left(\mathbf{R}s \begin{bmatrix} S_x' & 0 & 0 \\ 0 & S_y' & 0 \\ 0 & 0 & S_z' \end{bmatrix} \mathbf{M}_1^j + \mathbf{T} - \mathbf{M}_2^j \right) \right\|^2. \tag{6.20}$$

Denote by

$$\mathbf{P}_2^j = \frac{1}{s} \mathbf{R}^{-1} (\mathbf{M}_2^j - \mathbf{T}). \tag{6.21}$$

Step 1.   Initialize $S_x' = 1$, $S_y' = 1$, and $S_z' = 1$.
Step 2.   Given S_x', S_y', and S_z', estimate the isotropic similarity transformation $\mathbf{T}, \mathbf{R}, s$, using Eq. (6.15).
Step 3.   Given $\mathbf{T}, \mathbf{R}, s$, estimate the anisotropic scaling factors S_x', S_y', and S_z', using Eq. (6.23).
Step 4.   Repeat steps 2 and 3 until it converges.

Fig. 6.2 Algorithm to align two 3D shapes under the similarity transformation with anisotropic scaling

The optimization problem is then simplified as,

$$\hat{S}_x', \hat{S}_y', \hat{S}_z' = arg \min_{S_x', S_y', S_z'} \sum_{j=1}^{J} \left\| \begin{bmatrix} S_x' & 0 & 0 \\ 0 & S_y' & 0 \\ 0 & 0 & S_z' \end{bmatrix} \mathbf{M}_1^j - \mathbf{P}_2^j \right\|^2 . \tag{6.22}$$

Simple mathematic derivation will give us the following solution,

$$\hat{S}_x' = \frac{\sum_{j=1}^{J} \mathbf{M}_1^j(x) \mathbf{P}_2^j(x)}{\sum_{j=1}^{J} \mathbf{M}_1^j(x)^2},$$

$$\hat{S}_y' = \frac{\sum_{j=1}^{J} \mathbf{M}_1^j(y) \mathbf{P}_2^j(y)}{\sum_{j=1}^{J} \mathbf{M}_1^j(y)^2},$$

$$\hat{S}_z' = \frac{\sum_{j=1}^{J} \mathbf{M}_1^j(z) \mathbf{P}_2^j(z)}{\sum_{j=1}^{J} \mathbf{M}_1^j(z)^2}. \tag{6.23}$$

The above two steps need to be iterated a few times until the process converges. Figure 6.2 shows a brief summary of the algorithm to align two 3D shapes under the similarity transformation with anisotropic scaling.

6.3.4 Generalized Procrustes Analysis to Align a Group of Shapes Under Anisotropic Similarity Transformation

Having now a module to solve the anisotropic similarity transformation between two shapes, we can plug it into the Generalized Procrustes Analysis (GPA) to search for the optimal mean shape $\bar{\mathbf{m}}$ in Eq. (6.4). Figure 6.3 shows the algorithm for the GPA under the anisotropic similarity transformation. In our approach, besides the optimal mean shape, the optimal alignment $\mathcal{T}_i$ of the mean shape towards each example shape is also calculated. The transformation parameters of the optimal alignment provide the pose ground truth that the MSL can learn to estimate.

Step 1.   Randomly pick an example shape as a reference shape.
Step 2.   Calculate the optimal anisotropic similarity transformation $\mathscr{T}_i$ from the reference shape to each example shape i using the algorithm in Fig. 6.2.
Step 3.   Normalize each example shape i using the inverse transformation $\mathscr{T}_i^{-1}$.
Step 4.   Compute the mean (which is a simple average) of the normalized shapes.
Step 5.   Set the new mean shape as the reference shape.
Step 6.   Go to step 2 until the procedure converges.

Fig. 6.3   Generalized Procrustes analysis to align a group of shapes under the anisotropic similarity transformation

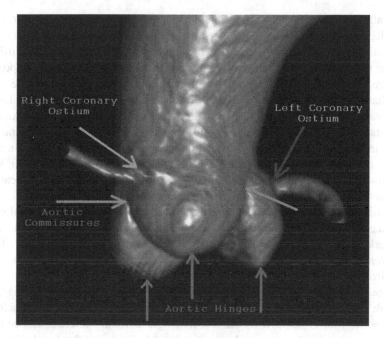

Fig. 6.4   The anatomy of the aortic valve with aortic hinges, aortic commissures, and left/right coronary ostium. Note: The third aortic commissure is at the back of the valve and blocked in this view. ©2012 IEEE. Reprinted, with permission, from Zheng, Y., John, M., Liao, R., Nottling, A., Boese, J., Kempfert, J., Walther, T., Brockmann, G., Comaniciu, D.: Automatic aorta segmentation and valve landmark detection in C-arm CT for transcatheter aortic valve implantation. *IEEE Trans. Medical Imaging* **31**(12), 2307–2321 (2012)

6.4   Application to Aortic Valve Landmark Detection

The method described in the previous section is generic, therefore it can be applied to determine the optimal pose parameters, together with the optimal mean shape, of any nonrigid object during the training procedure. For example, we applied it to determine the optimal pose of a global object composed of eight aortic valve landmarks in a hierarchical landmark detection framework. In addition, we use it for the whole-heart segmentation, a task often called heart isolation in the literature

[6, 26, 29, 30], to distinguish it from heart chamber segmentation. In this section, we focus on the application of landmark detection for the aortic valve. The whole-heart segmentation will be presented in the next section.

6.4.1   Aortic Valve Landmark Detection for Transcatheter Aortic Valve Implantation

Transcatheter Aortic Valve Implantation (TAVI), also known as Transcatheter Aortic Valve Replacement (TAVR), is an emerging, less invasive procedure to treat severe aortic valve stenosis, where the prosthetic valve is inserted and deployed using a catheter through a small puncture of the femoral artery (the transfemoral approach) or a small cut at the heart apex (the transapical approach). Before the TAVI procedure, several important parameters of the aortic valve (see Fig. 6.4 for the aortic valve anatomy) need to be measured for surgical planning. For example, the distance between the coronary ostia and the aortic valve hinge plane (the lowest level of the valve cusps) is a critical parameter for patient selection since a short distance increases the risk of blocking coronary circulation after valve deployment [13, 27, 28]. The diameter of aortic valve annulus needs to be measured accurately to select a prosthetic valve with an appropriate size.

Aortic valve landmarks play an important role in the surgical planning and visual guidance for TAVI. However, there is very limited work on automatic aortic valve landmark detection, except coronary ostium detection in CT Angiography (CTA) for coronary analysis [9, 18, 19, 22, 23]. The coronary ostia detection process often starts from segmenting the ascending aorta and a coronary artery is detected as a thin tubular structure attached to the aorta. The position of the attachment is taken as the detected ostium. For example, the largest connected component on each side of the aortic root is selected as the left and right coronary arteries, respectively, in [9]. However, simple connected component analysis is not robust under imaging noise, resulting in a success rate of only 57 %. Alternatively, coronary centerlines can be tracked from the aorta surface in order to detect coronary ostia [19]. Since the computationally expensive centerline tracing algorithm needs to run on the whole aorta surface, it is more time consuming. Compared to coronary ostium detection, there is less work on the detection of other aortic valve landmarks, i.e., the aortic hinges and commissures in this case. More recently Ionasec et al. [11, 12] presented a comprehensive aortic valve model, including all eight valve landmarks.

In this section, we present a hierarchical approach to landmark detection, by first detecting a global object comprised of all eight valve landmarks. The global object is detected efficiently using the MSL. From the position, orientation, and scale of this global object, we can infer the rough position of individual landmarks. We calculate the optimal mean shape and corresponding transformations using the GPA under anisotropic similarity transformation as described in the previous section.

After inferring the initial landmark position from the pose of the detected global object, each landmark is then refined in a small region (e.g., a cube of 10 mm centered on the initial position) under the guidance of its own specific landmark detector. Trained with the probabilistic boosting-tree classifier [20], the current landmark detector is similar to the detector used in [12], but using the steerable features [25] that can be efficiently extracted from the original volume. On the contrary, the method of [12] needs to re-sample the original volume to an isotropic resolution to use the Haar wavelet features.

6.4.2 Unique Mean Shape for Aortic Valve Landmarks

Observe that the optimal mean shape $\bar{\mathbf{m}}$ is not unique. Any translation, rotation, and scaling of $\bar{\mathbf{m}}$ is also an optimum since the transformation of the mean shape can be compensated by the individual transformation $\mathcal{T}_i$ in Eq. (6.4). We remove the unnecessary flexibility of the mean shape using the oriented bounding box based approach as follows. We first define a unique orientation. Suppose three aortic hinges are denoted as $\mathbf{H}_1$, $\mathbf{H}_2$, and $\mathbf{H}_3$; three aortic commissures are denoted as $\mathbf{C}_1$, $\mathbf{C}_2$, and $\mathbf{C}_3$; and $\mathbf{O}_l$ and $\mathbf{O}_r$ represent the left and right coronary ostium, respectively. Let $\mathbf{H}_c = (\mathbf{H}_1 + \mathbf{H}_2 + \mathbf{H}_3)/3$ be the mass center of three aortic hinges and $\mathbf{C}_c = (\mathbf{C}_1 + \mathbf{C}_2 + \mathbf{C}_3)/3$ be the mass center of three aortic commissures. The $\mathbf{z}$ axis is defined as a unit vector pointing from the hinge center $\mathbf{H}_c$ to the commissure center $\mathbf{C}_c$

$$\mathbf{z} = \frac{\mathbf{C}_c - \mathbf{H}_c}{\|\mathbf{C}_c - \mathbf{H}_c\|}. \tag{6.24}$$

The $\mathbf{x}$ axis is derived as follows

$$\mathbf{x}_1 = \frac{\mathbf{O}_r - \mathbf{O}_l}{\|\mathbf{O}_r - \mathbf{O}_l\|}, \tag{6.25}$$

$$\mathbf{x}_2 = (\mathbf{z} \times \mathbf{x}_1) \times \mathbf{z}, \tag{6.26}$$

$$\mathbf{x} = \frac{\mathbf{x}_2}{\|\mathbf{x}_2\|}. \tag{6.27}$$

Here, initial axis $\mathbf{x}_1$ is defined as a unit vector pointing from the left coronary ostium $\mathbf{O}_l$ to the right coronary ostium $\mathbf{O}_r$. We then rotate the $\mathbf{x}_1$ axis inside the plane spanned by the $\mathbf{x}_1$ and $\mathbf{z}$ axes to make it perpendicular to the $\mathbf{z}$ axis, arriving at axis $\mathbf{x}_2$. The final $\mathbf{x}$ axis is achieved by normalizing $\mathbf{x}_2$ to a unit vector. The $\mathbf{y}$ axis is then a cross product of the $\mathbf{z}$ and $\mathbf{x}$ axes, $\mathbf{y} = \mathbf{z} \times \mathbf{x}$.

After defining the orientation of the global shape, we calculate an oriented bounding box for the eight landmarks. We set the origin of the object-centered coordinate system to the center of the box and scale the bounding box anisotropically to make it a cube of 1 mm in length. The optimal mean shape $\bar{m}$ is tightly bounded in the cube. After each iteration of the generalized Procrustes analysis, $\bar{m}$ is normalized using the above procedure, therefore uniquely defined. We emphasize that such normalization of the mean shape $\bar{m}$ does not change its optimality, but helps achieving a unique solution.

6.4.3   Experiments on Aortic Valve Landmark Detection

We collected a dataset of 319 C-arm CT volumes of 276 patients from multiple clinical sites, worldwide. To evaluate the aortic valve landmark detection accuracy, the post-deployment C-arm CT scans (15 volumes) are excluded since the native aortic hinges and commissures have been significantly affected by the implant. The patients with prosthetic valves implanted from previous open-heart surgery are excluded for the same reason (6 volumes). We also exclude a few volumes (20 volumes) with extremely poor image quality, for which the landmarks cannot be identified even by an expert, although the aorta can be successfully segmented on these volumes. In total, we get 278 C-arm CT volumes useful for aortic valve landmark detection. The size of each slice in a volume is 256×256 or 512×512 pixels. A volume contains around 200–300 slices. The image resolution is isotropic and varies from volume to volume in the range of [0.70, 0.84] mm.

We first evaluate the alignment errors using different mean shapes by assuming the pose of the global landmark object can be estimated perfectly. This is the lower bound of the landmark initialization error that can be achieved. The landmark accuracy is measured using the Euclidean distance from the inferred landmark to the

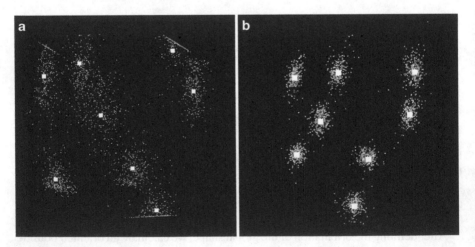

Fig. 6.5 The aligned aortic valve landmarks and mean shape (represented as *big rectangles*) using (a) the oriented bounding box based approach and (b) the GPA-based optimization approach. The distribution of the aligned landmarks is more compact using the GPA-based optimization

Table 6.1 Aortic valve landmark detection errors based on a fourfold cross-validation on 278 volumes. The mean, standard deviation (STD), and median of the errors are reported (measured in millimeters)

	Aortic hinges			Coronary ostia			Aortic commissures		
	Mean	STD	Median	Mean	STD	Median	Mean	STD	Median
Global pose estimation	3.38	1.27	3.16	4.26	1.78	4.01	3.35	1.31	3.18
Local refinement	2.09	1.18	1.82	2.07	1.53	1.61	2.17	1.31	1.88

ground truth. On our evaluation dataset with 278 volumes, the mean landmark error inferred from the aligned mean shape is about 2.77 mm using the oriented bounding box based approach. The GPA converges after three iterations and the mean landmark error is significantly reduced to 1.90 mm. This experiment demonstrates that the optimal mean shape derived using the proposed method can better represent the whole shape population. Figure 6.5a and b show the distribution of the aligned landmarks using the bounding box based approach and the proposed optimization approach, respectively. It is clear that the distribution is more compact using the proposed method.

We then evaluate the accuracy of automatic landmark detection. A fourfold cross-validation is performed to evaluate our algorithm. The whole dataset is randomly split into four roughly equal sets. Three sets are used to train the system and the remaining set is reserved for testing. The configuration is rotated, until each set has been tested once. Table 6.1 shows the landmark detection errors. After global landmark object pose estimation, we can get a good initial estimate of the landmark position. The mean errors range from 3.35 to 4.26 mm for different landmarks. Compared to the aortic hinges and commissures, the initial coronary ostia have a larger mean error of 4.26 mm due to the larger variations in the origin of a coronary artery. After local refinement for each landmark, the errors are significantly reduced. For example, the mean error of the aortic hinges reduces from 3.38 to 2.09 mm. The coronary ostia achieve the largest reduction in detection error, from 4.26 to 2.07 mm. Figure 6.6 shows the detected valve landmarks in two typical volumes.

Multiple 3D valve measurements can be derived from the detected landmarks. Due to the space limit, we only evaluate the errors in measuring the distance from the left and right coronary ostia to the aortic hinge plane. As shown in Table 6.2, the mean error for measuring the left coronary ostium to hinge plane distance is 2.10 mm. The right coronary ostium has a larger mean error of 2.51 mm. The overall distance measurement error is only slightly larger than the landmark detection errors (2.07 mm for the coronary ostia and 2.09 mm for the aortic hinges). The normal of aortic hinge plane (determined by three aortic hinges) plays an important role in selecting a proper C-arm angulation, which can affect the tilting of the deployed prosthetic valve; therefore, it needs to be estimated accurately. We calculate the angle between the estimated hinge plane normal and its true value derived from the ground truth. As shown in Table 6.2, the mean angle is 3.68°. A tilting error of 5° is regarded by physicians as almost perfect, our error being within this range.

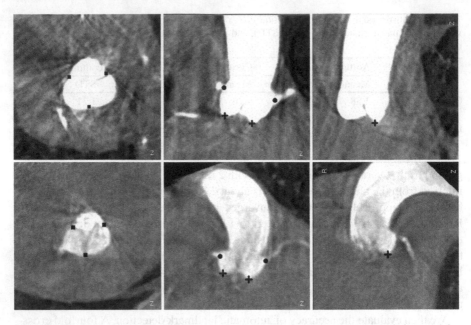

Fig. 6.6 The aortic valve landmark detection results on two example data with '*filled square*' for the commissures, '*plus symbol*' for the hinges, and '*filled circle*' for the left and right coronary ostia. Each row shows three orthogonal cuts of a volume

Table 6.2 Errors of automatic 3D measurements based on a fourfold cross-validation on 278 volumes, including the error of the distance measurement (in millimeters) from coronary ostia to the aortic hinge plane, and the angle (in degrees) between the detected and true aortic hinge plane normals

	Left ostium to hinge			Right ostium to hinge			Hinge plane normal		
	Mean	STD	Median	Mean	STD	Median	Mean	STD	Median
Errors	2.10	1.86	1.73	2.51	2.03	2.11	3.68°	3.61°	2.73°

6.5   Application to Whole-Heart Segmentation

In this section, we apply the GPA-based optimal mean shape estimation to the whole-heart segmentation [26] and perform a quantitative comparison with the bounding box based mean shape.

6.5.1   Whole-Heart Segmentation

While most previous work on heart segmentation is focused on segmenting heart chambers [25], segmenting the heart as a whole from CT data has clinical value

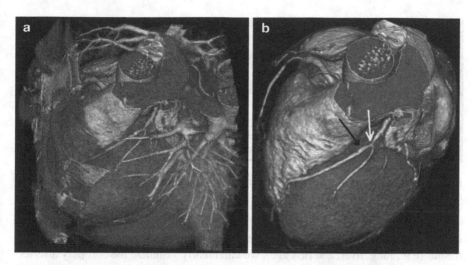

Fig. 6.7 Whole-heart segmentation for 3D visualization of the coronary arteries. (**a**) Before heart segmentation. (**b**) After heart segmentation. *Arrows* indicate suspicious regions in the left anterior descending artery (black for a calcified plaque and white for a soft plaque)

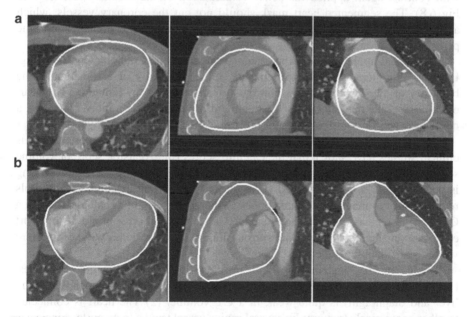

Fig. 6.8 Whole-heart segmentation (white contour) for a contrasted CT scan. (**a**) Initialization with the optimal mean shape mesh. (**b**) After final boundary delineation. From left to right: transaxial, sagittal, and coronal views

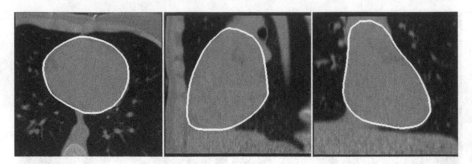

Fig. 6.9 Whole-heart segmentation (white contour) for a non-contrasted CT scan. From left to right: transaxial, sagittal, and coronal views

in several applications. For example, after separating the heart from the proximity tissues (e.g., lung, liver, and rib cage), we can clearly visualize the coronary arteries in 3D, as shown in Fig. 6.7. Such 3D visualization provides an intuitive view for physicians to diagnose suspicious coronary segments (as indicated by the black and white arrows in Fig. 6.7). For this application, generally, the patient is scanned with contrast agent applied for better visualization of the coronary arteries (see Fig. 6.8). The segmented heart mask should not cut the coronary vessels, which are located on the surface of the heart chambers. This presents a challenge to the prior segmentation algorithms.

The second application of whole-heart segmentation is radiotherapy planning. Usually, radiotherapists need to delineate, either manually or automatically, the boundary of the sensitive organs that must not be affected by radiation. The heart often needs to be masked out for the treatment of lung or liver tumors. Normally, a non-contrasted CT scan, as shown in Fig. 6.9, is used for radiotherapy planning.

The third application is for automatic calculation of the calcium scores. Various clinical studies have shown that the calcium scores (the Agatston score or volume score) are a good risk indicator for major future heart events [1, 7]. Calcium scoring is performed on a non-contrasted CT scan and the current calcium scoring tools require a user to manually exclude bones (which are as bright as calcifications in a CT scan) in the calculation. The procedure is tedious and error prone. If the heart can be automatically isolated from surrounding tissues, the bones will not interfere with the calculation of calcium scores.

Whole-heart segmentation is a hard problem due to the following challenges. (1) The boundary between the heart and some of the neighboring tissues (e.g., liver and diaphragm) is quite weak in a CT volume. (2) The heart is connected to other anatomical structures by several major vessel trunks (e.g., aorta, vena cava, pulmonary veins, and pulmonary arteries). To build a heart representation, we must cut those trunks somewhere, normally at the position where the vessels connect to the heart, although no image boundary is present. (3) The shape variation of the whole heart across patients is more complicated than each individual chamber. This brings a large variation in the heart shape. Furthermore, there are quite a few scans with a part of the heart missing in the captured volume, especially at the top or bottom of the heart, which introduces extra shape variations. (4) We are targeting at both contrasted and non-contrasted data, instead of just one homogeneous set (e.g., [6] for contrasted data and [15] for non-contrasted data). This presents an increase in appearance variability.

Previous work on whole-heart segmentation is limited. The atlas based methods are often used to segment the heart. For example, Rikvoort et al. [17] presented an adaptive local multi-atlas based approach. It took about 30 min to segment a scan. Lelieveldt et al. [14] proposed another atlas based approach, segmenting several organs (e.g., lung, heart, and liver) in a thoracic scan using a hierarchical organ model. Their approach only provided a rough segmentation and an error as large as 10 mm was regarded as a correct segmentation. It took 5–20 min to process one volume. Gregson et al. [8] proposed to segment the lungs first and the heart was approximated as a sphere between the left and right lungs. Moreno et al. [15] presented a more thorough model for the geometric relationship between lungs and the heart. Funka-Lea et al. [6] proposed an automatic approach based on graph cuts. They used the volumetric barycenter weighted by intensity as an initial estimate of the heart center. A small ellipsoid was put at the estimated heart center and progressively grown until it touched the transition between the heart and lung (which was easy to detect in a CT volume). The graph cuts technique was then applied to achieve the final detailed boundary delineation. Overall, it took about 20 s to process one volume.

We apply Marginal Space Learning (MSL) to whole-heart segmentation. Due to the large shape variation and presence of weak boundaries, the optimal mean shape presented in this chapter is used to improve the shape initialization accuracy. After shape initialization, we use the Active Shape Model (ASM) [4] to deform the mesh under the guidance of a learning based boundary detector. The sternum and rib cage are explicitly excluded in a post-processing step to further improve the boundary delineation accuracy. Please refer to [26] for more details of the boundary delineation in whole-heart segmentation.

6.5.2   Experiments on Whole-Heart Segmentation

The proposed method has been tested on 589 volumes from 288 patients (including 485 contrasted and 104 non-contrasted volumes). The scanning protocols are heterogeneous with different capture ranges and resolutions. Each volume contains 80–350 slices and the slice size is 512×512 pixels. The resolution inside a slice is isotropic and varies from 0.28 to 0.74 mm, while slice thickness is generally larger than the in-slice resolution and varies from 0.4 to 2.0 mm.

The out-most surface of the heart is annotated using a triangulated mesh with 514 mesh points and 1,024 triangles. The rotation axis based resampling method presented in Chap. 7 is used to establish the mesh point correspondence. A heart coordinate system based on three landmarks, namely, the aortic valve center, the

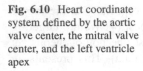

Fig. 6.10 Heart coordinate system defined by the aortic valve center, the mitral valve center, and the left ventricle apex

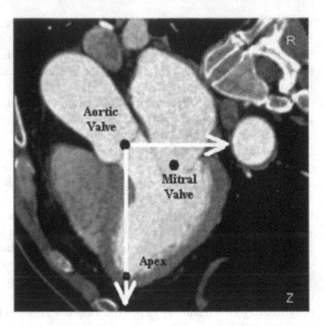

mitral valve center, and the left ventricle endocardium apex, is used to determine the rotation axis for resampling. These three landmarks determine a plane, on which the z and x axes lie. As shown in Fig. 6.10, the z axis is defined as the direction pointing from the aortic valve center to the left ventricle apex. The x axis is another vector on the plane that is perpendicular to the z axis and points toward the mitral valve center. The y axis is the cross product of the z and x axes.

We evaluate the shape initialization error of the GPA-based optimal mean shape and the heuristic bounding box based mean shape. In the bounding box based approach, the orientation ground truth is defined as the orientation of the bounding box, which is aligned with the heart coordinate system as shown in Fig. 6.10. The center of the bounding box is taken as the position ground truth of the training sample and sizes of the box along different directions are taken as the scale ground truth. The pose ground truth parameters in the GPA-based method are calculated according to the optimization of Eq. (6.4).

The point-to-mesh error, E_{p2m}, is used to evaluate the segmentation accuracy. For each point in a mesh, we search for the closest point in the other mesh to calculate the minimum distance. We calculate the point-to-mesh distance from the detected mesh to the ground truth mesh and vice versa to make the measurement symmetric.

We perform a fourfold cross-validation to evaluate the performance of the algorithm. After the MSL based heart pose estimation, we align the mean shape to the estimated position, orientation, and anisotropic scales, then calculate E_{p2m} of the aligned mean shape w.r.t. the ground truth mesh. The optimal mean shape is much more accurate than the heuristic bounding box based mean shape. It reduces

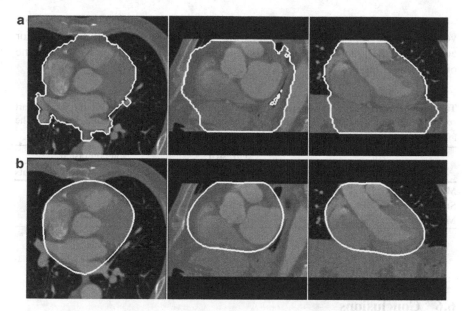

Fig. 6.11 Comparison of whole-heart segmentation of (**a**) the graph cuts based method [6] and (**b**) the proposed method. From left the right are three orthogonal cuts of the volume with white contours showing the automatically segmented heart surface mesh

the mean E_{p2m} error from 4.26 to 3.09 mm (about 27 % reduction), compared to the bounding box based approach.

After shape initialization, we use the ASM to deform the mesh under the guidance of a learning based boundary detector for final refinement. As shown in Table 6.3, we achieve the mean and median errors of 1.81 mm and 1.66 mm, respectively. The segmentation results on contrasted data are moderately better than the non-contrasted data (the mean error of 1.75 mm for the contrasted vs. 2.10 mm for the non-contrasted). Figure 6.8a shows the initialization of whole-heart segmentation using the optimal mean shape on a contrasted CT volume. The initial shape is quite close to the true boundary and final refinement using the learning based boundary detector results in accurate whole-heart segmentation, as shown in Fig. 6.8. Figure 6.9 shows another example of whole-heart segmentation on non-contrasted CT data. Due to the missing boundary between the heart and surrounding tissues (the liver and diaphragm) at the bottom, an accurate shape initialization is important for the success of our algorithm to avoid segmentation leakage.

In Table 6.3, we also compare our approach with a graph cuts based approach proposed in [6]. A binary program was provided by authors of [6], therefore avoiding the performance difference introduced in re-implementation of the algorithm. As shown in Table 6.3, the mean and median errors for the graph cuts based approach are 4.60 mm and 4.00 mm, higher than the proposed method. The performance of the graph cuts based approach degrades significantly on non-contrasted data. It tends to include more tissues into the heart mask, as shown in Fig. 6.11a.

Our approach is computationally efficient with a processing time of 1.5 s per volume on a computer with dual-core 3.2 GHz CPUs and 3 GB memory. For comparison, the graph cuts based approach takes about 20 s to process a volume on the same computer.

Table 6.3 Comparison of our approach and a graph cuts based approach [6] for whole-heart segmentation on 589 volumes (including 485 contrasted and 104 non-contrasted volumes). The point-to-mesh error (in millimeters) is used to measure the accuracy in boundary delineation

	All		Contrasted		Non-contrasted	
	Our method	Graph cuts	Our method	Graph cuts	Our method	Graph cuts
Mean error	1.81	4.60	1.75	3.94	2.10	7.65
Std deviation	0.70	2.61	0.69	1.62	0.67	3.87
Median error	1.66	4.00	1.63	3.69	2.01	6.91

6.6 Conclusions

In this chapter, we presented a method to improve the shape initialization accuracy for nonrigid object segmentation using an optimal mean shape calculated from the training set. We only change the training step and there is no computation overhead during object detection on unseen data. Our approach also generates an optimal anisotropic similarity transformation to align the mean shape to each individual training shape. This transformation provides the pose ground truth of each training sample for the MSL to learn the intrinsic relationships between the image data and the target object pose. The effectiveness of the method is demonstrated on the problems of landmark detection for the aortic valve and whole-heart segmentation.

References

1. Agatston, A.S., Janowitz, W.R., Hildner, F.J., Zusmer, N.R., Viamonte Jr., M., Detrano, R.: Quantification of coronary artery calcium using ultrafast computed tomography. Journal of the American College of Cardiology **15**(4), 827–832 (1990)
2. Arun, K.S., Huang, T.S., Blostein, S.D.: Least-squares fitting of two 3-D point sets. IEEE Trans. Pattern Anal. Machine Intell. **9**(5), 698–700 (1987)
3. Batchelor, P.G., West, J.B., Fitzpatrick, J.M.: Scalings and similarity transforms: Maximum likelihood estimations. In: Proc. Medical Image Understanding and Analysis (2002)
4. Cootes, T.F., Taylor, C.J., Cooper, D.H., Graham, J.: Active shape models—their training and application. Computer Vision and Image Understanding **61**(1), 38–59 (1995)
5. Dryden, I.L., Mardia, K.V.: Statistical Shape Analysis. John Wiley, Chichester (1998)
6. Funka-Lea, G., Boykov, Y., Florin, C., Jolly, M.P., Moreau-Gobard, R., Ramaraj, R., Rinck, D.: Automatic heart isolation for CT coronary visualization using graph-cuts. In: Proc. IEEE Int'l Sym. Biomedical Imaging, pp. 614–617 (2006)

7. Glodny, B., Helmel, B., Trieb, T., Schenk, C., Taferner, B., Unterholzner, V., Strasak, A., Petersen, J.: A method for calcium quantification by means of CT coronary angiography using 64-multidetector CT: Very high correlation with Agatston and volume scores. European Radiology 19(7), 1661–1668 (2009)
8. Gregson, P.H.: Automatic segmentation of the heart in 3D MR images. In: Canadian Conf. Eletrical and Computer Engineering, pp. 584–587 (1994)
9. Hennemuth, A., Boskamp, T., Fritz, D., Kühnel, C., Bock, S., Rinck, D., Scheuering, M., Peitgen, H.O.: One-click coronary tree segmentation in CT angiographic images. In: Proc. Computer Assisted Radiology and Surgery, pp. 317–321 (2005)
10. Horn, B.K.P.: Closed-form solution of absolute orientation using orthonormal matrices. Journal of Optical Society of American 5(7), 1127–1135 (1987)
11. Ionasec, R.I., Georgescu, B., Gassner, E., Vogt, S., Kutter, O., Scheuering, M., Navab, N., Comaniciu, D.: Dynamic model-driven quantitative and visual evaluation of the aortic valve from 4D CT. In: Proc. Int'l Conf. Medical Image Computing and Computer Assisted Intervention, vol. 1, pp. 686–694 (2008)
12. Ionasec, R.I., Voigt, I., Georgescu, B., Wang, Y., Houle, H., Vega-Higuera, F., Navab, N., Comaniciu, D.: Patient-specific modeling and quantification of the aortic and mitral valves from 4D cardiac CT and TEE. IEEE Trans. Medical Imaging 29(9), 1636–1651 (2010)
13. John, M., Liao, R., Zheng, Y., Nottling, A., Boese, J., Kirschstein, U., Kempfert, J., Walther, T.: System to guide transcatheter aortic valve implantations based on interventional 3D C-arm CT imaging. In: Proc. Int'l Conf. Medical Image Computing and Computer Assisted Intervention, vol. 1, pp. 375–382 (2010)
14. Lelieveldt, B.P.F., van der Geest, R.J., Rezaee, M.R., Bosch, J.G., Reiber, J.H.C.: Anatomical model matching with fuzzy implicit surfaces for segmentation of thoracic volume scans. IEEE Trans. Medical Imaging 18(3), 218–230 (1999)
15. Moreno, A., Takemura, C.M., Colliot, O., Camara, O., Bloch, I.: Using anatomical knowledge expressed as fuzzy constraints to segment the heart in CT images. Pattern Recognition 41(8), 2525–2540 (2008)
16. Pizarro, D., Bartoli, A.: Global optimization for optimal generalized Procrustes analysis. In: Proc. IEEE Conf. Computer Vision and Pattern Recognition, pp. 2409–2415 (2011)
17. van Rikxoort, E.M., Isgum, I., Staring, M., Klein, S., van Ginneken, B.: Adaptive local multi-atlas segmentation: Application to heart segmentation in chest CT scans. In: Proc. of SPIE Medical Imaging, pp. 1–6 (2008)
18. Saur, S.C., Kühnel, C., Boskamp, T., Székely, G., Cattin, P.: Automatic ascending aorta detection in CTA datasets. In: Proc. Workshop Bildverarbeitung für der Medizin, pp. 323–327 (2008)
19. Tek, H., Gulsun, M.A., Laguitton, S., Grady, L., Lesage, D., Funka-Lea, G.: Automatic coronary tree modeling. The Insight Journal pp. 1–8 (2008)
20. Tu, Z.: Probabilistic boosting-tree: Learning discriminative methods for classification, recognition, and clustering. In: Proc. Int'l Conf. Computer Vision, pp. 1589–1596 (2005)
21. Umeyama, S.: Least-squares estimation of transformation parameters between two point patterns. IEEE Trans. Pattern Anal. Machine Intell. 13(4), 376–380 (1991)
22. Wang, C., Smedby, O.: An automatic seeding method for coronary artery segmentation and skeletonization in CTA. The Insight Journal pp. 1–8 (2008)
23. Wang, S., Fu, L., Yue, Y., Kang, Y., Liu, J.: Fast and automatic segmentation of ascending aorta in MSCT volume data. In: Proc. Int'l Conf. Image and Signal Processing, pp. 1–5 (2009)
24. Zheng, Y., Barbu, A., Georgescu, B., Scheuering, M., Comaniciu, D.: Fast automatic heart chamber segmentation from 3D CT data using marginal space learning and steerable features. In: Proc. Int'l Conf. Computer Vision, pp. 1–8 (2007)
25. Zheng, Y., Barbu, A., Georgescu, B., Scheuering, M., Comaniciu, D.: Four-chamber heart modeling and automatic segmentation for 3D cardiac CT volumes using marginal space learning and steerable features. IEEE Trans. Medical Imaging 27(11), 1668–1681 (2008)

26. Zheng, Y., Georgescu, B., Vega-Higuera, F., Zhou, S.K., Comaniciu, D.: Fast and automatic heart isolation in 3D CT volumes: Optimal shape initialization. In: Proc. MICCAI Workshop Machine Learning in Medical Imaging, pp. 84–91 (2010)
27. Zheng, Y., John, M., Liao, R., Boese, J., Kirschstein, U., Georgescu, B., Zhou, S.K., Kempfert, J., Walther, T., Brockmann, G., Comaniciu, D.: Automatic aorta segmentation and valve landmark detection in C-arm CT: Application to aortic valve implantation. In: Proc. Int'l Conf. Medical Image Computing and Computer Assisted Intervention, vol. 1, pp. 476–483 (2010)
28. Zheng, Y., John, M., Liao, R., Nottling, A., Boese, J., Kempfert, J., Walther, T., Brockmann, G., Comaniciu, D.: Automatic aorta segmentation and valve landmark detection in C-arm CT for transcatheter aortic valve implantation. IEEE Trans. Medical Imaging 31(12), 2307–2321 (2012)
29. Zhong, H., Zheng, Y., Funka-Lea, G., Vega-Higuera, F.: Segmentation and removal of pulmonary arteries, veins and left atrial appendage for visualizing coronary and bypass arteries. In: Proc. Workshop on Medical Computer Vision (In conjunction with CVPR), pp. 24–30 (2012)
30. Zhong, H., Zheng, Y., Funka-Lea, G., Vega-Higuera, F.: Automatic heart isolation in 3D CT images. In: B. Menze, G. Langs, L. Lu, A. Montillo, Z. Tu, A. Criminisi (eds.) Medical Computer Vision, pp. 165–180. Springer (2013)

Chapter 7
Nonrigid Object Segmentation: Application to Four-Chamber Heart Segmentation

7.1 Introduction

Marginal Space Learning (MSL) is an effective tool to detect the pose of an anatomical structure in medical imaging. Examples of such applications are: detecting the brain mid-sagittal plane [41] or the spinal intervertebral disks [27, 28] for automatic alignment of MRI slice stacks, detecting the bounding box of the left ventricle in 2D MRI images [57], and detecting standard cardiac planes in 3D echocardiographic data [34]. In all the above applications, we only want to estimate the position, orientation, and scale of the target anatomical structures. However, in many other applications, the goal is segmenting the target anatomical structure from the surrounding tissues. Detailed and accurate boundary delineation is required. In this scenario, after detecting the pose with MSL, we align a mean shape with respect to the estimated position, orientation, and scale. If applicable, a few nonrigid deformation parameters are also estimated using nonrigid MSL [53]. Such aligned mean shape provides an initial estimate of the true shape and will be further refined during the subsequent boundary evolution.

In this chapter, we discuss an automatic object detection and segmentation framework based on the MSL. Its training procedure is composed of the following steps:

1. Build an anatomically accurate mesh model to represent the boundary of the target anatomy. If the shape is simple, use a closed mesh to enclose the whole structure. If the shape is complex (e.g., the right ventricle that has separate inflow and outflow tracts), use a parts based model [56, 58, 59] (see Chap. 5).
2. Build an annotation tool and annotate enough number of training volumes, at least 50 datasets to start with for 3D problems.
3. Establish mesh point correspondence across volumes. For a few geometrically simple shapes (e.g., a tube, a parabola, and other rotation symmetric shapes), we will show two mesh resampling methods to establish mesh correspondence. For more complicated shapes, Minimum Description Length (MDL) based

Y. Zheng and D. Comaniciu, *Marginal Space Learning for Medical Image Analysis:*   159
Efficient Detection and Segmentation of Anatomical Structures,
DOI 10.1007/978-1-4939-0600-0_7, © Springer Science+Business Media New York 2014

approaches [11] can be used. Note that such optimization based approaches are often too computationally expensive to be practical.

4. Calculate the mean shape and the corresponding pose ground truth for the training samples [55] (see Chap. 6).
5. Calculate the constrained searching range and the testing hypothesis set for translation, rotation, and scale, respectively [53, 54] (see Chap. 4).
6. Build a statistical shape model using principal component analysis [9].
7. Train the MSL pose detectors using the image data and the corresponding pose ground truth of the target anatomical structure (see Chap. 2).
8. Train a machine learning based boundary detector.

The detection and segmentation process on unseen data is composed of the following major steps.

1. Use the MSL to generate the best pose candidates. If the object exhibits large shape variability, nonrigid MSL may also be exploited to estimate a few nonrigid deformation parameters (see Chap. 2).
2. Aggregate the best pose candidates into the final estimate. If it is a prior known that there is only one object instance in the data, a simple average of the top candidates provides a good estimate. If there may be multiple instances of the same object type in the data, clustering should be used to select the final detections [27, 28].
3. Align the mean shape with respect to the estimated pose to get an initial shape.
4. Adjust each mesh point along the mesh surface normal to the optimal position where the response of the boundary detector is the largest.
5. Enforce the prior shape constraint by projecting the adjusted mesh into a shape subspace.
6. Repeat steps 4 and 5 a few iterations to improve the segmentation accuracy.

The object detection and segmentation framework presented in this chapter integrate the components described in the previous chapters. We also present a few methods that are integral part of the segmentation framework, but only briefly mentioned in the previous chapters. For example, in Chap. 6, we presented an optimization based method to calculate the optimal mean shape from a training set. There, we assumed that the annotated meshes had intrinsic anatomical correspondence across volumes. The mesh resampling based methods presented in this chapter are exemplar techniques to establish mesh point correspondence, being simple and efficient. Another topic presented in this chapter covers the boundary delineation, built upon learning based boundary detectors and a statistical shape model.

We will use four-chamber heart segmentation in cardiac Computed Tomography (CT) data as an example to illustrate the segmentation framework. This was in fact one of the first applications of the MSL [51, 52]. Most of the technologies developed for heart chamber segmentation are generic, therefore can be directly applied or easily adapted to segment other anatomies in different imaging modalities. On the other hand, different applications may have different clinical requirements, demanding some adaptation. For example, in left ventricle endocardium segmentation, it is preferred to have a smooth mesh tightly enclosing the blood pool (i.e., including the papillary muscles and trabeculation in the endocardium mesh). We therefore developed a special mesh refinement process that improves the left ventricle endocardium segmentation accuracy to meet the clinical requirements.

The remainder of this chapter is organized as follows. In Sect. 7.2, we review the previous work on heart chamber modeling and segmentation. The four-chamber heart model is presented in Sect. 7.3. In this section, we also present two mesh resampling based methods to establish point correspondence and the statistical shape model to enforce shape constraint. The process of nonrigid deformation estimation for boundary delineation is described in details in Sect. 7.4. A special mesh refinement process is developed in Sect. 7.5 to search for an optimal smooth left ventricle endocardium mesh to tightly enclose the blood pool. Quantitative evaluation on a large dataset in Sect. 7.6 demonstrates the efficiency and accuracy of the MSL based heart chamber segmentation method. This chapter concludes with Sect. 7.7.

7.2 Related Work on Heart Modeling and Segmentation

This section provides a brief review of the previous work on heart modeling and segmentation.

7.2.1 Heart Modeling

Geometric heart modeling is not a trivial task since the heart is a complex nonrigid organ, with multiple moving parts. The model must be anatomically accurate, accept manual editing, and provide sufficient information to guide automatic detection and segmentation. Except for a four-chamber heart model from [14] and [31], most of the previous work was focused on the Left Ventricle (LV) and/or the Right Ventricle (RV). A closed mesh was often used to represent heart chambers [18, 24, 33]. Nevertheless, it is not clear how the atria interacted with the ventricles around the mitral and tricuspid valves in [33]. The heart model in [31] was more accurate in anatomy and it also included trunks of the major vessels connected to heart chambers. However, artificial patches were added at all valves to close the chamber meshes. These artificial patches were not processed with a special care in the segmentation algorithm; therefore, they could not be delineated accurately [14]. In our heart model, we keep the mesh open at a valve. Mesh points at the valve rim are labeled as control points, being treated differently to the normal mesh points during automatic segmentation.

The statistical shape model [9] is used in nonrigid object segmentation to enforce shape constraints and to make the system more robust. However, to build a statistical shape model, it is necessary to establish point correspondence among a group of shapes [9]. There are a few papers on building a 3D statistical shape model automatically using pair-wise or group-wise registration based approaches [16, 32], which are time consuming. Another approach is to establish correspondence among shapes through mesh resampling. Although this is difficult for a generic 3D shape, we can consistently resample the surface to establish correspondence for a few simple shapes (e.g., a tube and a parabola) [19, 24].

7.2.2   Heart Segmentation

Given the heart model, the segmentation task is to fit the model onto an unseen volume. Since the heart is a nonrigid shape, the model fitting (or heart segmentation) procedure can be divided into two steps: object localization and boundary delineation. Most of the previous approaches were focused on boundary delineation using Active Shape Models (ASM) [2], Active Appearance Models (AAM) [1, 37], or deformable models [3, 10, 14, 20, 36, 40]. The above segmentation technologies suffer from two limitations: (1) Most of them are semi-automatic and proper manual initialization is demanded. (2) Gradient descending based search in some of the approaches are likely to converge to a sub-optimal solution.

   Object localization, a task largely ignored by early work in heart segmentation, is required for an automatic segmentation system. The MSL computational framework for object detection and pose estimation thus fills an important gap in a 3D heart segmentation pipeline, by efficiently providing automatic detection of the heart parts, and estimating their 3D pose and initial mean shape.

7.3   Four-Chamber Heart Modeling

In this section, we describe our four-chamber heart model. As part of the model, some mesh points are special and correspond to distinctive anatomical structures, such as those around the valve annulus. We label these points as control points. They are integral part of the mesh model in the sense that they are also connected to other mesh points with mesh triangles.

7.3.1   Left Ventricle and Left Atrium Models

A closed mesh has been used to represent the Left Ventricle (LV) [18, 24, 33]. Due to the lack of object boundary on the image, it is hard to consistently delineate the interfaces among the LV main body, the Left Ventricular Outflow Tract (LVOT), and the basal area around the mitral valve. The mesh often cuts the LVOT and the

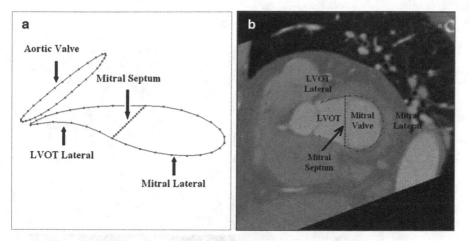

Fig. 7.1 Delineating the mitral and aortic valves. (**a**) A 3D view of the control points around the mitral and aortic valves. (**b**) Control points around the mitral valve embedded in a CT volume. Since the curves are 3D, they are only partially visible on a specific plane

mitral valve at an arbitrary position [18, 24, 33]. In our heart model, the mitral valve is explicitly represented as a closed contour along its border. Since we exclude the moving valve leaflets (which are hardly visible) from the model, the basal area can be delineated more consistently. Both the endo- and epi-cardiums are delineated for the LV. The commissure contour of both surfaces corresponds to the mitral valve annulus on one side and the aortic valve annulus (lying at the bottom edge of the Valsalva sinuses) on the other side, as shown in Fig. 7.2d. Three curves are formed by control points around the mitral valve, namely, the mitral lateral (16 points), the mitral septum (15 points), and the LVOT lateral (16 points). As shown in Fig. 7.1a, they define two closed regions, one for the interface between the LV and the Left Atrium (LA), and the other for the LV and the LVOT. The aortic valve (annotated with 32 points) is approximated as a plane, which cuts the valve at the bottom of the Valsalva sinuses. The LA is represented as an open mesh with an open area enclosed by the mitral septum and the mitral lateral control points (as shown in Fig. 7.1b). Figure 7.2 shows the LV/LA meshes with the control points (dots that are connected appropriately to form contours in the figure). The LV endocardium, epicardium, and LA meshes are represented with 545 points and 1,056 triangles each. The LVOT mesh is represented with 64 points and 64 triangles.

7.3.2   *Right Ventricle and Right Atrium Models*

The Right Ventricle (RV) has a complicated shape with separate inflow and outflow portions. Using a plane (indicated by a horizontal black line in Fig. 7.3a) passing the divergence point of the inflow and outflow tracts, we can naturally split the RV

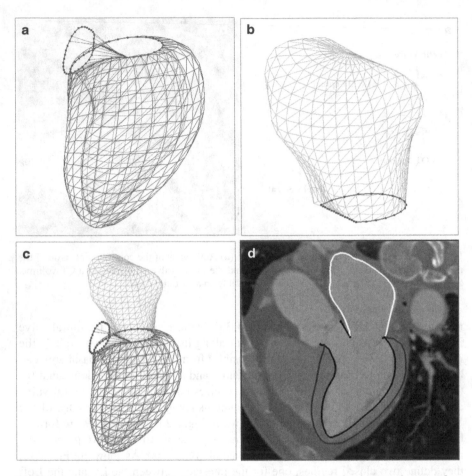

Fig. 7.2 Left Ventricle (LV) and Left Atrium (LA) meshes. The control points are shown as *dots* and connected appropriately to form contours. (**a**) LV mesh. The inner mesh is endocardium; the outer mesh is epicardium; and Left Ventricular Outflow Tract (LVOT) is a short region connecting the aortic valve and mitral valve. (**b**) LA mesh. (**c**) Combined mesh of the LV and LA. (**d**) LV/LA meshes embedded in a CT volume

into three parts with the RV main body lying below the cutting plane. We call this plane "the RV divergence plane." During the manual labeling of ground truth, the RV divergence plane is determined in the following way. We first determine the tricuspid valve, which is approximated as a plane. We then move the plane toward the RV apex to a position where the RV inflow and outflow tracts diverge. As shown in Fig. 7.3b, two curves, tricuspid lateral (23 points) and Right Ventricular Outflow Tract (RVOT) lateral (15 points), are annotated on the RV divergence plane to define the inflow and outflow connections. On a short axis view, the RV main body is a crescent (as shown in Fig. 7.3b and c). Two cusp points on the intersection are important landmarks, and an automatic detection algorithm is able to detect them

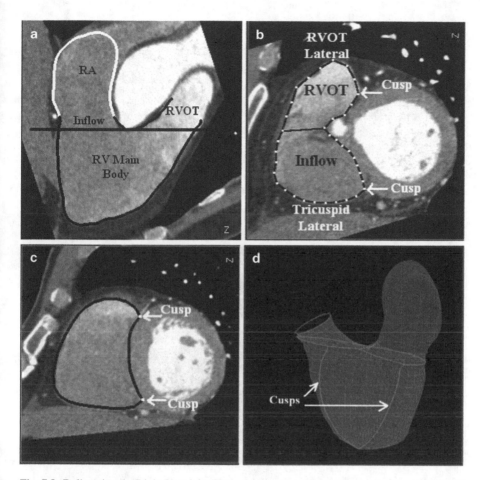

Fig. 7.3 Delineating the Right Ventricle (RV) control points. (**a**) The divergence plane (indicated by the *horizontal line*) of the RV inflow and outflow tracts splits the RV into three parts. (**b**) Delineating the divergence plane. (**c**) Inter-ventricular septum cusps labeled on a short-axis slice. (**d**) 3D visualization of the RV and Right Atrium (RA) meshes with inter-ventricular septum cusps indicated

reliably. They are explicitly represented in our model (Fig. 7.3d). The tricuspid (28 points) and pulmonary (18 points) valves are approximated as a plane. Similar to the LA, the Right Atrium (RA) is represented as an open mesh with the open area defined by the tricuspid valve. Figure 7.4 shows the RV/RA meshes with the control points (dots that are connected appropriately to form contours in the figure). In our model, the RV is represented with 761 points and 1,476 triangles and the RA is represented with 545 points and 1,056 triangles.

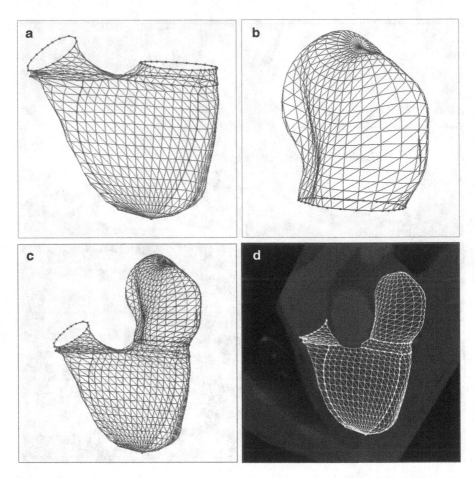

Fig. 7.4 Right Ventricle (RV) and Right Atrium (RA) meshes. The control points are shown as *dots* and connected appropriately to form contours. (**a**) RV mesh. (**b**) RA mesh (**c**) Combined mesh of the RV and RA. (**d**) 3D visualization of the RV/RA meshes embedded in a CT volume

7.3.3 Establishing Point Correspondence

After object pose estimation, we use the aligned mean shape as an initial estimate of the true shape. To calculate the mean shape, we demand the annotated training meshes to have intrinsic anatomical correspondence across volumes. Furthermore, we use the Active Shape Model (ASM) to enforce the shape constraint during boundary evolution. To build the statistical shape model of the ASM, we also need the point correspondence. Establishing mesh point correspondence is a difficult task for a generic 3D shape. Fortunately, for a few simple shapes, such as a tube or a parabola, we can consistently resample the surface to establish this correspondence. Since it is much easier to consistently resample a 2D curve, we use a few planes to

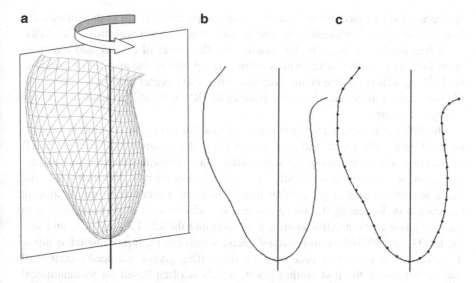

Fig. 7.5 The rotation-axis based resampling method demonstrated for the Left Ventricle (LV) endocardium mesh. (**a**) The LV endocardium mesh with its long axis. A cutting plane passing the long axis is also illustrated. (**b**) The intersection of the mesh with the cutting plane. (**c**) Resampled points indicated as *dots*. ©2008 IEEE. Reprinted, with permission, from Zheng, Y., Barbu, A., Georgescu, B., Scheuering, M., Comaniciu, D.: Four-chamber heart modeling and automatic segmentation for 3D cardiac CT volumes using marginal space learning and steerable features. *IEEE Trans. Medical Imaging* **27**(11), 1668–1681 (2008)

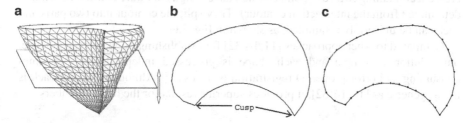

Fig. 7.6 The parallel-slice based resampling method for the Right Ventricle (RV) main body. (**a**) The RV main body mesh. A cutting plane perpendicular to the RV long axis is also illustrated. (**b**) The crescent-shaped intersection of the mesh with the cutting plane. Two cusps separate the intersection into two parts and each can be uniformly resampled independently. (**c**) Resampled points indicated as *dots*. ©2008 IEEE. Reprinted, with permission, from Zheng, Y., Barbu, A., Georgescu, B., Scheuering, M., Comaniciu, D.: Four-chamber heart modeling and automatic segmentation for 3D cardiac CT volumes using marginal space learning and steerable features. *IEEE Trans. Medical Imaging* **27**(11), 1668–1681 (2008)

cut the 3D mesh to get a set of 2D intersection curves. The resulting 2D curves are uniformly sampled to get a point set with built-in correspondence. Using different methods to select cutting planes, we develop two resampling schemes, the rotation-axis based method for simple parabola-like shapes such as the LV, LA, and RA, and parallel-slice based method for the more complicated RV. In both methods, the long axis of a chamber needs to be determined from the annotated mesh. Generally, we define the long axis as the line connecting the center of a valve and the mesh point farthest from the valve (which often corresponds to the apex). For example, the LV long axis is the line connecting the mitral valve center and the LV apex. The RV long axis is determined as a line passing the RV apex and perpendicular to the divergence plane.

The rotation-axis based method is appropriate for a roughly rotation symmetric shape. Cutting the mesh with a plane passing the rotation axis, we get a 2D intersection. As shown in Fig. 7.5b, the rotation axis separates the intersection into two parts, which can be uniformly resampled independently. We then rotate the plane around the axis to get another intersection and resample the intersection in the same way. Repeating the above process, we achieve a set of points with built-in correspondence. We use this approach to resample the LV, LA, and RA, and also the LVOT, and RV inflow and outflow tracts, which can be approximated as tubes. To establish the correspondence between the cutting planes, we need a consistent way to determine the first cutting plane, which is often based on an anatomical landmark. Different chambers may use different landmarks. For the LV, we pick the cutting plane passing the aortic valve center as the first cutting plane.

The rotation-axis based method is not applicable to the RV main body since it is not rotation symmetric. Instead, a parallel-slice based method is developed for the RV, where we use a plane perpendicular to the RV long axis to cut the 3D mesh, as shown in Fig. 7.6a. The shape of an RV short-axis intersection is a crescent containing two cusp points (which have a high curvature and can be reliably determined from the intersection contour). They split the contour into two parts and each can be uniformly resampled, as shown in Fig. 7.6c.

Compared to other approaches [11, 16, 32] for establishing point correspondence, our solution is simple and each shape is processed independently. No time-consuming and error-prone 3D registration is necessary. Although our approach is not as generic as [11, 16, 32], it provides superior results for the heart chambers.

7.3.4 Statistical Shape Model

The statistical shape model [9] (a.k.a., the point distribution model) is widely used in computer vision and medical image analysis to enforce prior shape constraint during the segmentation of a nonrigid object. The statistical shape model is learned from a set of training shapes, $M_1, M_2, \ldots, M_N$. Each shape M_i is composed of the same number of points J and can be represented as $M_i^j, j = 1, \ldots, J$. Point M_i^j is assumed to have correspondence across volumes. That means it represents the same anatomical position in different volumes. The point correspondence can be established by various methods, such as the mesh resampling techniques presented in the previous section.

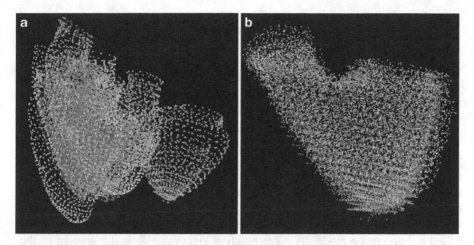

Fig. 7.7 Generalized Procrustes analysis of the right ventricle meshes (761 points). (a) Before alignment. (b) After alignment

Before performing shape analysis, the external transformations of the training shapes need to be compensated. That means we need to transform the shapes to the same coordinate system. This process, called Generalized Procrustes Analysis (GPA) [13], searches for a mean shape $\bar{\mathbf{m}}$ and an optimal transformation T_i^o for each individual shape $\mathbf{M}_i$ to minimize the sum of residual errors after alignment,

$$\bar{\mathbf{m}}, T_i^o = arg \min_{\mathbf{m}, T_i} \sum_{i=1}^{N} \|T_i(\mathbf{m}) - \mathbf{M}_i\|^2. \tag{7.1}$$

The similarity transformation is used as T in GPA and is often solved using an iterative approach. Please refer to Sect. 6.3.2 of Chap. 6 for an in-depth discussion on GPA. Figure 7.7 shows the RV shapes before and after the GPA.

Suppose after alignment a training shape $\mathbf{M}_i$ is transferred to $\mathbf{m}_i$. The mean shape $\bar{\mathbf{m}}$ over the whole training set after alignment is

$$\bar{\mathbf{m}} = \frac{1}{N} \sum_{i=1}^{N} \mathbf{m}_i. \tag{7.2}$$

The residual, $d\mathbf{m}_i$, of each shape to the mean shape is

$$d\mathbf{m}_i = \mathbf{m}_i - \bar{\mathbf{m}}. \tag{7.3}$$

The covariance matrix Φ, which is a $3J \times 3J$ symmetric matrix, of the aligned shapes is calculated as

$$\Phi = \frac{1}{N} \sum_{i=1}^{N} d\mathbf{m_i} d\mathbf{m_i}^T. \tag{7.4}$$

Using eigen-decomposition, the covariance matrix Φ can be decomposed as

$$\Phi = \mathbf{P}\Lambda\mathbf{P}^T$$
$$= [\mathbf{P}_1, \mathbf{P}_2, \ldots, \mathbf{P}_{3J}] diag(\lambda_1, \lambda_2, \ldots, \lambda_{3J}) [\mathbf{P}_1, \mathbf{P}_2, \ldots, \mathbf{P}_{3J}]^T, \tag{7.5}$$

where λ_i is an eigenvalue and $\mathbf{P}_i$ is the corresponding eigenvector. Since Φ is a real symmetric matrix that is semi-positive definite, all of its eigenvalues are non-negative real numbers. Without loss of generality, suppose the eigenvalues are ordered as $\lambda_1 \geq \lambda_2, \ldots, \geq \lambda_{3J} \geq 0$. In the statistical shape model, the linear space represented by $\mathbf{P}$ is often called the shape space and each axis of the space, $\mathbf{P}_i$, is called a deformation mode. Its corresponding eigenvalue λ_i is the amount of the variation of this deformation mode. The total variation λ_T is

$$\lambda_T = \sum_{i=1}^{3J} \lambda_i. \tag{7.6}$$

A shape in the training set can be presented as the mean shape plus a weighted sum of the deformation modes,

$$\mathbf{m} = \bar{\mathbf{m}} + \mathbf{Pw}, \tag{7.7}$$

where $\mathbf{w} = (w_1, w_2, \ldots, w_{3J})^T$ is a vector of weights. Since eigenvectors $\mathbf{P}_i$ are orthonormal to each other, the weight w_i can be easily calculated by the dot product of vectors $\mathbf{m}$ and $\mathbf{P}_i$,

$$w_i = \mathbf{m}.\mathbf{P}_i. \tag{7.8}$$

In general, a shape out of the training set cannot be represented exactly with Eq. (7.7). However, if the training set is large enough and can well represent the diversity of the whole shape population of the target object, the representation residual error is small.

In practice, we do not want to use the full shape space learned from a training set. The first t deformation modes explain most amount of the shape variation and the remaining modes mainly correspond to noise in the data. Therefore, a shape $\mathbf{m}$ is often approximated as

$$\tilde{\mathbf{m}} = \bar{\mathbf{m}} + \sum_{i=1}^{t} w_i \mathbf{P}_i. \tag{7.9}$$

This process is often called a *projection* into a shape subspace. The shape space is often truncated such that a certain amount α (e.g., $\alpha = 98\%$) of variation is preserved. Therefore, t is the minimum integer such that

$$\sum_{i=1}^{t} \lambda_i \geq \alpha \lambda_T. \tag{7.10}$$

By varying the weights w_i in Eq. (7.9), a new shape can be generated. To make the generated shape similar to those in the training set, we often enforce a limit to the weights,

$$-3\sqrt{\lambda_i} \leq w_i \leq 3\sqrt{\lambda_i}. \tag{7.11}$$

The covariance matrix Φ in Eq. (7.4) has a dimension of $3J \times 3J$. In most of our applications, a shape is represented as a dense mesh to achieve a detailed segmentation of the object. For example, our whole heart model is represented as 3,005 points. The corresponding covariance matrix has a dimension of 9,015 $\times$ 9,015, which consumes a lot of memory (310 MB if the values are represented as 4-byte 'double' variables) and eigen-decomposition of such a huge matrix can be quite slow. Fortunately, the rank of the covariance matrix Φ is bounded,

$$rank(\Phi) \leq \min\{3J - 1, N - 1\}. \tag{7.12}$$

In practice, the number of training shapes, N, is much smaller than the number of points in a shape, therefore $N << 3J$. For example, our heart chamber detectors are trained on no more than 500 volumes. That means most eigenvalues of Φ are zero. To enforce statistical shape constraint, the deformation modes with small (or zero) eigenvalues are discarded. It is not necessary to calculate those eigenvectors at all.

In the following, we present two efficient methods to calculate the eigenvectors $\mathbf{P}_i$ of Φ based on the fact that Φ has a low rank. We can write the residual vectors of aligned training shapes $d\mathbf{m}_i$ into a matrix,

$$\mathbf{D} = [d\mathbf{m}_1, d\mathbf{m}_2, \ldots, d\mathbf{m}_N]. \tag{7.13}$$

The dimension of matrix $\mathbf{D}$ is $3J \times N$. We then perform Singular Value Decomposition (SVD) of matrix $\mathbf{D}$ directly, without calculating the covariance matrix Φ at all. Suppose matrix $\mathbf{D}$ can be decomposed as

$$\mathbf{D} = \mathbf{U\Sigma V}^T, \tag{7.14}$$

where $\mathbf{U}$ is a $3J \times 3J$ matrix; Σ is a $3J \times N$ rectangular matrix with nonzero eigenvalues $\sigma_1, \sigma_2, \ldots, \sigma_N$ at the diagonal; and $\mathbf{V}$ is an $N \times N$ matrix. Here, $\mathbf{U}$ and $\mathbf{V}$ are orthonormal, $\mathbf{UU}^T = \mathbf{I}_{3J \times 3J}$ and $\mathbf{VV}^T = \mathbf{I}_{N \times N}$. Then, Φ can be represented as follows,

$$\Phi = \frac{1}{N}\mathbf{D}\mathbf{D}^T$$

$$= \frac{1}{N}\mathbf{U}\Sigma\mathbf{V}^T\mathbf{V}\Sigma^T\mathbf{U}^T$$

$$= \frac{1}{N}\mathbf{U}\Sigma\Sigma^T\mathbf{U}^T$$

$$= \mathbf{U}diag\left(\frac{\sigma_1^2}{N},\ldots,\frac{\sigma_N^2}{N},0,\ldots,0\right)\mathbf{U}^T. \qquad (7.15)$$

The above equation is an eigen-decomposition of Φ. The largest N eigenvalues λ_i of Φ is related to the eigenvalues σ_i of $\mathbf{D}$ as

$$\lambda_i = \frac{\sigma_i^2}{N}. \qquad (7.16)$$

The remaining eigenvalues are zero. Eigenvector $\mathbf{P}_i$ of Φ is a left-eigenvector of $\mathbf{D}$, $\mathbf{P}_i = \mathbf{U}_i$. The SVD of $\mathbf{D}$ is much faster than eigen-decomposition of Φ since matrix $\mathbf{D}$ has a lower dimension.

Alternatively, we can calculate another covariance matrix Ψ as

$$\Psi = \frac{1}{N}\mathbf{D}^T\mathbf{D}. \qquad (7.17)$$

The dimension of matrix Ψ is $N \times N$, which is much smaller than that of Φ. Suppose the eigen-decomposition of Ψ is

$$\Psi = \mathbf{Q}\mathbf{S}\mathbf{Q}^T$$

$$= [\mathbf{Q}_1,\mathbf{Q}_2,\ldots,\mathbf{Q}_N]diag(s_1,s_2,\ldots,s_N)[\mathbf{Q}_1,\mathbf{Q}_2,\ldots,\mathbf{Q}_N]^T. \qquad (7.18)$$

That means

$$\Psi\mathbf{Q}_i = s_i\mathbf{Q}_i. \qquad (7.19)$$

Left multiply both sides of the equation with $\mathbf{D}$, we get

$$\mathbf{D}\Psi\mathbf{Q}_i = s_i\mathbf{D}\mathbf{Q}_i$$

$$\mathbf{D}\frac{1}{N}\mathbf{D}^T\mathbf{D}\mathbf{Q}_i = s_i\mathbf{D}\mathbf{Q}_i$$

$$\Phi\mathbf{D}\mathbf{Q}_i = s_i\mathbf{D}\mathbf{Q}_i. \qquad (7.20)$$

That means Ψ has the same eigenvalues as Φ, ($s_i = \lambda_i$); and for an eigenvector $\mathbf{Q}_i$ of Φ, if we left multiple it with $\mathbf{D}$, it is an eigenvector of Φ, ($\mathbf{P}_i = \mathbf{D}\mathbf{Q}_i$).

Both alternative methods presented here are much more efficient to calculate the eigenvalues and eigenvectors of Φ than working directly on Φ. Among all three methods, the one based on the eigen-decomposition of the covariance matrix Ψ is the most efficient in our applications since Ψ has the smallest dimension of $N \times N$ when $N < 3J$.

7.4 Nonrigid Deformation Estimation for Heart Chambers

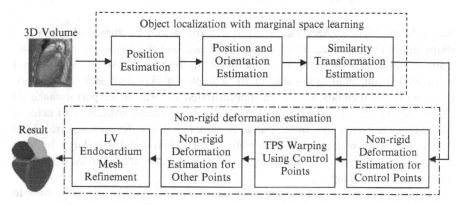

Fig. 7.8 Diagram for 3D heart chamber detection and segmentation. ©2008 IEEE. Reprinted, with permission, from Zheng, Y., Barbu, A., Georgescu, B., Scheuering, M., Comaniciu, D.: Four-chamber heart modeling and automatic segmentation for 3D cardiac CT volumes using marginal space learning and steerable features. *IEEE Trans. Medical Imaging* **27**(11), 1668–1681 (2008)

In this section, we present the MSL based heart chamber detection and segmentation method. The system diagram is shown in Fig. 7.8. We first automatically estimate the pose of heart chambers using the MSL and the mean shape is aligned with respect to the estimated pose to get an initial shape. The initial shape is further deformed to fit the object boundary under the guidance of a learning based boundary detector and a statistical shape model. Since the MSL based object pose estimation has been discussed in detail in the previous chapters, in the following we will skip this step. Instead, we focus this section on nonrigid deformation estimation.

The control points in our heart model represent specific image characteristics and should be specially treated. As shown in [14], without special processing, the connection of different chambers around the mitral or tricuspid valve cannot be delineated well. The boundary delineation process is composed of four steps (as shown in Fig. 7.8). We first estimate the deformation of control points. The Thin-Plate Spline (TPS) model [6] is then used to warp the initial mesh toward the refined control points for better alignment. The normal mesh points are further deformed to fit the image boundary. Note that, at this step, the control points are kept unchanged. Last, the LV endocardium mesh is refined to tightly enclose the blood pool.

In the following, we first present the learning based boundary detector and the thin-plate spline model, followed by a more detailed description of the heart chamber boundary delineation process. The first three steps of boundary delineation are generic and can be applied to almost all 3D object segmentation problems. The last step is special for LV endocardium segmentation and will be presented in Sect. 7.5.

7.4.1   Learning Based Boundary Detector

Active Shape Models (ASM) are used to deform an initial estimate of a nonrigid shape under the guidance of the image evidence and the shape prior. The non-learning based generic boundary detector in the original ASM [9, 19] does not work well in our application due to the complex background and weak edges. Learning based methods have been demonstrated to have better performance on 2D images [12, 21, 35] since they can exploit more image evidences to achieve robust boundary detection. In the previous work [12, 35], a detector was trained to detect a boundary with a specific orientation (e.g., a horizontal boundary). In order to detect boundaries with different orientations, detection needed to be performed on a set of rotated images.

In this work, we extend the learning based methods to 3D and show how to avoid the time-consuming volume rotation using our efficient steerable features. Here, boundary detection is formulated as a classification problem: whether there is a boundary passing point (X, Y, Z) with orientation (O_x, O_y, O_z). This problem is similar to the classification problem we solve for position-orientation estimation in MSL: whether there is an object centered at (X, Y, Z) with orientation (ψ, ϕ, θ). Similarly, the boundary detector is trained using the Probabilistic Boosting-Tree (PBT) [45] and steerable features.

It is sufficient to represent the orientation of a boundary point using the normal of boundary surface (n_x, n_y, n_z). To determine the sampling points of steerable features, we need to define a local coordinate system with three orthogonal axes. We take the boundary normal as the $\mathbf{z}'$ axis of the local coordinate system, $\mathbf{z}' = (n_x, n_y, n_z)$. We then need to pick an axis inside a plane perpendicular to the $\mathbf{z}'$ axis as the $\mathbf{x}'$ axis. This can be accomplished by randomly picking a vector $\mathbf{v}$ and calculate its cross product with $\mathbf{z}'$,

$$\mathbf{x}' = \frac{\mathbf{v} \times \mathbf{z}'}{\|\mathbf{v} \times \mathbf{z}'\|}. \tag{7.21}$$

Normalization is performed to make the $\mathbf{x}'$ axis a unit vector. The $\mathbf{y}'$ axis is then determined as the cross product of the $\mathbf{z}'$ and $\mathbf{x}'$ axes, $\mathbf{y}' = \mathbf{z}' \times \mathbf{x}'$. The initially picked vector $\mathbf{v}$ should not be parallel to the $\mathbf{z}'$ axis; otherwise, its cross product with $\mathbf{z}'$ is ill-defined. To increase the stability of the arithmetic calculation, we also want to avoid picking a vector close to parallel to the $\mathbf{z}'$ axis. To accomplish this, we start from three axes $\mathbf{x} = (1,0,0)$, $\mathbf{y} = (0,1,0)$, and $\mathbf{z} = (0,0,1)$ of the world coordinate system and then select the one most perpendicular to the $\mathbf{z}'$ axis (whose dot product with the $\mathbf{z}'$ axis has the smallest absolute value) as $\mathbf{v}$,

$$\mathbf{v} = arg \min_{\mathbf{u} \in \{\mathbf{x}, \mathbf{y}, \mathbf{z}\}} |\mathbf{u}.\mathbf{z}'|. \tag{7.22}$$

With the local coordinate system fully defined, we can determine the sampling points and extract steerable features from the sampling points.

Another difference to position-orientation estimation in MSL is that we do not search for the orientation in the boundary detection problem. In position-orientation estimation, all possible orientation hypotheses are determined from the training set using an example-based sampling strategy. For each position candidate obtained after position estimation, we search for all possible orientation hypotheses. This increases the calculation time. In boundary delineation, we start from an initial shape using the aligned mean shape. For each mesh point, we search along the mesh surface normal in a certain range (e.g., ± 12 mm). The mesh surface normal is used to test all candidate positions of that mesh point. We assume the initial shape is close to the true shape; therefore, the initial estimate of the boundary surface normal is also close to the true normal. Since the initial shape is quite accurate, this simplification does not introduce noticeable degradation in segmentation accuracy, especially since the boundary delineation process is iterated a few times.

The positive and negative samples are generated from the annotated mesh to train the boundary detector. Suppose $\mathbf{p} = (p_x, p_y, p_z)$ is a mesh point and the mesh normal at point $\mathbf{p}$ is $\mathbf{n}^{\mathbf{p}} = (n_x^p, n_y^p, n_z^p)$. A positive training sample is generated as $(p_x, p_y, p_z, n_x^p, n_y^p, n_z^p)$. For most of our applications, the search ranges inside and outside of the mesh are both set to 12 mm. Intuitively, any point $\mathbf{q}$ inside the search range that is different to $\mathbf{p}$ can be taken as a negative training sample. However, to avoid confusing the classifier, a negative training sample is required to be with a certain distance away from the true boundary. Here, we set the distance threshold to 5 mm. Therefore, the negative samples are generated in the range [5, 12] mm (outside of the mesh) or [−12, −5] mm (inside of the mesh), as shown in Fig. 7.9.

7.4.2 TPS Deformation Model

The Thin-Plate Spline (TPS) model is often used for representing flexible coordinate transformations because it has a physical explanation and closed-form solutions in both transformation and parameter estimation [6]. It is widely used for nonrigid shape matching [4,7]. Three TPS deformation fields are used for the 3-D coordinate transformation. Suppose point (x_i, y_i, z_i) is matched to (u_i, v_i, w_i) for $i = 1, 2, \cdots, n$. Here, points (x_i, y_i, z_i) and (u_i, v_i, w_i) are often called anchor points. Let $f_i = f(x_i, y_i, z_i)$ be the target function value at location (x_i, y_i, z_i). We set f_i equal to u_i, v_i, and w_i in turn to obtain one continuous transformation for each coordinate.

Fig. 7.9 Generating positive and negative samples to train the boundary detector. Positive samples are composed of true boundary points. Negative samples are generated inside a searching range (R2) after excluding the region (R1) too close to the true boundary

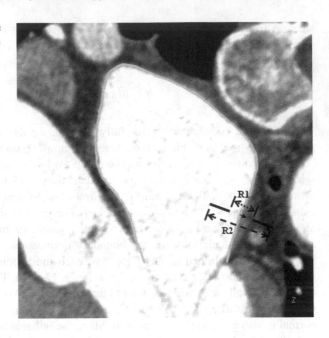

The TPS interpolant $f(x,y,z)$ minimizes the bending energy of a thin plate

$$I_f = \int\int\int_{\mathscr{R}^3} \left(\frac{\partial^2 f}{\partial x^2}\right)^2 + \left(\frac{\partial^2 f}{\partial y^2}\right)^2 + \left(\frac{\partial^2 f}{\partial z^2}\right)^2 + 2\left(\frac{\partial^2 f}{\partial x\partial y}\right)^2 + 2\left(\frac{\partial^2 f}{\partial x\partial z}\right)^2 + 2\left(\frac{\partial^2 f}{\partial y\partial z}\right)^2 dxdydz \tag{7.23}$$

and has the solution of the form

$$f(x,y,z) = a_0 + a_x x + a_y y + a_z z + \sum_{i=1}^{n} w_i r_i, \tag{7.24}$$

where $r_i = -\sqrt{(x-x_i)^2 + (y-y_i)^2 + (z-z_i)^2}$ is the kernel function. The parameters of the TPS models $\mathbf{w} = (w_1, w_2, \ldots, w_n)^T$ and $\mathbf{a} = (a_0, a_x, a_y, a_z)^T$ are the solution of the following linear equation

$$\begin{bmatrix} \mathbf{K} & \mathbf{P} \\ \mathbf{P}^T & \mathbf{0} \end{bmatrix} \begin{bmatrix} \mathbf{w} \\ \mathbf{a} \end{bmatrix} = \begin{bmatrix} \mathbf{f} \\ \mathbf{0} \end{bmatrix} \tag{7.25}$$

where $\mathbf{K}_{ij} = -\sqrt{(x_i-x_j)^2 + (y_i-y_j)^2 + (z_i-z_j)^2}$; the ith row of $\mathbf{P}$ is $(1, x_i, y_i, z_i)$; and $\mathbf{f}$ is a column vector formed by f_i.

Using the above TPS deformation field, an anchor point (x_i, y_i, z_i) is transformed exactly to a target point (u_i, v_i, w_i). If errors are expected in the matching results, we can use regularization to get a trade-off between exact interpolation and minimizing the bending energy as follows

$$H_f = \sum_{i=1}^{n} [f_i - f(x_i, y_i, z_i)]^2 + \lambda I_f, \qquad (7.26)$$

where λ is the regularization parameter, controlling the amount of smoothing. The regularized TPS can be solved by replacing $\mathbf{K}$ in Eq. (7.25) with $\mathbf{K} + \lambda \mathbf{I}$, where $\mathbf{I}$ is an $n \times n$ identity matrix [22, 46]. For our applications, the control points are used as anchor points (x_i, y_i, z_i) to estimate a deformation field, which is then used to transform normal mesh points. We set λ to zero since we want to have exact warping of the control points.

7.4.3   Boundary Delineation

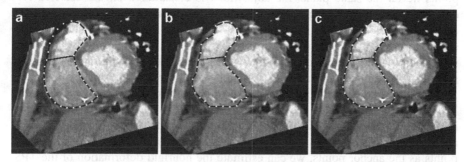

Fig. 7.10 Nonrigid deformation estimation for control points (the tricuspid lateral and the right ventricular outflow tract lateral) on the RV divergence plane. (**a**) Detected mean shape. (**b**) After boundary adjustment. (**c**) Final result by projecting the adjusted shape onto a shape subspace with 25 dimensions

As stated before, the control points in our mesh representation correspond to specific image characteristics and should be specially treated. As shown in [14], it is difficult to represent the connection of different chambers around the mitral or tricuspid valve without special processing. Our boundary delineation process starts from the detection of control points. Each group of control points has its own boundary detector and a statistical shape model. In the following we illustrate the refinement of the control points on the RV divergence plane. All other control points are refined in a similar way.

First, all control points on the RV divergence plane are extracted from the initial RV mesh. The initial pose (position, orientation, and scale) of the object composed of these control points is determined. The MSL is then used to refine the pose estimate, e.g., moving the RV divergence plane a bit higher or lower, tilting it slightly, and stretching/compressing the contour formed by control points. After that, we get an aligned mean shape for the control points. Figure 7.10a shows the aligned mean shape under the estimated pose. The boundary detectors are then used to move each control point along the normal direction to the optimal position,

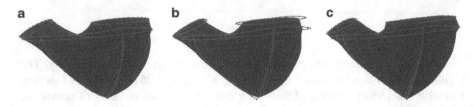

Fig. 7.11 Right Ventricle (RV) mesh warping using control points (which are connected appropriately to form contours). (**a**) Mean shape using the estimated RV pose. (**b**) After control point refinement, the mesh is not consistent. (**c**) Warped mesh, where the control points and the mesh are consistent again

where the score from the boundary detector is the highest. Since all these control points lie on the same plane, the adjustment is constrained on the detected RV divergence plane. After adjustment, the control points fit the boundary well, but the contour is not smooth (Fig. 7.10b). Finally, we project the deformed shape onto a shape subspace [9]. In all our experiments, to determine the dimension of the shape subspace, we demand it to capture 98 % of variations. As shown in Fig. 7.10c, the statistical shape model is very effective to enforce the prior shape constraint.

The refined control points can be used to warp a mesh and make it fit the image better. Figure 7.11a shows the mean shape aligned with the detected RV pose. Figure 7.11b shows the refinement of the control points, which fit the data more accurately, but inconsistent with the mesh. Using the original and refined control points as the anchor points, we can estimate the nonrigid deformation of the TPS model and use it to warp the mesh points. As shown in Fig. 7.11c, the mesh points and the control points are consistent again after warping.

To estimate the 3D deformation field accurately, the TPS anchor points are required to distribute over the whole mesh. This is the case for the RV, but not for the other three chambers. Since the control points are clustered around the aortic and mitral valves for the LV, if we use only the valve control points as TPS anchor points, the estimated deformation field around the LV apex may exhibit a large distortion. To fix this issue, we add the point farthest from the mitral valve (which is the LV apex) as an additional anchor point in the TPS model to warp the LV. A similar treatment is applied to warp both atria.

Due to the large variation introduced by cardiac motion, each chamber is processed separately since the variation of a chamber is smaller than that of a whole heart. However, after chamber pose estimation, the initial mesh of atria and ventricles have conflict around the mitral and tricuspid valves. Using the control points around the valves as anchor points in TPS warping, we can resolve such mesh conflict. After the whole segmentation procedure, further mesh conflict can be resolved through a post-processing step.

After TPS warping, the mesh points are closer to the chamber boundary. To further reduce the error, we train a boundary detector for each mesh surface. The boundary detectors are then used to adjust each point (the control points are kept

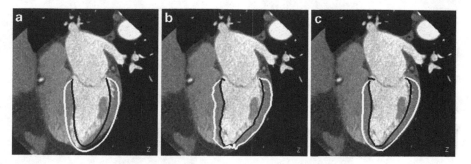

Fig. 7.12 Nonrigid deformation estimation for the Left Ventricle (LV) with black for the endo-cardium and white for the epicardium. (**a**) Mean shape. (**b**) After boundary adjustment. (**c**) Final delineation by projecting the adjusted shape onto a shape subspace with 50 dimensions

unchanged in this step). Figure 7.12a shows the aligned LV in a cardiac CT volume. Figure 7.12b shows the adjusted shape. Shape constraint is enforced by projecting the adjusted shape onto a shape subspace to get the final result, as shown in Fig. 7.12c. The above steps can be iterated a few times. Based on the trade-off between speed and accuracy, we use one iteration for the LV/LA, and two iterations for the RV/RA since the right side of the heart has typically much lower contrast and more iterations are required to get an accurate segmentation result.

7.5 Optimal Smooth Surface for Left Ventricle Endocardium Segmentation

7.5.1 Clinical Requirements

The segmentation method presented in the last section works well on an object with smooth boundary. However, the LV endocardium surface is not smooth due to the presence of trabeculation and papillary muscles. Different clinical applications may require to delineate the LV endocardium surface differently. For example, there are various preferences among cardiologists on whether to include or exclude the papillary muscles and trabeculation in measuring the LV volume. Therefore, there are two ways to delineate the LV endocardium surface. One approach is to delineate the detailed boundary between the LV blood pool and myocardium, as shown in Fig. 7.13a. The other approach is to use a smooth mesh to tightly enclose the whole blood pool (indicated by the black contour in Fig. 7.13c), including the papillary muscles and trabeculation. A smooth surface segmentation of the LV endocardium is required for LV myocardium wall motion analysis, e.g., measuring wall thickness, myocardium stress, and motion dyssynchrony. In this section, we present a method based on an optimal smooth surface to generate accurate segmentation tightly

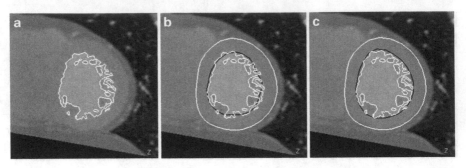

Fig. 7.13 Illustration of left ventricle endocardium segmentation by using a smooth mesh to tightly enclose the whole blood pool. (**a**) Original data with blood pool labeled (the region enclosed by the contour). (**b**) Segmentation result using a learning based boundary detector and a statistical shape model. Here, the segmented endocardium is shown as a black contour and the epicardium is shown as a smooth white contour. (**c**) After further refinement using an optimal smooth surface

enclosing the whole LV blood pool. If the separation between the blood pool and myocardium is required, we can then perform thresholding for all voxels enclosed in the smooth surface to make further distinction. Therefore, our approach can generate two different segmentations of the LV endocardium.

In the ASM based segmentation method, the mesh smoothness is enforced by projecting the mesh onto a subspace of the statistical shape model defined by a set of training shapes based on Principal Component Analysis (PCA) [9]. The segmentation result is quite good and robust even for volumes with low contrast and severe streak artifacts. However, for volumes with high contrast, a small error in boundary delineation can be easily observed. Therefore, the accuracy requirement for these volumes is much higher than those with low contrast, where we cannot clearly see the boundary. Figure 7.13b shows such an example where the segmented LV endocardium may traverse blood pool, instead of enclosing whole blood pool. Although the errors are quite small, they are clearly visible.

Here, we present an optimization based approach to searching for an optimal smooth surface that tightly encloses the whole blood pool. Given the initial segmentation results for both LV endocardium and epicardium, we extract the blood pool using histogram-based optimal adaptive thresholding (as shown in Fig. 7.13a), which minimizes the tissue classification error for blood pool and myocardium. We project the endocardium mesh onto the extracted blood pool, resulting in a zigzagged shape that tightly encloses the whole blood pool. The endocardium mesh is further adjusted to maximize an explicit mesh smoothness measurement under the constraint that the mesh should tightly enclose the whole blood pool, as shown in Fig. 7.13c. We prove that our objective function is a strictly convex quadratic function with a unique global optimal solution. Therefore, a set of efficient methods [23, 38] are readily available in the literature to solve the optimization problem.

7.5.2   Left Ventricle Blood Pool Extraction

Voxel intensity thresholding is commonly used in the previous work [17, 25] to extract blood pool since normally blood pool has a higher intensity than papillary muscles and myocardium. However, a preset threshold does not work well due to variations in the use of contrast agents. An optimal threshold should be tuned for each volume. Here, we present an automatic scheme to determine the optimal threshold based on the initial segmentation of LV endocardium and epicardium using the approach discussed in Sect. 7.4. We calculate two histograms of the voxel intensity, one for all voxels enclosed by the endocardium surface (most of them from blood pool with a few from papillary muscles) and the other for all voxels enclosed between endocardium and epicardium surfaces, denoting the myocardium. As shown in Fig. 7.14a, for volumes with high contrast, these histograms are well separated with slight overlapping in the middle. The optimal threshold (which is 212 HU for this volume) can be quickly searched for to minimize the overall voxel classification error. We do observe that histograms of the blood pool and myocardium may have large overlap for volumes with low contrast and the extracted blood pool may contain some errors (see Fig. 7.14b). Therefore, if the tissue classification error is larger than a threshold, we stick with the initial learning based segmentation without applying any further refinement.

After getting the optimal threshold, we can easily classify those voxels enclosed by the endocardium surface as blood pool or papillary muscles. One issue is that the automatic segmentation algorithm is not perfect around the boundary: a portion of blood pool may be segmented as myocardium and vice versa. We can correct such minor segmentation errors by expanding the endocardium mesh a little bit (e.g., 5 mm) before voxel intensity thresholding. After thresholding, connected component analysis is performed for voxels with intensity larger than the threshold. Only the largest component is preserved as blood pool and small isolated pieces are discarded. Figure 7.15 shows the region of the extracted blood pool overlaid with the original segmentation results of LV endocardium and epicardium. We can see that small segmentation errors are corrected. After that, we project the LV endocardium mesh onto the extracted blood pool as follows. At each mesh point, a line along the mesh surface normal is determined and it may intersect the blood pool boundary multiple times. The mesh point is adjusted to the outer-most intersection; therefore, the resulted mesh tightly encloses the whole blood pool. However, the mesh after adjustment is not smooth. In the next section, we present an optimization based approach to searching for an optimal mesh satisfying both the smoothness and tightness constraints.

As a by-product of blood pool extraction, we can easily calculate LV volumes for both including and excluding papillary muscles. For the former, we just need to calculate the volume enclosed by LV endocardium surface. For the latter, we count the number of voxels of the extracted blood pool and convert it to a volume measurement since we know the CT scanning resolutions.

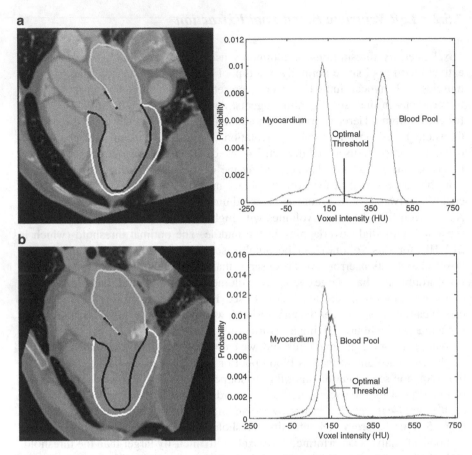

Fig. 7.14 Voxel intensity histograms of blood pool and myocardium for (**a**) a volume with sufficient contrast in the blood pool and (**b**) a volume with low contrast. The *left column* shows the image data and the *right column* shows the corresponding histograms together with the optimal threshold to distinguish blood pool and myocardium. ©2009 SPIE. Reprinted, with permission, from Zheng, Y., Lu, X., Georgescu, B., Littmann, A., Mueller, E., Comaniciu, D.: Automatic left ventricle detection in MRI images using marginal space learning and component-based voting. In: *Proc. of SPIE Medical Imaging*, vol. 7259, pp. 1–12 (2009)

7.5.3   Optimization Based Surface Smoothing

The smoothness of a surface, S, is often measured by the sum of squares of derivative as

$$SM(S) = \int \|\nabla \mathbf{S}\|^2 ds. \tag{7.27}$$

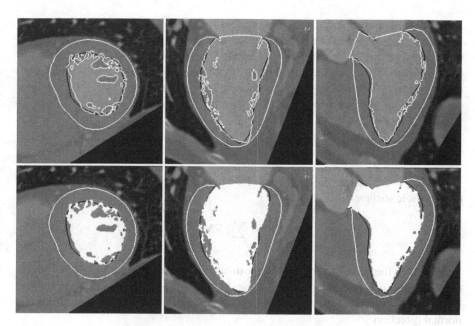

Fig. 7.15 An example of Left Ventricle (LV) blood pool extraction. The extracted blood pool is overlaid with the initial segmentation of LV endocardium and epicardium. Three orthogonal views from the same volume are shown in each row. The *top row* visualizes the blood pool as an unfilled region and the *bottom row* visualizes the same blood pool as a filled region

A smaller *SM* represents a smoother surface. In practice, a discrete surface (e.g., a polyhedral surface) is often used to represent the boundary of a 3D object. We represent a polyhedral surface as a graph $\mathbf{S} = \{\mathbf{V}, \mathbf{F}\}$, where $\mathbf{V}$ is an array of vertices and $\mathbf{F}$ is an array of faces. Triangulated surfaces are the most common representation, where all faces are triangles. For each vertex $\mathbf{V}_i$ on the surface, we can define a neighborhood $\mathcal{N}_i$. Normally, a first order neighborhood is used, meaning that vertex j is a neighbor of vertex i if they are on the same face. The smoothness around a vertex is often defined as [43, 44]

$$\nabla \mathbf{V}_i = \sum_{j \in \mathcal{N}_i} w_{ij}(\mathbf{V}_j - \mathbf{V}_i), \tag{7.28}$$

where the weights w_{ij} are positive numbers that add up to one for each vertex

$$\sum_{j \in \mathcal{N}_i} w_{ij} = 1. \tag{7.29}$$

Therefore, Eq. (7.28) can be written as

$$\nabla \mathbf{V}_i = \mathbf{V}_i - \sum_{j \in \mathcal{N}_i} w_{ij} \mathbf{V}_j, \tag{7.30}$$

In this form, the meaning of this smoothness measurement is clear. A vertex on a smooth surface (a plane) can be represented as a weighted average of its neighbors, therefore with zero ∇V_i. On the other hand, a vertex at the tip of a bump cannot be represented by a weighted average of its neighbors if the weights are required to be positive. The weights can be chosen in many different ways taking into consideration of the neighborhoods. The simplest way is to set w_{ij} to be uniform

$$w_{ij} = \frac{1}{\#\mathcal{N}_i},$$ (7.31)

where $\#\mathcal{N}_i$ is the number of neighbors of vertex i. Given Eq. (7.28), the smoothness of the whole surface is

$$SM(\mathbf{S}) = \sum_i \|\nabla \mathbf{V}_i\|^2.$$ (7.32)

We adjust the mesh to generate a smooth surface by minimizing Eq. (7.32). Since there is too much freedom to adjust a mesh, similar to the well accepted practice in the active contours [26] and ASM [9], we only allow the adjustment along the normal direction

$$\mathbf{V}_i' = \mathbf{V}_i + \delta_i \mathbf{N}_i,$$ (7.33)

where δ_i is a scalar and $\mathbf{N}_i$ is the surface normal at vertex i. We can further limit the adjustment of each vertex by enforcing the following constraints,

$$l_i \leq \delta_i \leq u_i,$$ (7.34)

where l_i and u_i are the lower and upper bound of the adjustment for vertex i. For example, in the following application on left ventricle endocardium segmentation, we enforce $\delta_i \geq 0$ to guarantee that the mesh encloses the whole blood pool. Note that the surface normal is pointing outside of the mesh.

We also want to get a trade-off between smoothness and the amount of adjustment (which affects the tightness of the enclosure). Our final optimization problem is

$$\min F = \sum_i \left\| \sum_{j \in \mathcal{N}_i} w_{ij}(\mathbf{V}_j' - \mathbf{V}_i') \right\|^2 + \alpha \sum_i \delta_i^2,$$ (7.35)

subject to the bound constraint of Eq. (7.34). Here, $\alpha \geq 0$ is a scalar for the above trade-off.

It turns out that our optimization problem is a classical quadratic programming problem. In the following we will prove that the objective function defined in Eq. (7.35) is a strictly convex function for $\alpha > 0$. Therefore, it has a unique global optimal solution.

Theorem 7.1. *For $\alpha \geq 0$, the objective function defined in (7.35) is a convex function. If $\alpha > 0$, it is a strictly convex function.*

Proof. The second term of the objective function, $\sum \delta_i^2$, is a strictly convex function. We only need to prove the first term, F_1, is convex. Substituting (7.33) into (7.35) and after re-organizing, we can get

$$F_1 = \delta^T Q \delta + c^T \delta + c_0, \tag{7.36}$$

where δ is a vector formed by δ_i; Q is a symmetric square matrix; c is a vector; and c_0 is a constant. To prove F_1 is a convex function, we only need to prove all eigenvalues of matrix Q is nonnegative. Q can be represented as

$$Q = W^T \Lambda W, \tag{7.37}$$

where W is a matrix with each column corresponding to an eigenvector of Q and Λ is a diagonal matrix composed of the eigenvalues of Q. Therefore,

$$F_1 = \delta^T W^T \Lambda W \delta + c^T \delta + c_0, \tag{7.38}$$

Suppose Q has a negative eigenvalue, without loss of generality, suppose the first eigenvalue, λ_1, of Q is less than zero. Let $e_1 = [1, 0, \ldots, 0]$ be a vector with the first element being 1 and all the other elements being 0. Let $\delta = bW^{-1}e_1$. Here, b is a scalar. Substituting δ into F_1, we get

$$F_1 = \lambda_1 b^2 + c^T W^{-1} e_1 b + c_0. \tag{7.39}$$

F_1 is a quadratic function of b and its value is dominated by the first term $\lambda_1 b^2$. Since $\lambda_1 < 0$, we get $F_1 < 0$ for a sufficient large b. From Eq. (7.35), we know F_1 is a sum of squares and always no less than zero. Therefore, matrix Q has no negative eigenvalue. It is well-known that all eigenvalues of a real symmetric matrix are real. Therefore, all eigenvalues of Q are real and nonnegative. Therefore, F_1 is a convex function. This completes the proof. $\square$

For a strictly convex quadratic programming problem, there is a unique global optimal solution and many algorithms have been proposed in the literature to search for the optimal solution [23]. With a bound constraint as in our case, a more efficient and specialized method is available [38]. The optimization process takes less than 0.2 s in our case for a mesh with 545 points.

7.5.4 Comparison with Previous Work

There are a few mesh smoothing techniques proposed in the literature. The Laplacian smoothing method is an iterative approach where, in each iteration, a vertex is updated with a weighted average of itself and its neighbors [43]. Laplacian smoothing acts as a low pass filter, therefore it suffers from the shrinkage problem: when the smoothing method is applied iteratively a large number of times, a shape eventually collapses to a point. Another issue with the mesh smoothing methods is that the resulting mesh cannot be guaranteed to tightly enclose the whole blood pool (which is a hard constraint from the clinical requirements).

In practice, smooth segmentation can also be enforced by projecting a shape into a shape subspace [9], which also incorporates prior shape constraint. However, similar to the mesh smoothing methods, the resulting mesh cannot guarantee to be tight. Instead, the mesh may transverse the LV blood pool, as shown in Fig. 7.13b. Another limitation is that the shape space cannot cover all shape variations encountered in real applications especially when the training set is not large enough.

The active balloon model is a variation of active contours, where an outward force is applied to each point to inflate the evolving contour [8]. If all forces and parameters are properly set, it may result in a smooth mesh enclosing the blood pool. However, our approach has several advantages over the active balloon model. First, it guarantees to achieve the global optimum. By contrary, the active balloon model only converges to a local optimum. Second, there are many free parameters in the active balloon, especially the balloon force, which is hard to tune. For comparison, there is only one regularization parameter α in our approach. Last, the final surface achieved by the active balloon model generally cannot tightly enclose the blood pool.

Recently, Li et al. [29] proposed a graph-cut based approach to searching for an optimal surface. Similar to ours, they also search for an optimal adjustment along the surface normal for each point. However, the adjustment in their approach is restricted to discretized positions. Instead, we use continuous optimization and can achieve finer adjustments. Another major drawback of their approach is that their objective function lacks an explicit smoothness measurement. Smoothness is enforced as hard constraints: the difference in the adjustments of neighboring points should be less than a threshold, which is an application dependent parameter. Therefore, their method is limited to handling terrain-like (height-field) and cylindrical surfaces. For a rough object (e.g., LV endocardium in our case), their method may generate a non-smooth mesh. For comparison, with an explicit smoothness measurement, we guarantee to achieve the smoothest mesh under the constraints.

7.6   Experiments on Four-Chamber Heart Segmentation

7.6.1   Data Sets

Under the guidance of cardiologists, we manually annotated all four chambers in 323 cardiac CT volumes (representing various cardiac phases) from 137 patients with different cardiovascular diseases. The specific disease information for a patient has not been captured. Since the LV is clinically more important than other

Table 7.1 Mean and standard deviation (in parentheses) of the point-to-mesh error (in millimeters) for the segmentation of heart chambers based on cross-validation

	After rigid localization	After control point alignment	Baseline ASM [9]	Proposed approach
Left ventricle endocardium	3.17 (1.10)	3.00 (1.11)	2.24 (1.21)	**1.13 (0.55)**
Left ventricle epicardium	2.51 (0.78)	2.35 (0.73)	2.45 (1.02)	**1.21 (0.41)**
Left atrium	2.78 (0.98)	2.67 (1.01)	1.89 (1.43)	**1.32 (0.42)**
Right ventricle	2.93 (0.75)	2.40 (0.82)	2.69 (1.10)	**1.55 (0.38)**
Right atrium	3.09 (0.86)	2.90 (0.92)	2.81 (1.15)	**1.57 (0.48)**

chambers, to improve the system performance on LV detection and segmentation, we annotated extra 134 volumes. In total, we have 457 volumes from 186 patients for the LV. The annotation is done by multiple experts. However, for each volume, there is only one annotation. Therefore, we cannot study the intra- and inter-observer variabilities, this being a limitation of the dataset. The number of patients used in our experiments is significantly larger than those reported in the literature, for example, 13 in [14], 18 in [25], 27 in [31], and 30 in [19].

The data was collected from 27 institutes, mostly from Germany, the USA, and China using Siemens Somatom Sensation or Definition scanners. The imaging protocols are heterogeneous with different capture ranges and resolutions. A volume may contain 80–350 slices, while the size of each slice is the same with 512×512 pixels. The resolution inside a slice is isotropic and varies from 0.28 to 0.74 mm for different volumes. The slice thickness (distance between neighboring slices) is larger than the in-slice resolution and varies from 0.4 to 2.0 mm for different volumes.

We use a fourfold cross-validation to evaluate our algorithm. Data from the same patient may have similar shapes and image characteristics since they were often captured on the same CT scanner with the same scanning parameters. If such data appears in both the training and test sets during cross-validation, the result is biased toward a lower segmentation error. To remove such bias, we enforce the constraint that the volumes from the same patient can only appear in either the training or test set, but not in both.

7.6.2 Experiments on Boundary Delineation

The symmetric point-to-mesh distance [14, 19, 31] E_{p2m} is selected to measure the accuracy in surface boundary delineation. For each point on a mesh, we search for the closest point (not necessarily at mesh triangle vertices) on the other mesh to calculate the minimum Euclidean distance. We calculate the point-to-mesh distance from the detected mesh to the ground truth and vice versa to make the measurement symmetric.

Table 7.2 Mean and standard deviation (in parentheses) of the point-to-mesh error E_{p2m} (in millimeters) for left ventricle endocardium segmentation using an optimal smooth surface. A fourfold cross-validation is performed on 457 volumes

	Initialization	Subspace projection [9]	Generic smoothing [43]	Our approach
E_{p2m}	1.13 (0.55)	1.31 (0.55)	1.39 (0.60)	**0.84 (0.47)**

In our experiments, we estimate the pose of each chamber separately. Therefore, we use $4 \times 9 = 36$ pose parameters to align the mean shapes. As shown in the second column of Table 7.1, the mean E_{p2m} error after heart localization is 3.17 mm for the LV endocardium, 2.51 mm for the LV epicardium, 2.78 mm for the LA, 2.93 mm for the RV, and 3.09 mm for the RA. Alternatively, we can treat the whole heart as one object in heart localization, then we use only nine pose parameters. In this way, the mean E_{p2m} error achieved is 3.52 mm for the LV endocardium, 3.07 mm for the LV epicardium, 3.95 mm for LA, 3.94 mm for the RV, and 4.64 mm for the RA. Obviously, treating each chamber separately, we can obtain a better initialization.

In our nonrigid deformation estimation, control points and normal mesh points are treated differently. We first estimate the deformation of control points and use TPS transformation to make the mesh consistent after warping. As shown in the third column in Table 7.1, after control point based alignment, we slightly reduce the error for the LV, LA, and RA by 5 % and significantly reduce the error by 17 % for the RV since the control points are more uniformly distributed in the RV mesh. After deformation estimation of all mesh points under the guidance of a learning based boundary detector and a statistical shape model (as presented in Sect. 7.4), the final segmentation error ranges from 1.13 to 1.57 mm for different chambers. The LV and LA have smaller errors than the RV and RA due to the use of contrast agent in the left heart in most of our data.

We compare our approach to the baseline ASM using non-learning based boundary detection scheme [9]. The comparison is limited to the last step on normal mesh point deformation. Input to both algorithms are the same initialized mesh. The iteration number in the baseline ASM is tuned to give the best performance. As shown in Table 7.1, the baseline ASM actually increase the error for weak boundaries (e.g., the LV epicardium and RV). It performs well for strong boundaries, such as the LV endocardium and the LA, but it is still significantly worse than the proposed method.

Most clinical applications require to generate a smooth surface mesh tightly enclosing the papillary muscles and trabeculation for LV endocardium segmentation. We further search for an optimal smooth surface to improve the LV endocardium segmentation accuracy, using the technology presented in Sect. 7.5. As shown in Table 7.2, the initial error of LV endocardium is 1.13 mm. Using the proposed approach, we reduce the mean error by 22 % to 0.84 mm. We compare our approach with two alternative methods, the shape subspace projection [9] and the generic mesh smoothing approach [43]. Starting from the same extracted blood pool, these generic approaches generate a smooth mesh traversing the blood pool

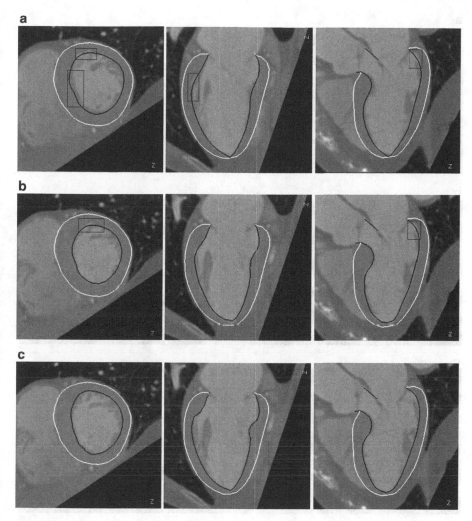

Fig. 7.16 Left Ventricle (LV) segmentation by (**a**) shape subspace projection [9], (**b**) generic mesh smoothing [43], and (**c**) the proposed optimal smooth surface approach. Three orthogonal views are shown at each row, with black for endocardium and white for epicardium. *Black boxes* indicate regions with noticeable errors. ©2009 SPIE. Reprinted, with permission, from Zheng, Y., Lu, X., Georgescu, B., Littmann, A., Mueller, E., Comaniciu, D.: Automatic left ventricle detection in MRI images using marginal space learning and component-based voting. In: *Proc. of SPIE Medical Imaging*, vol. 7259, pp. 1–12 (2009)

and actually increase the error, as shown in Table 7.2. The segmentation results using different approaches on a volume are shown in Fig. 7.16.

Figure 7.17 shows several examples of heart chamber segmentation using the proposed approach. Since our system is trained on volumes from all phases of a cardiac cycle, we can process volumes from the end-systolic phase (which has

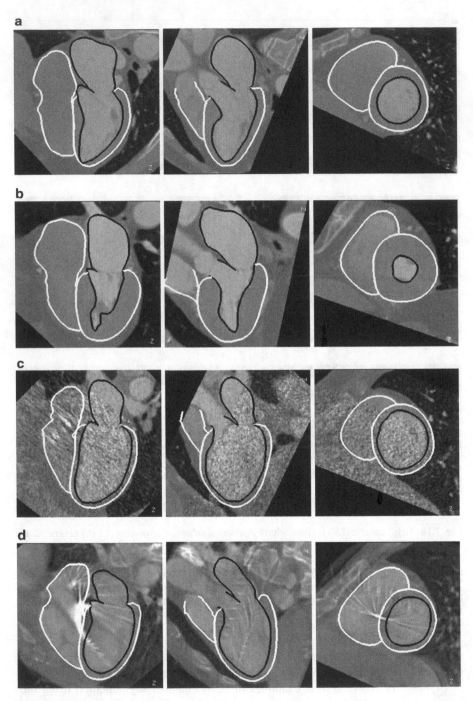

Fig. 7.17 Examples of heart chamber segmentation in 3D CT volumes. Each row represents three orthogonal views of a volume

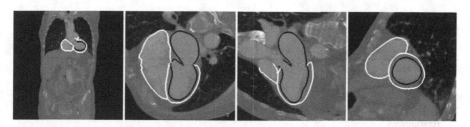

Fig. 7.18 Heart chamber segmentation result for a low-contrast full-torso CT volume. The first column shows a full torso view and the right three columns show close-up views

a significantly small blood pool for the LV) without any difficulty, as shown in Fig. 7.17b. It performs well on noisy volumes (as shown in Fig. 7.17c) and it is robust even under severe streak artifacts (as shown in Fig. 7.17d). Figure 7.18 shows the segmentation result of a full torso CT volume, where no contrast agent nor electrocardiogram-based gating is applied. This volume is challenging for thresholding based region growing techniques [19, 25]. However, our machine learning based approach can deal with this case quite well.

With some amount of code optimization and using multi-threading techniques, we achieve an average speed of 4.0 s for the automatic segmentation of all four chambers on a computer with a dual-core 3.2 GHz processor and 3 GB memory. The computation time is roughly equally split on the MSL based similarity transformation estimation and the nonrigid deformation estimation.

In Table 7.3, we present a brief summary of the previous work on heart segmentation in 3D CT volumes. Our approach is clearly faster than other algorithms, e.g., 5 s for left ventricle segmentation in [25], 15 s for nonrigid deformation in [5], and more than 1 min in [36, 39]. Compared with segmentation methods on other imaging modalities [24, 37], to the best of our knowledge, our approach is also the fastest. Most of the previous approaches are semi-automatic, except [14]. In general, we cannot compare error measures reported in different papers directly due to the difference in heart models and datasets. In the literature, we noticed two papers [14, 31] reporting smaller segmentation errors (on much smaller datasets) than ours. Both used the same heart model, one automatic [14] and one semi-automatic [31]. After blood pool based post-processing, we achieve a segmentation error of 0.84 mm for the LV endocardium, which is equivalent to theirs. However, our segmentation errors of the RV and RA (which have much lower contrast than the left heart in a CT volume) seem to be higher. Different from our four-chamber model, the heart model used in [14] and [31] also included major vessel trunks. Both papers only gave overall errors for the whole heart model (including the major vessel trunks), without any break-down error measure for each chamber.

Some care needs to be taken to compare our approach with these two papers. (1) Ecabert et al. [14] mentioned that it was hard to distinguish the boundary of different chambers. For example, it was likely to include a part of the LA in the segmented LV mesh and vice verse. Such errors were only partially penalized in

Table 7.3 Comparison with previous work on heart chamber segmentation in 3D CT volumes

	Patients/ Subjects	Volumes	Chambers	Automatic	Speed	Error (mm)
Neubauer and Wegenkiltl [39]	N/A	N/A	Left ventricle	No	>1 min	N/A
McInerney and Terzopoulos [36]	1	16	Left ventricle	No	100 min[a]	N/A
Fritz et al. [19]	30	30	Left ventricle	No	N/A	1.5
Jolly [25]	18	36	Left ventricle	No[b]	~5 s	N/A
Ecabert et al. [14]	13	28	Four chambers and vessel trunks	Yes[c]	N/A	0.85[d]
Lorenz and von Berg [31]	27	27	Four chambers and vessel trunks	No	N/A	0.81–1.19
von Berg and Lorenz [5]	6	60	Four chambers and vessel trunks	No	15 s	N/A
Our approach	137+	323+	Four chambers	Yes	4.0 s	0.84–1.57

[a] This was the time used to process the whole sequence of 16 volumes
[b] The long axis of the left ventricle needed to be manually aligned. All other steps were automatic
[c] The success rate of automatic heart localization was about 90 %
[d] Gross failures in heart localization were excluded from evaluation

both [14] and [31] since they did not provide break-down error measure for each chamber. However, in our evaluation, we fully penalize such errors. (2) About 8 % mesh points around the connection of vessel trunks to heart chambers were excluded for evaluation in [14]. In their model, all chambers and vessel trunks were artificially closed. Since there are no image features around these artificial caps, these regions cannot be delineated accurately even by an expert. Based on this consideration, they were removed from evaluation. In our model, all valves are represented as contours along their borders in our heart model. We only need to delineate the border of the valves and this can be done more accurately. Therefore, no mesh part is excluded from evaluation. (3) In [14], the automatic heart localization module failed on about 10 % volumes and such gross failures were also excluded for evaluation. (4) In [31], only volumes from the end-diastolic phase were used for experiments. However, our dataset contains 323+ volumes from all cardiac phases. The size and shape of a chamber change significantly from the end-diastolic phase to the end-systolic phase. Therefore, there is much more variability in our dataset.

7.6.3   Heart Chamber Tracking

Table 7.4 The Ejection Fraction (EF) estimation accuracy for all six dynamic sequences in our dataset

	P #1	P #2	P #3	P #4	P #5	P #6	Mean error (Std)
Ground truth (%)	68.7	49.7	45.8	62.9	47.4	38.9	
Estimation (%)	66.8	51.8	42.8	64.4	42.3	38.5	2.3 (1.6)

The size and shape of a heart chamber (especially, the LV) change significantly from an expansion phase to a contraction phase. Since our system is trained on volumes from all phases in a cardiac cycle, we can reliably detect and segment the heart from any cardiac phase. By performing heart segmentation frame by frame, the heart motion is tracked in the robust tracking-by-detection framework. To make the motion more consistent, mild motion smoothing is applied after the segmentation of each frame. Figure 7.19 shows the tracking results on one sequence. To further improve the system performance, we can exploit a motion model learned from an annotated dataset [48–50], but this is out of the scope of this work.

The motion pattern of a chamber during a cardiac cycle provides many important clinical measurements of its functionality, e.g., the Ejection Fraction (EF), myocardium wall thickness, and dyssynchrony within a chamber or between different chambers [15]. Among all these measurements, the EF is the most important since it reflects the overall functionality of a heart chamber. Given the tracking result, we can calculate the EF as follows,

$$EF = \frac{Volume_{ED} - Volume_{ES}}{Volume_{ED}}, \tag{7.40}$$

where $Volume_{ED}$ and $Volume_{ES}$ are the volume measures of the End-Diastolic (ED) and End-Systolic (ES) phases, respectively. In our dataset, there are six patients each with 10 frames from the whole cardiac cycle. Figure 7.20 shows the LV volume-time curves for two dynamic sequences. Table 7.4 shows the EF estimation accuracy for all six sequences. The estimated EFs are close to the ground truth with a mean error of 2.3 %.

In Fig. 7.20, we calculate the EF by using the volume enclosed by the smooth LV endocardium surface (which includes both the LV blood pool, papillary muscles, and trabeculation). We can also calculate the LV blood pool volume (excluding papillary muscles and trabeculation from the measurement). Using the proposed adaptive intensity thresholding presented in Sect. 7.5.2, we can extract the LV blood pool. After that, we count the number of voxels of the extracted blood pool and convert it to a volume measurement using the scan resolution information. Figure 7.21a shows the ground truth of the volume curves (both including and excluding papillary muscles/trabeculation) for a dynamic 3D sequences with 10 frames. Figure 7.21b and c compare the volume measures automatically generated

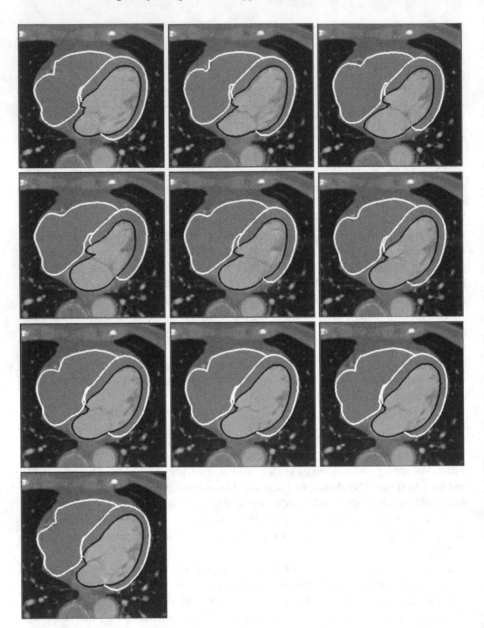

Fig. 7.19 Tracking results for the heart chambers on a dynamic 3D sequence with 10 frames

by our system against the ground truth for including and excluding papillary muscles/trabeculation, respectively. For the sequence shown in Fig. 7.21, the errors in EF estimation are quite small, no more than 2 %.

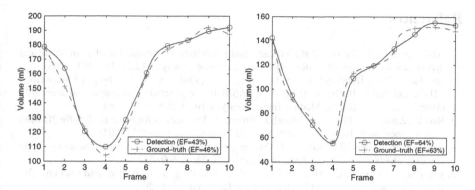

Fig. 7.20 The left ventricle volume-time curves for two dynamic 3D sequences

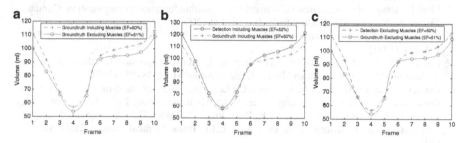

Fig. 7.21 The left ventricle volume-time curves for one dynamic 3D sequence with 10 frames.
(**a**) Ground truth including and excluding papillary muscles/trabeculation from the volume
measurements. (**b**) Detection vs. ground truth by including the papillary muscles/trabeculation.
(**c**) Detection vs. ground truth by excluding the papillary muscles/trabeculation

7.7 Conclusions

In this chapter, we used four-chamber heart segmentation in 3D CT volumes as
an example to illustrate a learning based segmentation framework. Our approach
is both efficient and robust. The efficiency comes from marginal space learning
based object pose estimation. We achieved an average speed of 4.0 s per volume
to segment all four chambers. The robustness is obtained by using recent advances
in learning discriminative models and exploiting a large annotated dataset. All
major steps in our approach are learning-based, therefore minimizing the use of
assumptions. The presented segmentation approach is generic and we have tested it
on other challenging 3D segmentation tasks in various medical imaging modalities,
e.g., liver segmentation in abdominal CT [30], brain tissue segmentation in MRI
images [47], heart chamber segmentation in ultrasound images [34,49], and multiple
organ segmentation in full torso CT [42].

References

1. Andreopoulos, A., Tsotsos, J.K.: Efficient and generalizable statistical models of shape and appearance for analysis of cardiac MRI. Medical Image Analysis **12**(3), 335–357 (2008)
2. van Assen, H.C., Danilouchkine, M.G., Frangi, A.F., Ordas, S., Westernberg, J.J.M., Reiber, J.H.C., Lelieveldt, B.P.F.: SPASM: A 3D-ASM for segmentation of sparse and arbitrarily oriented cardiac MRI data. Medical Image Analysis **10**(2), 286–303 (2006)
3. Bao, Z., Zhukov, L., Guskov, I., Wood, J., Breen, D.: Dynamic deformable models for 3D MRI heart segmentation. In: Proc. of SPIE Medical Imaging, pp. 398–405 (2002)
4. Belongie, S., Malik, J., Puzicha, J.: Shape matching and object recognition using shape contexts. IEEE Trans. Pattern Anal. Machine Intell. **24**(4), 509–522 (2002)
5. von Berg, J., Lorenz, C.: Multi-surface cardiac modelling, segmentation, and tracking. In: Proc. Functional Imaging and Modeling of the Heart, pp. 1–11 (2005)
6. Bookstein, F.L.: Principal warps: Thin-plate splines and the decomposition of deformation. IEEE Trans. Pattern Anal. Machine Intell. **11**(6), 567–585 (1989)
7. Chui, H., Rangarajan, A.: A new point matching algorithm for non-rigid registration. Computer Vision and Image Understanding **89**(2–3), 114–141 (2003)
8. Cohen, L.D.: On active contour models and balloons. CVGIP: Image Understanding **53**(2), 211–218 (1991)
9. Cootes, T.F., Taylor, C.J., Cooper, D.H., Graham, J.: Active shape models—their training and application. Computer Vision and Image Understanding **61**(1), 38–59 (1995)
10. Corsi, C., Saracino, G., Sarti, A., Lamberti, C.: Left ventricular volume estimation for real-time three-dimensional echocardiography. IEEE Trans. Medical Imaging **21**(9), 1202–1208 (2002)
11. Davies, R.H., Twining, C.J., Cootes, T.F., Waterton, J.C., Taylor, C.J.: A minimum description length approach to statistical shape modeling. IEEE Trans. Medical Imaging **21**(5), 525–537 (2002)
12. Dollár, P., Tu, Z., Belongie, S.: Supervised learning of edges and object boundaries. In: Proc. IEEE Conf. Computer Vision and Pattern Recognition, pp. 1964–1971 (2006)
13. Dryden, I.L., Mardia, K.V.: Statistical Shape Analysis. John Wiley, Chichester (1998)
14. Ecabert, O., Peters, J., Weese, J.: Modeling shape variability for full heart segmentation in cardiac computed-tomography images. In: Proc. of SPIE Medical Imaging, pp. 1199–1210 (2006)
15. Frangi, A.F., Niessen, W.J., Viergever, M.A.: Three-dimensional modeling for functional analysis of cardiac images: A review. IEEE Trans. Medical Imaging **20**(1), 2–25 (2001)
16. Frangi, A.F., Rueckert, D., Schnabel, J.A., Niessen, W.J.: Automatic construction of multiple-object three-dimensional statistical shape models: Application to cardiac modeling. IEEE Trans. Medical Imaging **21**(9), 1151–1166 (2002)
17. Fritz, D., Krolla, J., Dillmann, R., Scheuring, M.: Automatic 4D-segmentation of the left ventricle in cardiac-CT-data. In: Proc. of SPIE Medical Imaging, pp. 1–11 (2007)
18. Fritz, D., Rinck, D., Dillmann, R., Scheuring, M.: Segmentation of the left and right cardiac ventricle using a combined bi-temporal statistical model. In: Proc. of SPIE Medical Imaging, pp. 605–614 (2006)
19. Fritz, D., Rinck, D., Unterhinninghofen, R., Dillmann, R., Scheuring, M.: Automatic segmentation of the left ventricle and computation of diagnostic parameters using regiongrowing and a statistical model. In: Proc. of SPIE Medical Imaging, pp. 1844–1854 (2005)
20. Gerard, O., Billon, A.C., Rouet, J.M., Jacob, M., Fradkin, M., Allouche, C.: Efficient model-based quantification of left ventricular function in 3-D echocardiography. IEEE Trans. Medical Imaging **21**(9), 1059–1068 (2002)
21. van Ginneken, B., Frangi, A.F., Staal, J.J., ter Haar Romeny, B.M., Viergever, M.A.: Active shape model segmentation with optimal features. IEEE Trans. Medical Imaging **21**(8), 924–933 (2002)
22. Girosi, F., Jones, M., Poggio, T.: Regularization theory and neural networks architectures. Neural Computation **7**(2), 219–269 (1995)

23. Goldfarb, G., Idnani, A.: A numerically stable dual method for solving strictly convex quadratic programs. Mathematical Programming **27**(1), 1–33 (1983)
24. Hong, W., Georgescu, B., Zhou, X.S., Krishnan, S., Ma, Y., Comaniciu, D.: Database-guided simultaneous multi-slice 3D segmentation for volumetric data. In: Proc. European Conf. Computer Vision, pp. 397–409 (2006)
25. Jolly, M.P.: Automatic segmentation of the left ventricle in cardiac MR and CT images. Int. J. Computer Vision **70**(2), 151–163 (2006)
26. Kass, M., Witkin, A., Terzopoulos, D.: Snakes: Active contour models. Int. J. Computer Vision **1**(4), 321–331 (1988)
27. Kelm, B.M., Wels, M., Zhou, S.K., Seifert, S., Suehling, M., Zheng, Y., Comaniciu, D.: Spine detection in CT and MR using iterated marginal space learning. Medical Image Analysis **17**(8), 1283–1292 (2013)
28. Kelm, B.M., Zhou, S.K., Suehling, M., Zheng, Y., Wels, M., Comaniciu, D.: Detection of 3D spinal geometry using iterated marginal space learning. In: Proc. MICCAI Workshop Medical Computer Vision — Recognition Techniques and Applications in Medical Imaging, pp. 96–105 (2010)
29. Li, K., Wu, X., Chen, D.Z., Sonka, M.: Optimal surface segmentation in volumetric images—A graph-theoretic approach. IEEE Trans. Pattern Anal. Machine Intell. **28**(1), 119–134 (2006)
30. Ling, H., Zhou, S.K., Zheng, Y., Georgescu, B., Suehling, M., Comaniciu, D.: Hierarchical, learning-based automatic liver segmentation. In: Proc. IEEE Conf. Computer Vision and Pattern Recognition, pp. 1–8 (2008)
31. Lorenz, C., von Berg, J.: A comprehensive shape model of the heart. Medical Image Analysis **10**(4), 657–670 (2006)
32. Lorenz, C., Krahnstover, N.: Generation of point based 3D statistical shape models for anatomical objects. Computer Vision and Image Understanding **77**(2), 175–191 (2000)
33. Lötjönen, J., Kivistö, S., Koikkalainen, J., Smutek, D., Lauerma, K.: Statistical shape model of atria, ventricles and epicardium from short- and long-axis MR images. Medical Image Analysis **8**(3), 371–386 (2004)
34. Lu, X., Georgescu, B., Zheng, Y., Otsuki, J., Bennett, R., Comaniciu, D.: AutoMPR: Automatic detection of standard planes from three dimensional echocardiographic data. In: Proc. IEEE Int'l Sym. Biomedical Imaging, pp. 1279–1282 (2008)
35. Martin, D., Fowlkes, C., Malik, J.: Learning to detect natural image boundaries using local brightness, color and texture cues. IEEE Trans. Pattern Anal. Machine Intell. **26**(5), 530–549 (2004)
36. McInerney, T., Terzopoulos, D.: A dynamic finite element surface model for segmentation and tracking in multidimensional medical images with application to cardiac 4D image analysis. Computerized Medical Imaging and Graphics **19**(1), 69–83 (1995)
37. Mitchell, S.C., Bosch, J.G., Lelieveldt, B.P.F., van Geest, R.J., Reiber, J.H.C., Sonka, M.: 3-D active appearance models: Segmentation of cardiac MR and ultrasound images. IEEE Trans. Medical Imaging **21**(9), 1167–1178 (2002)
38. Moré, J.J., Toraldo, G.: On the solutions of large quadratic programming problems with bound constraints. SIAM J. Optimization **1**(1), 93–113 (1991)
39. Neubauer, A., Wegenkiltl, R.: Analysis of four-dimensional cardiac data sets using skeleton-based segmentation. In: Proc. Int'l Conf. in Central Europe on Computer Graphics and Visualization, pp. 330–337 (2003)
40. Park, K., Montillo, A., Metaxas, D., Axel, L.: Volumetric heart modeling and analysis. Communications of the ACM **48**(2), 43–48 (2005)
41. Schwing, A., Zheng, Y.: Reliable extraction of the mid-sagittal plane in 3D brain MRI via hierarchical landmark detection. In: Proc. IEEE Int'l Sym. Biomedical Imaging, pp. 1–4 (2014)
42. Seifert, S., Barbu, A., Zhou, K., Liu, D., Feulner, J., Huber, M., Suehling, M., Cavallaro, A., Comaniciu, D.: Hierarchical parsing and semantic navigation of full body CT data. In: Proc. of SPIE Medical Imaging, pp: 1–8 (2009)
43. Taubin, G.: Curve and surface smoothing without shrinkage. In: Proc. Int'l Conf. Computer Vision, pp. 852–857 (1995)

44. Taubin, G.: Optimal surface smoothing as filter design. In: Proc. European Conf. Computer Vision, pp. 283–292 (1996)
45. Tu, Z.: Probabilistic boosting-tree: Learning discriminative methods for classification, recognition, and clustering. In: Proc. Int'l Conf. Computer Vision, pp. 1589–1596 (2005)
46. Wahba, G.: Spline Models for Observational Data. Soc. Industrial and Applied Math. (1990)
47. Wels, M., Zheng, Y., Carneiro, G., Huber, M., Hornegger, J., Comaniciu, D.: Fast and robust 3-D MRI brain structure segmentation. In: Proc. Int'l Conf. Medical Image Computing and Computer Assisted Intervention, vol. 2, pp. 575–583 (2009)
48. Yang, L., Georgescu, B., Zheng, Y., Foran, D.J., Comaniciu, D.: A fast and accurate tracking algorithm of left ventricles in 3D echocardiography. In: Proc. IEEE Int'l Sym. Biomedical Imaging, pp. 221–224 (2008)
49. Yang, L., Georgescu, B., Zheng, Y., Meer, P., Comaniciu, D.: 3D ultrasound tracking of the left ventricles using one-step forward prediction and data fusion of collaborative trackers. In: Proc. IEEE Conf. Computer Vision and Pattern Recognition, pp. 1–8 (2008)
50. Yang, L., Georgescu, B., Zheng, Y., Wang, Y., Meer, P., Comaniciu, D.: Prediction based collaborative trackers (PCT): A robust and accurate approach toward 3D medical object tracking. IEEE Trans. Medical Imaging **30**(11), 1921–1932 (2011)
51. Zheng, Y., Barbu, A., Georgescu, B., Scheuering, M., Comaniciu, D.: Fast automatic heart chamber segmentation from 3D CT data using marginal space learning and steerable features. In: Proc. Int'l Conf. Computer Vision, pp. 1–8 (2007)
52. Zheng, Y., Barbu, A., Georgescu, B., Scheuering, M., Comaniciu, D.: Four-chamber heart modeling and automatic segmentation for 3D cardiac CT volumes using marginal space learning and steerable features. IEEE Trans. Medical Imaging **27**(11), 1668–1681 (2008)
53. Zheng, Y., Georgescu, B., Comaniciu, D.: Marginal space learning for efficient detection of 2D/3D anatomical structures in medical images. In: Proc. Information Processing in Medical Imaging, pp. 411–422 (2009)
54. Zheng, Y., Georgescu, B., Ling, H., Zhou, S.K., Scheuering, M., Comaniciu, D.: Constrained marginal space learning for efficient 3D anatomical structure detection in medical images. In: Proc. IEEE Conf. Computer Vision and Pattern Recognition, pp. 194–201 (2009)
55. Zheng, Y., Georgescu, B., Vega-Higuera, F., Zhou, S.K., Comaniciu, D.: Fast and automatic heart isolation in 3D CT volumes: Optimal shape initialization. In: Proc. MICCAI Workshop Machine Learning in Medical Imaging, pp. 84–91 (2010)
56. Zheng, Y., John, M., Liao, R., Nottling, A., Boese, J., Kempfert, J., Walther, T., Brockmann, G., Comaniciu, D.: Automatic aorta segmentation and valve landmark detection in C-arm CT for transcatheter aortic valve implantation. IEEE Trans. Medical Imaging **31**(12), 2307–2321 (2012)
57. Zheng, Y., Lu, X., Georgescu, B., Littmann, A., Mueller, E., Comaniciu, D.: Robust object detection using marginal space learning and ranking-based multi-detector aggregation: Application to automatic left ventricle detection in 2D MRI images. In: Proc. IEEE Conf. Computer Vision and Pattern Recognition, pp. 1343–1350 (2009)
58. Zheng, Y., Wang, T., John, M., Zhou, S.K., Boese, J., Comaniciu, D.: Multi-part left atrium modeling and segmentation in C-arm CT volumes for atrial fibrillation ablation. In: Proc. Int'l Conf. Medical Image Computing and Computer Assisted Intervention, vol. 3, pp. 487–495 (2011)
59. Zheng, Y., Yang, D., John, M., Comaniciu, D.: Multi-part modeling and segmentation of left atrium in C-arm CT for image-guided ablation of atrial fibrillation. IEEE Trans. Medical Imaging (2014). In Press

Chapter 8
Applications of Marginal Space Learning in Medical Imaging

8.1 Introduction

Marginal Space Learning (MSL) is a generic and open framework for efficient object detection and segmentation. It has been extensively tested on multiple anatomical structure detection/segmentation problems in different medical imaging modalities. In this chapter, we provide a literature review of the MSL applications in medical imaging. In principle, the MSL can also be applied to detect objects in non-medical images, however, such potential applications are not the focus of this book.

A few of the applications have already been discussed in the previous chapters to illustrate various developments of the MSL. To make this chapter self-contained, these applications are included. In some applications, variants of MSL are developed to further improve the detection speed and robustness. For example, iterated MSL is presented in Sect. 8.2.9 to extend MSL to the detection of multiple instances of the same object type (e.g., intervertebral disks). Hierarchical Detection Network (HDN) (a.k.a. hierarchical MSL) is presented in Sect. 8.2.17 to perform MSL based object detection at multiple resolutions on an image pyramid. The detected object candidates at a lower resolution are propagated to a higher resolution to achieve more efficient and robust detection. Many imaging modalities can now generate a dynamic sequence of 3D volumes (3D+t) to analyze the motion of an anatomical structure. Section 8.3.7 presents a joint spatio-temporal MSL to detect the motion trajectory of the object across volumes. It is more robust than the independent detection and the traditional detection-followed-by-tracking approaches. In other applications, the MSL is only a component, for example, by providing an estimate of the bounding box of a structure, and the major contributions of those publications may be on other tasks, such as the segmentation and tracking of the target structure. We include such work in this review solely to illustrate the generalization capability of the MSL.

We first review applications on "pure" detection problems, followed by those combining detection, segmentation and tracking.

Y. Zheng and D. Comaniciu, *Marginal Space Learning for Medical Image Analysis: Efficient Detection and Segmentation of Anatomical Structures*, DOI 10.1007/978-1-4939-0600-0_8, © Springer Science+Business Media New York 2014

8.2   Detection of Devices and Anatomical Structures

8.2.1   Ultrasound Transducer Detection in Fluoroscopy

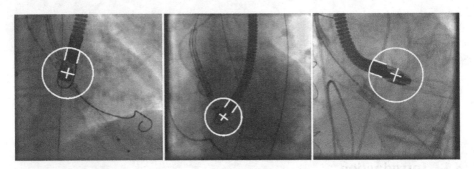

Fig. 8.1 Automatic transesophageal echocardiography transducer detection on 2D fluoroscopy images. The detected in-plane transformation (two translation, one rotation, and two anisotropic scaling parameters) is represented as an oriented *white circle*. Image courtesy of Tobias Heimann

X-ray fluoroscopy is an imaging modality used to guide minimally invasive transcatheter interventions, such as Transcatheter Aortic Valve Implantation (TAVI) and mitral valve repair. Although fluoroscopy provides a large view of the operating field, it has limitations due to the weak visibility of soft tissues and the overlapping of 3D structures on a 2D projection.

For cardiac interventions, 3D Transesophageal Echocardiography (TEE) is increasingly used as a supplementary imaging modality for its good capability to delineate soft tissues. Each imaging modality is captured in its own coordinate system and displayed separately. Fusion of both imaging modalities into a common coordinate system can provide a better visual guidance during cardiac interventions. Since the TEE probe is captured in fluoroscopy (Fig. 8.1), automatic estimation of its 3D pose helps to determine the transformation between two imaging modalities. The 3D pose of a TEE probe can be decomposed to in-plane transformation and out-of-plane rotation. In [42], the in-plane transformation of the TEE probe (which has five degrees of freedom and can be represented as an oriented bounding box) is estimated efficiently using the MSL. The out-of-plane rotation is then determined by matching against a library of pre-calculated 2D projects of the TEE probe along different orientations.

Since it is time consuming to collect and annotate a large training set necessary to build a robust detection system, synthesized data can be generated to enrich the training set [20].

Publications

- Mountney, P., Ionasec, R., Kaizer, M., Mamaghani, S., Wu, W., Chen, T., John, M., Boese, J., Comaniciu, D.: Ultrasound and fluoroscopic images fusion by autonomous ultrasound probe detection. In: *Proc. Int'l Conf. Medical Image Computing and Computer Assisted Intervention*, vol. 2, pp. 544–551 (2012)
- Heimann, T., Mountney, P., John, M., Ionasec, R.: Learning without labeling: Domain adaptation for ultrasound transducer localization. In: *Proc. Int'l Conf. Medical Image Computing and Computer Assisted Intervention*, vol. 3, pp. 49–56 (2013)

8.2.2 Balloon Marker Detection in Fluoroscopy for Stent Enhancement

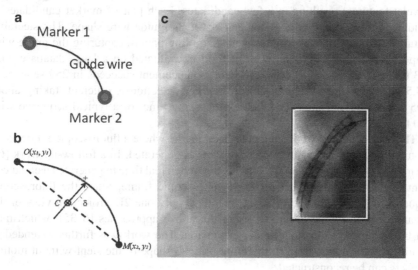

Fig. 8.2 Balloon marker detection in a fluoroscopy sequence for stent enhancement. (**a**) A simplified model composed of two balloon markers with a guide wire connecting them. (**b**) Representation of the model with five parameters $(x_1, y_1, x_2, y_2, \delta)$. (**c**) An image frame from a fluoroscopy sequence with an in-box showing the motion compensated enhancement of a stent. Image courtesy of Xiaoguang Lu. ©2011 IEEE. Reprinted, with permission, from Lu, X., Chen, T., Comaniciu, D.: Robust discriminative wire structure modeling with applications to stent enhancement in fluoroscopy. In: *Proc. IEEE Conf. Computer Vision and Pattern Recognition*, pp. 1121–1127 (2011)

Lu et al. [35] presented an interesting application of the MSL for stent enhancement from a fluoroscopy sequence. Stent thrombosis and re-stenosis are major complications for patients undergoing Percutaneous Coronary Intervention (PCI) and they are often associated with stent under-expansion. Real time fluoroscopy is the image modality to guide the deployment of a stent via a balloon. Due to motion artifacts (cardiac motion plus respiratory motion), a stent is barely visible as shown in Fig. 8.2c. Low visibility prevents confident quantification of stent under-expansion. If the motion can be estimated for each frame, the stent can be significantly enhanced by averaging multiple frames after motion compensation as shown in the in-box of Fig. 8.2c.

In [35], two balloon markers are automatically detected to provide motion estimation. As markers appear as tiny dots on fluoroscopy, independent detection often results in a lot of false positive detections from confounding structures. The two markers are connected by a guide wire; therefore, joint detection of markers and the guide wire can remove false positive detections. The whole object is parameterized as five parameters $(x_1, y_1, x_2, y_2, \delta)$, with (x_1, y_1) for the position of one marker, (x_2, y_2) for the other marker, and δ representing the shape of the guide wire, as shown in Fig. 8.2b. Since it is time consuming to estimate five parameters simultaneously, the MSL principle is applied to estimate the model parameters sequentially. First, the position of the balloon markers is detected (using 2D Haar wavelet features) resulting in a few candidates. Each pair of marker candidates is validated after incorporating parameter δ for the guide wire shape. The steerable features [70] are adapted with a special sampling pattern capturing the guide wire shape for the final validation. The method is evaluated on a large database with 263 fluoroscopic sequences and the stent enhancement succeeds in 259 sequences (98.5 %). Since the MSL is used, the marker detection is efficient, taking about 0.05 s for a single frame. The whole processing time for a typical sequence with 100 frames is about 5 s.

The above method works in a play-back mode, where a fluoroscopic sequence is captured and one static enhanced stent view is generated. In a follow-up work [6], the motion of detected balloon marker is tracked in real time to generate an enhanced stent in the original context for each fluoroscopic frame. Since the fluoroscopic sequence is captured with a fixed orientation, only one 2D projection view of the enhanced stent can be generated using the above approaches [6, 35], which may not be enough to exam stent under-expansion. The work was further extended to rotational fluoroscopy in [57]; therefore, the 3D shape of the stent without motion artifacts can be reconstructed.

Publications

- Lu, X., Chen, T., Comaniciu, D.: Robust discriminative wire structure modeling with applications to stent enhancement in fluoroscopy. In: *Proc. IEEE Conf. Computer Vision and Pattern Recognition*, pp. 1121–1127 (2011)
- Chen, T., Wang, Y., Durlak, P., Comaniciu, D.: Real time assistance for stent positioning and assessment by self-initialized tracking. In: *Proc. Int'l Conf. Medical Image Computing and Computer Assisted Intervention*, vol. 1, pp. 405–413 (2012)

- Wang, Y., Chen, T., Wang, P., Rohkohl, C., Comaniciu, D.: Automatic localization of balloon markers and guidewire in rotational fluoroscopy with application to 3D stent reconstruction. In: *Proc. European Conf. Computer Vision*,
  pp. 428–441 (2012)

8.2.3 Pigtail Catheter Tip Detection in Fluoroscopy

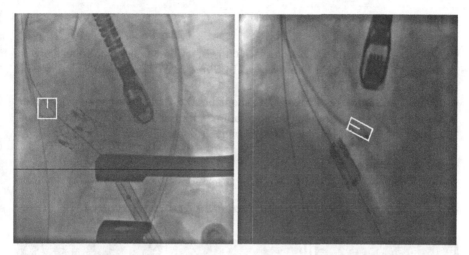

Fig. 8.3 Pigtail catheter tip detection results in two fluoroscopic images. Image courtesy of Stratis
Tzoumas. ©2012 SPIE. Reprinted, with permission, from Tzoumas, S., Wang, P., Zheng, Y., John,
M., Comaniciu, D.: Robust pigtail catheter tip detection in fluoroscopy. In: *Proc. of SPIE Medical
Imaging*, vol. 8316, pp. 1–8 (2012)

Motion compensated overlay of a 3D aorta model on fluoroscopy is helpful to
guide Transcatheter Aortic Valve Implantation (TAVI). A pigtail catheter is often
inserted into the aortic valve leaflet pocket for contrast agent injection to highlight
the valvular structure when necessary. Once the pigtail catheter tip is tightly attached
to the aortic valve, it has the same motion as the valve. Automatic detection and
tracking of the pigtail catheter tip can help to dynamically update the overlay of a 3D
aortic valve model, which is extracted from pre-operative Computed Tomography
(CT) or intra-operative C-arm CT [78]. MSL can be exploited to detect the catheter
tip on a 2D fluoroscopic frame as an oriented bounding box [50] and the tip position
in the following frames can be tracked via online learning [56].

A pigtail catheter tip forms a circular shape. However, depending on the
projection angle of fluoroscopy, the shape varies from a circular structure to an
elongated ellipse, or even degenerating to a line on a 2D projection view, as
shown in Fig. 8.3. Therefore, a direct application of MSL achieves a moderate
success rate. The MSL detection pipeline is revised in [50] to further improve the
detection rate by splitting the catheter tip into three shape categories: a circular

shape, an elongated ellipse, and a line. A combined position detector for all shape categories is trained for early rejection of easy negative samples. Different position-orientation and position-orientation-scale detectors are then trained for different shape categories. During detection, an estimated position candidate is forwarded to the detectors of each shape category. The final detection is achieved by cluster analysis of all estimated bounding-box candidates. Thus, by treating each shape category differently, the detection accuracy is increased.

Publications

- Tzoumas, S., Wang, P., Zheng, Y., John, M., Comaniciu, D.: Robust pigtail catheter tip detection in fluoroscopy. In: *Proc. of SPIE Medical Imaging*, vol. 8316, pp. 1–8 (2012)
- Wang, P., Zheng, Y., John, M., Comaniciu, D.: Catheter tracking via online learning for dynamic motion compensation in transcatheter aortic valve implantation. In: *Proc. Int'l Conf. Medical Image Computing and Computer Assisted Intervention*, vol. 2, pp. 17–24 (2012)

8.2.4   Catheter Detection and Tracking in Fluoroscopy

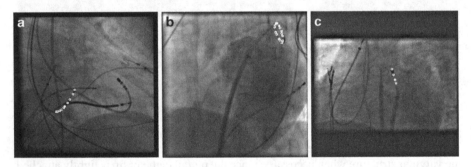

Fig. 8.4 Catheter tracking results in fluoroscopic image sequences. The tracked catheter tips and electrodes are indicated by *white circles*. (**a**) Coronary sinus catheter. (**b**) Circumferential mapping catheter. (**c**) Ablation catheter. Image courtesy of Wen Wu. ©2011 IEEE. Reprinted, with permission, from Wu, W., Chen, T., Barbu, A., Wang, P., Strobel, N., Zhou, S.K., Comaniciu, D.: Learning-based hypothesis fusion for robust catheter tracking in 2D X-ray fluoroscopy. In: *Proc. IEEE Conf. Computer Vision and Pattern Recognition*, pp. 1097–1104 (2011)

Atrial fibrillation is the most common cardiac arrhythmia, characterized by fast irregular heart beats of the atria. Catheter based ablation is used to treat atrial fibrillation when pharmaceutic therapy is not effective. During the ablation procedure, multiple catheters (e.g., coronary sinus catheter, circumferential mapping catheter, and ablation catheter as shown in Fig. 8.4) are inserted into the heart to facilitate the intervention. The intervention is guided under real time fluoroscopy. However, fluoroscopy is only good at visualizing bony and metal structures, while the heart tissues are hardly visible.

A 3D heart model extracted from 3D imaging modalities such as Computed Tomography (CT) and Magnetic Resonance Imaging (MRI), is often overlaid onto fluoroscopy for visual guidance. A static overlay only provides limited help since the operating scene is subject to cardiac and respiratory motion. When attached to a cardiac structure (e.g., coronary sinus), a catheter has a similar motion pattern as the heart; therefore, real time tracking of the catheter can be used to generate a dynamic overlay of the 3D heart model onto fluoroscopy for better visual guidance (similar to the pigtail catheter based motion compensation presented in Sect. 8.2.3).

Wu et al. [62] presented a robust system to track the tip and electrodes of a catheter. The initial position of the tip and electrodes is specified on the first frame and the motion is tracked in a tracking-by-detection framework in the following frames. Since the size of a catheter is less important, the tip and electrodes are detected as oriented points (x, y, θ). MSL is exploited to detect them in two steps, position estimation followed by position-orientation estimation. The MSL based oriented point detectors generate multiple candidates for the catheter tip and electrodes, which can be fused with other imaging cues to build a robust tracking system. Figure 8.4 shows tracking results of several catheters. The tracking speed is further increased using Graphics Processing Units (GPU) [63].

Publications

- Wu, W., Chen, T., Barbu, A., Wang, P., Strobel, N., Zhou, S.K., Comaniciu, D.: Learning-based hypothesis fusion for robust catheter tracking in 2D X-ray fluoroscopy. In: *Proc. IEEE Conf. Computer Vision and Pattern Recognition*, pp. 1097–1104 (2011)
- Wu, W., Chen, T., Strobel, N., Comaniciu, D.: Fast tracking of catheters in 2D fluoroscopic images using an integrated CPU-GPU framework. In: *Proc. IEEE Int'l Sym. Biomedical Imaging*, pp. 1184–1187 (2012)

8.2.5 Landmark Detection and Scan Range Delimitation in Topogram

A topogram is an X-ray image acquired in a CT scanner to define a precise scan range of a target anatomical structure for the following 3D scanning and image reconstruction. Traditionally, the scan range is manually determined by a clinician. Automatic detection of the scan range can reduce the scan time, therefore increasing the patient throughput. Furthermore, it can reduce the inter-user variability. Figure 8.5 shows five scan ranges for different body regions:

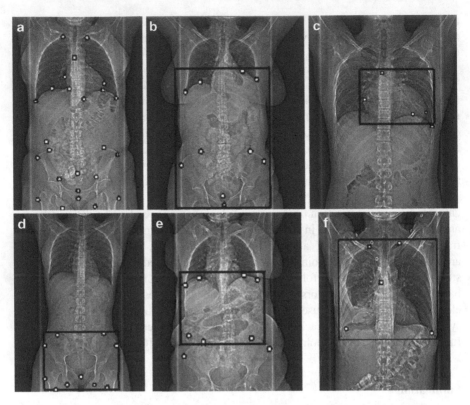

Fig. 8.5 Topogram images with predefined (**a**) anatomical landmarks (*black dots*) and five scan ranges for different body regions (*black boxes*): (**b**) abdomen, (**c**) heart, (**d**) pelvis, (**e**) liver, and (**f**) thorax. Image courtesy of Wei Zhang. ©2010 SPIE. Reprinted, with permission, from Zhang, W., Mantlic, F., Zhou, S.K.: Automatic landmark detection and scan range delimitation for topogram images using hierarchical network. In: *Proc. of SPIE Medical Imaging*, vol. 7623, pp. 1–8 (2010)

abdomen, heart, pelvis, liver, and thorax. However, automatic scan range detection is challenging because of (1) overlap of anatomical structures on a 2D projection image, (2) variations in patients' age, obesity, and pathology, (3) missing body part (up to half of the target body region may be out of the field of view), and (4) low signal-to-noise ratio (since a topogram is acquired with a low radiation dose).

Zhang et al. [68] proposed an automatic and efficient method to detect scan ranges using a hierarchical network with a combination of body region detection and landmark detection. Each body region is defined as an axially-aligned box with four pose parameters (two for position and two for scales). The MSL is exploited to detect the body region box in two steps: position estimation followed by position-scale estimation. Each body region detector generates multiple box candidates and a body region network is built and optimized to select the best candidate for each body region using the context information in the network. The body region detection is robust if more than 90 % of the region is inside the field of view.

However, the algorithm is demanded to tolerate up to 50% missing part. As a result, the solution has to exploit the local image context through which an anatomical landmark can be detected more robustly under occlusion. A set of landmarks are predefined (as shown in Fig. 8.5a) and associated with different body regions (as shown in Fig. 8.5b–f). The initial landmark position is inferred from the estimated body region and then refined under its own detector. Even though only the position of a landmark is needed, a landmark is detected as a box to exploit the embedded scale information in a local image patch, which is similar to the Left Ventricle (LV) landmark detection in [80]. Again, MSL is used to train the landmark detectors. Similar to the body region network, the landmarks associated with the same region also form a local network, which is then optimized to search for the optimal configuration of the landmarks. The proposed method is efficient, taking about four seconds to detect five body regions. Its robustness has been demonstrated with quantitative evaluation on about 1,000 topogram images.

Publication

- Zhang, W., Mantlic, F., Zhou, S.K.: Automatic landmark detection and scan range delimitation for topogram images using hierarchical network. In: *Proc. of SPIE Medical Imaging*, vol. 7623, pp. 1–8 (2010)

8.2.6   Left and Right Ventricle Detection in 2D MRI

The 2D Magnetic Resonance Imaging (MRI) technology is often used for Left Ventricle (LV) quantification. Detection of the LV in an MRI image is a prerequisite for functional measurement (e.g., measuring the LV volume and ejection fraction). However, due to the large variations in the orientation, size, shape, and image intensity of the LV, automatic detection of the LV on a long-axis MRI image is challenging. We adapted the MSL to detect the LV on a long-axis MRI image, by modeling it as an oriented bounding box (Fig. 8.6) [37, 79, 80]. This was the first application of the MSL on 2D object detection. The work was later on extended to detect Right Ventricle (RV) landmarks (e.g, the RV insertion points and RV lateral point) on short-axis MRI images [36].

The LV bounding box detector alone is not robust enough to accommodate variations in the 2D plane rotation around the LV axis, which translate into large variability of the LV appearance and shape, and variability in the surrounding tissue. Additionally, we also needed to detect several LV landmarks, such as the LV apex and two mitral valve annulus points. If we combine the detected candidates from the LV bounding box detector and landmark detectors, it is possible to further improve the system robustness. Initially, we proposed a simple voting based approach [79], which could improve the overall robustness, compared to a single LV detector. Later on, we developed a ranking-based strategy, more systematic and theoretically

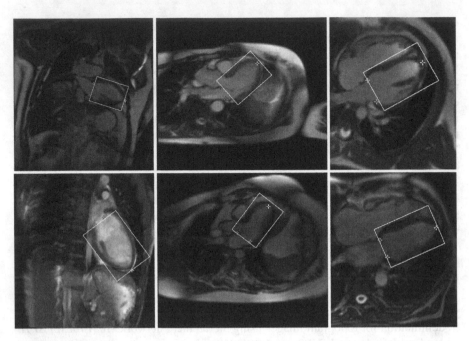

Fig. 8.6 Detection results of the left ventricle (the oriented bounding boxes) and its landmarks (*white stars* for the apex and *dark stars* for two annulus points on the mitral valve) on 2D MRI images

founded [80]. Experiments show that the ranking-based aggregation approach can significantly reduce the detection outliers.

Perfusion MRI is an important imaging modality for the diagnosis and quantification of myocardium infarction. In a typical perfusion protocol, a sequence of 2D short-axis images of the LV and RV are scanned to monitor the perfusion of the contrast agent. The short-axis images correspond to the same cardiac phase; therefore, the sequence is free of or with minimal cardiac motion. Automatic detection of the landmarks (e.g., the LV blood pool center and two RV insertion points) in a perfusion scan is challenging due to the variation of contrast. In addition, we also need to select two key frames that have the optimal amount of contrast to delineate the LV and RV, respectively. Lu et al. [41] proposed a method for joint spatio-temporal detection of key frames and landmarks. The 2D short-axis sequence is first stacked together to form a 3D volume (different to a normal 3D volume since the z-axis denotes the temporal dimension in this spatio-temporal volume). A 3D context box is defined, containing three position parameters (X, Y, Z), one rotation (θ), and three scales (S_x, S_y, S_z). Here, Z is the position of the key frame in the sequence and (X, Y) is the position of the landmarks on the key frame. The MSL is used to detect the 3D context box. Using joint spatio-temporal detection, the key frame and landmarks are detected simultaneously. The solution is more robust than

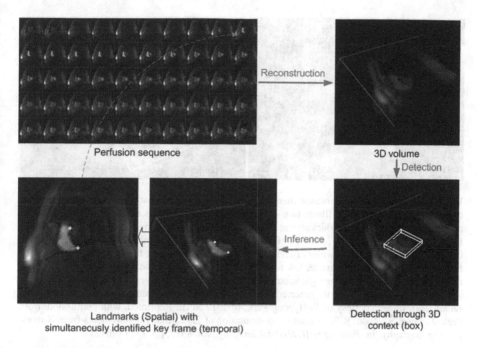

Fig. 8.7 Joint landmark detection and key-frame identification. RV insertion landmarks are used as an example. Image courtesy of Xiaoguang Lu. ©2011 SPIE. Reprinted, with permission, from Lu, X., Xue, H., Jolly, M.P., Guetter, C., Kellman, P., Hsu, L.Y., Arai, A., Zuehlsdorff, S., Littmann, A., Georgescu, B., Guehring, J.: Simultaneous detection of landmarks and key-frame in cardiac perfusion MRI using a joint spatial-temporal context model. In: *Proc. of SPIE Medical Imaging*, pp. 1–7 (2011)

independent landmark detection on each 2D images since the temporal information is also incorporated into the detection. Figure 8.7 shows the detection workflow.

Publications

- Zheng, Y., Lu, X., Georgescu, B., Littmann, A., Mueller, E., Comaniciu, D.: Automatic left ventricle detection in MRI images using marginal space learning and component-based voting. In: *Proc. of SPIE Medical Imaging*, vol. 7259, pp. 1–12 (2009)
- Zheng, Y., Lu, X., Georgescu, B., Littmann, A., Mueller, E., Comaniciu, D.: Robust object detection using marginal space learning and ranking-based multi-detector aggregation: Application to automatic left ventricle detection in 2D MRI images. In: *Proc. IEEE Conf. Computer Vision and Pattern Recognition*, pp. 1343–1350 (2009)

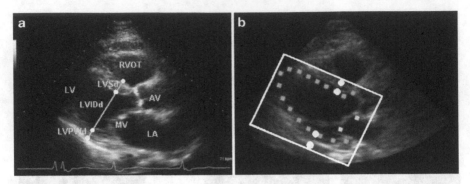

Fig. 8.8 Automatic cardiac measurements in a 2D ultrasound of a parasternal long-axis view of the Left Ventricle (LV). (**a**) Illustration of the cardiac measurements at the End-Diastolic (ED) phase, including LV septum thickness at ED (LVSd), LV internal dimension at ED (LVIDd), and LV posterior wall thickness at ED (LVPWd). All three measurements are calculated on a line defined by four landmarks (*white circles*). The meanings of the text labels on the image are as follows: LV for the left ventricle, LA for the left atrium, AV for the aortic valve, MV for the mitral valve, and RVOT for the right ventricular outflow tract, respectively. (**b**) Landmark detection (*white circles*) constrained by the detected LV box (*white*) and segmented endocardium (*small filled rectangles*). Image courtesy of JinHyeong Park. ©2012 SPIE. Reprinted, with permission, from Park, J., Feng, S., Zhou, K.S.: Automatic computation of 2D cardiac measurements from B-mode echocardiography. In: *Proc. of SPIE Medical Imaging*, vol. 8315, pp. 1–11 (2012)

- Lu, X., Georgescu, B., Jolly, M.P., Guehring, J., Young, A., Cowan, B., Littmann, A., Comaniciu, D.: Cardiac anchoring in MRI through context modeling. In: *Proc. Int'l Conf. Medical Image Computing and Computer Assisted Intervention*, vol. 1, pp. 383–390 (2010)
- Lu, X., Xue, H., Jolly, M.P., Guetter, C., Kellman, P., Hsu, L.Y., Arai, A., Zuehlsdorff, S., Littmann, A., Georgescu, B., Guehring, J.: Simultaneous detection of landmarks and key-frame in cardiac perfusion MRI using a joint spatial-temporal context model. In: *Proc. of SPIE Medical Imaging*, pp. 1–7 (2011)

8.2.7   Cardiac Measurements from 2D Ultrasound

Ultrasound is one of the main modalities to assess heart function since it is widely available, cost effective, real-time and free of radiation. Park et al. [43] presented a system to automatically calculate cardiac measurements of the Left Ventricle (LV), including LV septum thickness (LVS), LV internal dimension (LVID), and LV posterior wall thickness (LVPW), on a dynamic B-mode ultrasound sequence. Each measurement can be calculated separately on the End-Diastolic (ED) and End-Systolic (ES) phases, resulting in a total of six measurements. All are measured on a line defined by four landmarks, as shown in Fig. 8.8a. However, it is difficult to detect those four landmark points by only observing the local region around the points because an ultrasound image is subject to noise and signal dropout.

A hierarchical framework is presented to detect the landmarks by first examining a global context and then focusing on a local context. An oriented LV box is first detected using the MSL and then the LV endocardium is segmented using shape inference, as shown in Fig. 8.8b. The position of each landmark is estimated and refined, and the final landmark position is validated in a pseudo anatomic M-mode image generated by accumulating the same line image in a dynamic B-mode sequence to incorporate the temporal information.

Publication

* Park, J., Feng, S., Zhou, K.S.: Automatic computation of 2D cardiac measurements from B-mode echocardiography. In: *Proc. of SPIE Medical Imaging*, vol. 8315, pp. 1–11 (2012)

8.2.8 Mid-Sagittal Plane Detection in 3D MRI

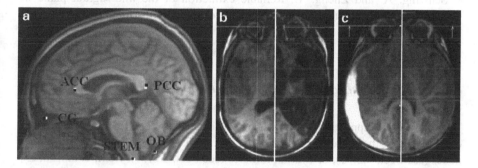

Fig. 8.9 Detection of the Mid-Sagittal Plane (MSP) and five plane landmarks in 3D MRI volumes. (a) Five landmarks on the MSP. The automatic detection and ground truth are shown in *white and black dots*, respectively. (b) and (c) Automatically detected MSP (white vertical lines) for two pathological cases. Image courtesy of Alexander Schwing

It is important to register the MRI datasets into a common coordinate system and establish correspondences between similar anatomical landmarks. This process of spatial normalization is required in neuro-science multi-subject studies or in oncology, for follow-up exams. Although the brain exhibits most of the time a regular structure, the presence of brain tumors and various deformations create a challenge for achieving a robust spatial normalization. Let us consider for example the Mid-Sagittal Plane (MSP) alignment. A maximum error of about 1° is often clinically required for MSP plane orientation estimation, which is quite restrictive.

In order to achieve such accuracy, we combine the pose estimation and refinement of the corresponding landmarks. In [45], we first use the MSL to roughly estimate the bounding box of five landmarks on the MSP plane, i.e., the Crista Galli

(CG), the tip of the Occipital Bone (OB), the Anterior of the Corpus Callosum (ACC), the Posterior of the Corpus Callosum (PCC) and a landmark in the brain stem (STEM), as shown in Fig. 8.9a. The MSP box detection results in a plane orientation error a bit larger than 3.0°. We then estimate the rough position of each landmark from the bounding box and each landmark is further refined in a small neighborhood around its initial position, using a dedicated landmark detector. Finally, a plane is fitted to the five detected landmarks using the least-squares method, which significantly improves the MSP detection accuracy.

To validate this approach, an experiment is conducted on 509 volumes (of $200 \times 200 \times 150$ voxels) coming from patients of different gender and ages with various neurological disorders. We achieve 1.09° error in determining the plane orientation, at the same level of the inter-observer variability. The center of the mid-sagittal plane represented by the mass center of the five landmarks is detected with an error less than 2 mm.

Publication

* Schwing, A. and Zheng, Y.: Reliable extraction of the mid-sagittal plane in 3D brain MRI via hierarchical landmark detection. In: *Proc. IEEE Int'l Sym. Biomedical Imaging*, pp. 1–4 (2014)

8.2.9 Intervertebral Disk Detection in 3D MRI/CT

There are a few applications for which we do need to detect a variable number of instances of the same anatomical structure, such as intervertebral disks, lymph nodes (see Sect. 8.2.11), or ovarian follicles (see Sect. 8.3.14). Kelm et al. [28, 29] presented an application of the MSL to detect the intervertebral disks in a 3D MRI or CT volume. A healthy subject has 24 vertebrae that can be grouped into three segments, called the cervical, thoracic, and lumbar segments. The shape of vertebrae changes gradually along the spinal column and neighboring vertebrae are similar to each other. It is challenging to distinguish and label neighboring vertebrae without considering the entire global structure of the spine, which may not be completely available in a volume with a limited field of view as shown in Fig. 8.11c. Therefore, instead of training 24 vertebrae detectors with one dedicated to each vertebra, three detectors are trained with one for each spinal segment (i.e., cervical, thoracic, and lumbar segments). The cervical spine disk detector should be able to detect all instances of the cervical vertebrae. The same is true for the other two disk detectors.

The MSL is subject to the *sample concentration* problem when applied for detecting multiple disk instances, the estimated candidates being concentrated to a few salient disks. Figure 8.10a shows the workflow of iterated MSL [28, 29], which elegantly solves the sample concentration problem. After position detection,

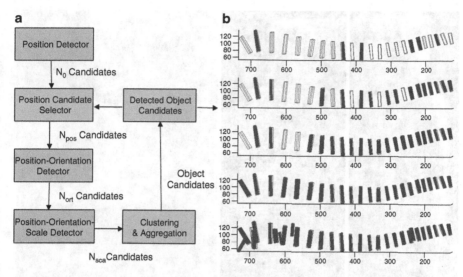

Fig. 8.10 Iterated marginal space learning for intervertebral disk detection. (**a**) Workflow. (**b**) Detected disks after each iteration. The ground truth is labeled as *empty boxes* and the detection is labeled as *filled boxes*. Image courtesy of Michael Kelm

we keep N_0 candidates and only the top $N_{pos} < N_0$ candidates are propagated to the following MSL detection pipeline to detect some object instances. The detected instances are then used to prune the remaining $N_0 - N_{pos}$ position candidates by removing those candidates close to the already detected instances. The top N_{pos} remaining position candidates are then propagated to detect more object instances. The process is iterated until there are no more position candidates. Iterated MSL overcomes the sample concentration issue of the original MSL and maintains its efficiency at the same time. As shown in Fig. 8.10b, more and more object instances are detected after each iteration.

Iterated MSL detects almost all true disks with a few false detections. A graph model is further used to remove false detections and assign a label to each disk by considering the anatomical constraint of the spine. Figure 8.11 shows a few examples of detected and labeled intervertebral disks in both MRI and CT. Experimental results based on 42 MR volumes show that the resulting system achieves superior accuracy, being also the fastest system of its kind in the literature. On average, the disks of a whole spine are detected in 11.5 s with 98.6 % sensitivity and 0.073 false positive detections per volume. An average position error of 2.4 mm and angular error of 3.9° are achieved. On the CT data a comparable sensitivity of 98.0 % with 0.267 false positives per volume is achieved.

Alternatively, the sample concentration problem can be solved by cluster analysis on the position candidates, as demonstrated for the detection of lymph nodes (Sect. 8.2.11) and ovarian follicles (Sect. 8.3.14).

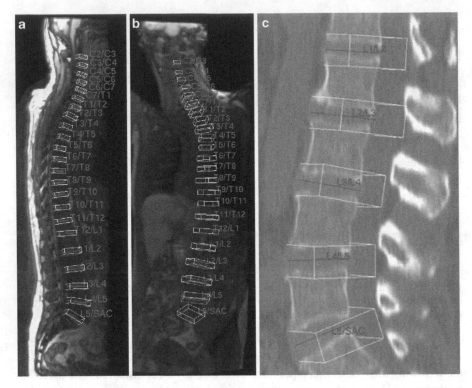

Fig. 8.11 Detected and labeled intervertebral disks. (**a**) MRI volume of a healthy subject. (**b**) MRI volume of a subject with a twisted spine. (**c**) CT volume of a lumbar spine. Image courtesy of Michael Kelm

Publications

- Kelm, B.M., Zhou, S.K., Suehling, M., Zheng, Y., Wels, M., Comaniciu, D.: Detection of 3D spinal geometry using iterated marginal space learning. In: *Proc. MICCAI Workshop Medical Computer Vision — Recognition Techniques and Applications in Medical Imaging*, pp. 96–105 (2010)
- Kelm, B.M., Wels, M., Zhou, S.K., Seifert, S., Suehling, M., Zheng, Y., Comaniciu, D.: Spine detection in CT and MR using iterated marginal space learning. *Medical Image Analysis* **17**(8), 1283–1292 (2013)

8.2.10 Osteolytic Spinal Bone Lesion Detection in CT

Wels et al. [59] presented an adapted MSL method for the detection of osteolytic spinal bone lesions in 3D CT. CT is an important imaging modality to detect and analyze spinal bone lesions, helping to quantify metastasis progression or response

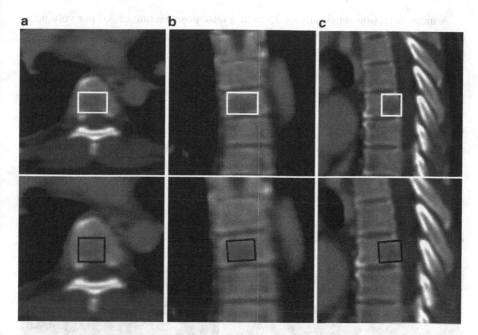

Fig. 8.12 Detection of an osteolytic spinal bone lesion in (**a**) axial, (**b**) coronal, and (**c**) sagittal views. The first row shows the ground-truth annotation in *white*. The second row shows the detection result in *black*. Image courtesy of Michael Wels. ©2012 SPIE. Reprinted, with permission, from Wels, M., Kelm, B.M., Tsymbal, A., Hammon, M., Soza, G., Suehling, M., Cavallero, A., Comaniciu, D.: Multi-stage osteolytic spinal bone lesion detection from CT data with internal sensitivity control. In: *Proc. of SPIE Medical Imaging*, vol. 8315, pp. 1–8 (2012)

to therapy over time. However, manual identification of spinal bone lesions from 3D CT data is a challenging and labor-intensive task even for experienced radiologists. The reading process is subject to intra- and inter-user variability. A computer aided detection system can improve sensitivity and reduce reading variability.

To reduce the false positive rate, the vertebral body is detected first to constrain the search for osteolytic spinal bone lesions. Furthermore, each vertebral body is normalized to a standard orientation to reduce the variations of the extracted image features for the following lesion detection. The vertebral body bounding box can be detected efficiently using MSL, although for evaluation of the lesion detection performance, a manually annotated bounding box is used in [59]. The orientation of a lesion is less important than the center and extension of the lesion; therefore, the adapted MSL detection pipeline has only two stages: position (center) estimation and position-scale estimation. Due to the large variations of a lesion in appearance and shape, the lesion center detector is further composed of three sequential classifiers trained with more and more descriptive (and also more computationally expensive) image features.

A mean detection sensitivity of 75 % at a false positive rate of 3.0 per volume is achieved, close to be clinically applicable for screening examinations. Figure 8.12 shows one exemplary detection result.

Publication

* Wels, M., Kelm, B.M., Tsymbal, A., Hammon, M., Soza, G., Suehling, M., Cavallero, A., Comaniciu, D.: Multi-stage osteolytic spinal bone lesion detection from CT data with internal sensitivity control. In: *Proc. of SPIE Medical Imaging*, vol. 8315, pp. 1–8 (2012)

8.2.11 Lymph Node Detection in CT

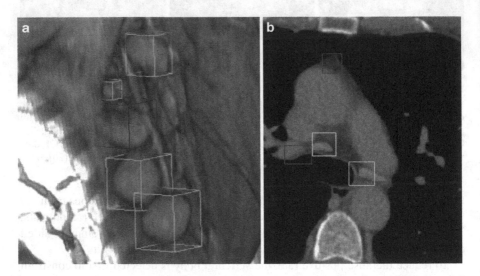

Fig. 8.13 Lymph node detection. (**a**) Axillary lymph nodes are marked with bounding boxes and labeled as solid (*light boxes*) and non-solid (*dark boxes*). Image courtesy of Adrian Barbu. (**b**) Detection results for mediastinal lymph nodes. Image courtesy of Johannes Feulner. ©2010 IEEE. Reprinted, with permission, from Feulner, J., Zhou, S.K., Huber, M., Hornegger, J., Comaniciu, D., Cavallaro, A.: Lymph node detection in 3-D chest CT using a spatial prior probability. In: *Proc. IEEE Conf. Computer Vision and Pattern Recognition*, pp. 2926–2932 (2010)

Lymph nodes play an important role in clinical practice. They routinely need to be considered during oncological examination, being related to multiple cancers, for instance lung cancer where metastases may settle in lymph nodes, but also lymphoma that is a cancer of the lymphatic system itself. However, lymph node detection is a challenging problem due to the similar intensity of the lymph nodes to the surrounding tissues and the large variation in shape and size of a lymph node. Feulner et al. [13, 16] presented an automatic lymph node detection method in the mediastinum. The bounding box of a lymph node was detected by using the MSL (Fig. 8.13). Since the orientation of a lymph node is of no interest and was ignored during detection, there were only two stages in the MSL pipeline, i.e., position detection and position-scale detection. Local and global spatial priors were integrated to prune the detected lymph nodes to further improve the detection accuracy.

Barbu et al. [1, 2] proposed a different method to detect the axillary lymph nodes. Similar to [16], the MSL was used to generate lymph node candidates. The region around a detected candidate was segmented and segmentation based features were extracted to enhance the detection. An extensive evaluation on 101 volumes containing 362 lymph nodes showed that this method obtained a 82.3 % detection rate at one false positive per volume, with a running time of 5–20 s per volume.

Publications

- Feulner, J., Zhou, S.K., Huber, M., Hornegger, J., Comaniciu, D., Cavallaro, A.: Lymph node detection in 3-D chest CT using a spatial prior probability. In: *Proc. IEEE Conf. Computer Vision and Pattern Recognition*, pp. 2926–2932 (2010)
- Feulner, J., Zhou, S.K., Hammon, M., Hornegger, J., Comaniciu, D.: Lymph node detection and segmentation in chest CT data using discriminative learning and a spatial prior. *Medical Image Analysis* **17**(2), 254–270 (2013)
- Barbu, A., Suehling, M., Xu, X., Liu, D., Zhou, S.K., Comaniciu, D.: Automatic detection and segmentation of axillary lymph nodes. In: *Proc. Int'l Conf. Medical Image Computing and Computer Assisted Intervention*, vol. 1, pp. 28–36 (2010)
- Barbu, A., Sü£¡hling, M., Xu, X., Liu, D., Zhou, S.K., Comaniciu, D.: Automatic detection and segmentation of lymph nodes from CT data. *IEEE Trans. Medical Imaging* **31**(2), 240–250 (2012)

8.2.12 *Ileocecal Valve Detection in CT*

The ileocecal valve is a muscle situated at the junction of the small intestine (ileum) and the large intestine (colon). Its main functionality is to restrict the movement of content from the colon back to the ileum. Automatic colon polyp detection and categorization is a prerequisite for computer-aided colon cancer diagnosis. Detection of the ileocecal valve can reduce the false positive detections generated from the small intestine. Nevertheless, the automatic detection of the ileocecal valve is challenging due to the large variations in its internal shape and appearance and variability of the surrounding tissue (Fig. 8.14).

Lu et al. [34] presented a method for ileocecal valve detection using the MSL. They achieved a detection rate of 94.4 % on a large diverse dataset and the computation time ranged from 4–10 s per volume, which was significantly faster than other published results.

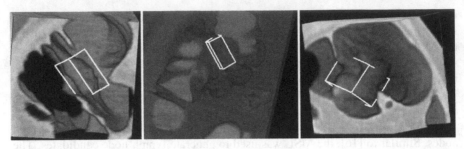

Fig. 8.14 Ileocecal valve detection results in three colonography CT volumes. Image courtesy of Le Lu

Publication

- Lu, L., Barbu, A., Wolf, M., Liang, J., Bogoni, L., Salganicoff, M., Comaniciu, D.: Simultaneous detection and registration for ileo-cecal valve detection in 3D CT colonography. In: *Proc. European Conf. Computer Vision*, pp. 465–478 (2008)

8.2.13   Aortic Valve Landmark Detection in C-arm CT

In [26, 77, 78], we presented an application of the MSL to aortic valve landmark detection and aorta segmentation in C-arm CT volumes to provide measurement and visual guidance for Transcatheter Aortic Valve Implantation (TAVI). The aorta segmentation is discussed in Sect. 8.3.6. Here we summarize the detection of eight aortic valve landmarks: three aortic hinge points, three aortic commissure points, and left and right coronary ostia (Fig. 8.15). These landmarks provide valuable 3D measurements for surgical planning, for instance, the distance between the coronary ostia and aortic hinge planes [26]. In addition, the detected aortic hinge points can guide the selection of a proper angulation of the C-arm system. Overlaying the detected landmarks onto 2D real time fluoroscopic images also provides critical visual guidance during the intervention. For example, the coronary ostia are particularly important for the proper positioning of the prosthetic valve to avoid blocking the blood flow to the coronary arteries after valve deployment.

We define a hierarchical approach by first detecting a global object composed of all eight valve landmarks. From the position, orientation, and scale of this global object, we can infer the rough position of individual landmarks. Each landmark is then refined in a small neighborhood, under the guidance of its own specific landmark detector. This is a similar approach to the one used to detect the five mid-sagittal plane landmarks in 3D MRI in Sect. 8.2.8. Again, the MSL contributes to efficiently detect the position, orientation, and scale of the global landmark object.

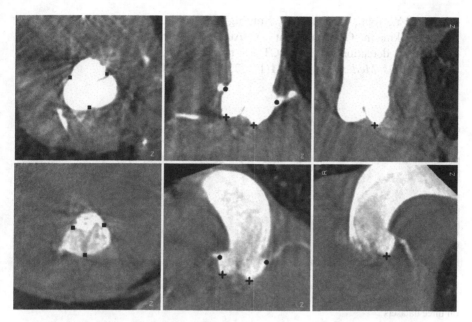

Fig. 8.15 Aortic valve landmark detection results on two example C-arm CT data with '*filled square*' for the commissures, '*plus*' for the hinges, and '*filled circle*' for the left and right coronary ostia. Each row shows three orthogonal cuts of a volume

A fourfold cross-validation is performed on 278 C-arm CT volumes for aortic valve landmark detection [78]. The landmark detection accuracy is measured using the Euclidean distance from the detected landmark to the ground truth. The mean errors are 2.09 mm for the aortic hinges, 2.07 mm for the coronary ostia, and 2.17 mm for the aortic commissure points. The detection of all eight aortic valve landmarks takes less than 0.5 s.

Publications

- Zheng, Y., John, M., Liao, R., Boese, J., Kirschstein, U., Georgescu, B., Zhou, S.K., Kempfert, J., Walther, T., Brockmann, G., Comaniciu, D.: Automatic aorta segmentation and valve landmark detection in C-arm CT: Application to aortic valve implantation. In: *Proc. Int'l Conf. Medical Image Computing and Computer Assisted Intervention*, vol. 1, pp. 476–483 (2010)
- John, M., Liao, R., Zheng, Y., Nottling, A., Boese, J., Kirschstein, U., Kempfert, J., Walther, T.: System to guide transcatheter aortic valve implantations based on interventional 3D C-arm CT imaging. In: *Proc. Int'l Conf. Medical Image Computing and Computer Assisted Intervention*, vol. 1, pp. 375–382 (2010)

- Zheng, Y., John, M., Liao, R., Nottling, A., Boese, J., Kempfert, J., Walther, T., Brockmann, G., Comaniciu, D.: Automatic aorta segmentation and valve landmark detection in C-arm CT for transcatheter aortic valve implantation. *IEEE Trans. Medical Imaging* **31**(12), 2307–2321 (2012)

8.2.14   Coronary Ostium Detection in CT

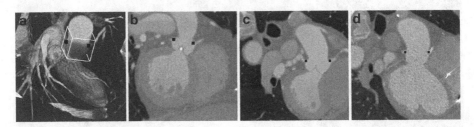

Fig. 8.16 Coronary ostium detection in CT angiography data. (**a**) Detected bounding box of the coronary ostia in a 3D volume visualization. (**b**)–(**d**) Coronary ostium detection results (*black dots*) on three datasets

Coronary stenosis (narrowing of the coronary artery) is the most common cardio-vascular disease. If the stenosis is too severe and medical therapy does not help, an artery or vein from elsewhere in the patient's body is often harvested and grafted to the coronary arteries to bypass the stenosis. Alternatively, a stent can be deployed via a catheter to open the blocked region. CT angiography is the primary imaging modality to diagnose coronary stenosis thanks to its superior image resolution. To facilitate the diagnosis, it is important to develop a robust system that can efficiently extract the coronary artery centerline, followed by vessel lumen segmentation, to provide quantification of the coronary stenosis (i.e., measuring the percentage of the lumen area blocked by plaques). Although various methods have been proposed for coronary artery segmentation, most of them rely on at least one user click to provide a seed point to initialize the centerline extraction. Since the coronary segmentation is a time consuming task, it is desirable to perform the segmentation automatically in a preprocessing step; therefore, when a physician starts the exam, the segmentation is readily available. Automatic detection of the coronary ostia creates the potential to make the whole workflow fully automatic, therefore increasing a physician's throughput.

Almost all previous methods on coronary ostium detection start with an explicit segmentation of the aorta. A coronary artery is detected as a tubular structure attached to the aorta and the position of the attachment is taken as the detected ostium. However, for Chronic Total Occlusion (CTO) patients, an artery originated from a coronary ostium may be completely obstructed thus not visible in a cardiac CT volume. Therefore, existing coronary ostium detection methods may be challenged. As an anatomical structure, the coronary ostium has strong constraints that facilitate the automatic detection. Even for CTO patients, the correct position of the ostium can still be inferred from the surrounding tissues.

Similar to the aortic valve landmarks in Sect. 8.2.13, coronary ostia are treated as a global object [81], detected using the MSL. The pose of the global object is defined in a special way so that the position of the coronary ostia can be easily inferred after box detection. As shown in Fig. 8.16a, a bounding box is defined as a cube with one side aligned with the direction connecting the left and right coronary ostia, and the second side aligned with the aortic root centerline. The coronary ostia are located at the centers of two opposite faces of the cube.

Different to the previous methods [22, 49, 55], no explicit aorta segmentation is necessary; therefore, our approach is efficient, taking a fraction of a second. Trained on 1,360 volumes, it is much more robust than the previously reported approaches. Based on a fourfold cross-validation, the Euclidean distance from the detected left coronary ostium to the corresponding ground truth has a mean of 1.66 mm (standard deviation of 1.15 mm) and a median of 1.45 mm. The corresponding errors of the right coronary ostium are 1.73 mm for the mean (standard deviation of 1.71 mm) and 1.31 mm for the median. Only about 0.8 % of datasets have a detection error larger than 5 mm (which is approximately the diameter of the coronary arteries around the ostia) and are treated as failures. Figure 8.16 shows examples of the detected coronary ostia.

Publication

- Zheng, Y., Tek, H., Funka-Lea, G., Zhou, S.K., Vega-Higuera, F., Comaniciu, D.: Efficient detection of native and bypass coronary ostia in cardiac CT volumes: Anatomical vs. pathological structures. In: *Proc. Int'l Conf. Medical Image Computing and Computer Assisted Intervention*, vol. 3, pp. 403–410 (2011)

8.2.15 Rib Detection in CT

It is tedious and time-consuming to find rib metastases and fractures in chest CT scans. Due to the curved shape of a rib, a physician typically needs to read hundreds of axial CT slices to visually track changes in rib cross-section area. Since a person has 24 ribs, a physician needs to go through the CT slices many times, often focusing on one rib at a time, especially when the rib anomalies are small. Unfolding a cursive 3D structure into one 2D image (as shown in Fig. 8.17) makes routine bone reading tasks much more efficient and effective for the radiologists.

To generate such an unfolded view, the rib centerlines have to be extracted. Wu et al. [61] proposed an efficient method to extract rib centerlines by fitting an articulated rib cage model to a chest CT scan. First, the ribs are enhanced using a classifier that can estimate a probability of a voxel to be inside ribs. The articulated rib cage model is then deformed to fit the probability map so that an objective function is maximized. Each rib is decomposed into four segments, each segment being subject to anisotropic similarity transformation, with nine degrees

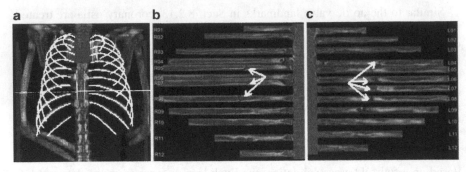

Fig. 8.17 Rib centerline extraction in CT. (**a**) 3D visualization of the extracted centerlines. (**b**) and (**c**) are unfolded ribs of the left and right cage, respectively. The *arrows* indicate fractures, which are clearly visible on the unfolded views. Image courtesy of Dijia Wu. ©2012 IEEE. Reprinted, with permission, from Wu, D., Liu, D., Puskas, Z., Lu, C., Wimmer, A., Tietjen, C., Soza, G., Zhou, S.K.: A learning based deformable template matching method for automatic rib centerline extraction and labeling in CT images. In: *Proc. IEEE Conf. Computer Vision and Pattern Recognition*, pp. 980–987 (2012)

of freedom. The MSL principle is exploited to efficiently search the pose space. Different to other MSL applications, there are no object pose classifiers in this work. A predefined objective function serves as a classifier to assign a score to each pose hypothesis. Since all rib centerlines are extracted simultaneously with a top-down fitting of an articulated rib cage model, this approach is robust to the presence of rib anomalies. Another advantage is that all ribs are already properly labeled after centerline extraction.

Publication

- Wu, D., Liu, D., Puskas, Z., Lu, C., Wimmer, A., Tietjen, C., Soza, G., Zhou, S.K.: A learning based deformable template matching method for automatic rib centerline extraction and labeling in CT images. In: *Proc. IEEE Conf. Computer Vision and Pattern Recognition*, pp. 980–987 (2012)

8.2.16 Standard Echocardiographic Plane Detection in 3D Ultrasound

Three-dimensional echocardiography is an emerging real-time imaging modality, increasingly used in clinical practice to assess cardiac function. It provides a more detailed heart representation in comparison to conventional 2D echocardiography. However, interpretation and quantitative analysis of the 3D volumetric data is more complex and time consuming than for conventional 2D echocardiography.

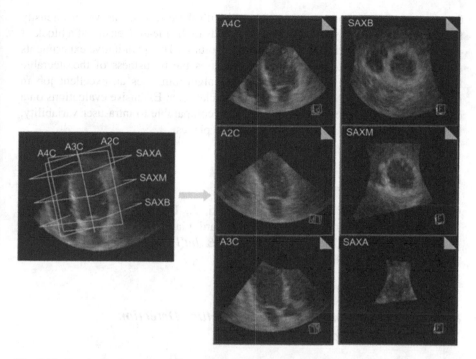

Fig. 8.18 Standard echocardiographic planes in a 3D ultrasound volume. Image courtesy of Xiaoguang Lu. ©2008 IEEE. Reprinted, with permission, from Lu, X., Georgescu, B., Zheng, Y., Otsuki, J., Bennett, R., Comaniciu, D.: AutoMPR: Automatic detection of standard planes from three dimensional echocardiographic data. In: *Proc. IEEE Int'l Sym. Biomedical Imaging*, pp. 1279–1282 (2008)

Standard views are often used to visualize the cardiac structures, being the starting point of many echocardiographic examinations. In a 3D volume, such views can be reconstructed as Multi-Planar Reformatted/Reconstruction (MPR) planes. Finding the standard 2D planes in a 3D volume can help improving the consistency among users and can be used to adjust the on-line acquisition parameters for a better image quality. As shown in Fig. 8.18, we are particularly interested in detecting the following standard views, apical four chamber view (A4C), apical two chamber view (A2C), apical three chamber view (A3C), and short axis views at basal (SAXB), middle (SAXM), and apex (SAXA) levels. Although a geometric plane has no size, we prefer to associate size to each standard plane using the target anatomy, i.e., the left ventricle; therefore, the automatically detected plane can be zoomed properly on the MPR view.

In [38], the MSL is used to detect these standard planes, as one of the first applications of the MSL to ultrasound data. Before the experiments, there was a concern on the robustness of steerable features which are composed of a set of local features (e.g., voxel intensity and gradient at a sampling point). Such local features have large variations on noisy ultrasound data. To increase their stability, we extract the steerable features on a volume pyramid with three levels. The voxel intensity feature at the coarsest pyramid level corresponds to the mean intensity of a block of $4 \times 4 \times 4$ voxels in the original high resolution volume. The quantitative experiments show that the pyramid based approach increases the robustness of the steerable features. Furthermore, the boosting learning algorithm does an excellent job in integrating the weak features to build a strong classifier. Extensive evaluations on a database of 326 volumes show a performance comparable to intra-user variability. It only takes about 2 s to detect all six standard planes.

Publication

- Lu, X., Georgescu, B., Zheng, Y., Otsuki, J., Bennett, R., Comaniciu, D.: AutoMPR: Automatic detection of standard planes from three dimensional echocardiographic data. In: *Proc. IEEE Int'l Sym. Biomedical Imaging*, pp. 1279–1282 (2008)

8.2.17 Fetal Brain Anatomical Structure Detection in 3D Ultrasound

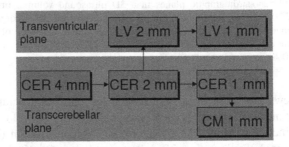

Fig. 8.19 The detection order and hierarchy of three brain structures: Cerebellum (CER), Cisterna Magna (CM), and Lateral Ventricles (LV). Image courtesy of Michal Sofka. ©2010 IEEE. Reprinted, with permission, from Sofka, M., Zhang, J., Zhou, S.K., Comaniciu, D.: Multiple object detection by sequential Monte Carlo and hierarchical detection network. In: *Proc. IEEE Conf. Computer Vision and Pattern Recognition*, pp. 1735–1742 (2010)

In [48], Sofka et al. presents a nice extension of MSL, namely Hierarchical Detection Network (HDN) (a.k.a. hierarchical MSL), where detectors are trained on multiple resolutions on an image pyramid and aggregated to achieve a robust detection. A larger object context is considered at a coarser image resolution resulting in robustness against noise, occlusions, and missing data. High detection accuracy is achieved by focusing the search in a smaller neighborhood at finer resolutions.

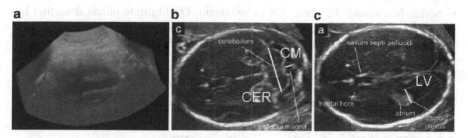

Fig. 8.20 Fetal brain anatomical structure detection in ultrasound. (**a**) A 3D volume. (**b**) and (**c**) Detection results of three brain structures: Cerebellum (CER), Cisterna Magna (CM), and Lateral Ventricle (LV). Image courtesy of Michal Sofka. ©2010 IEEE. Reprinted, with permission, from Sofka, M., Zhang, J., Zhou, S.K., Comaniciu, D.: Multiple object detection by sequential Monte Carlo and hierarchical detection network. In: *Proc. IEEE Conf. Computer Vision and Pattern Recognition*, pp. 1735–1742 (2010)

HDN has been demonstrated on several applications and the most challenging one is the detection of fetal brain anatomical structures, including cerebellum, cisterna magna, and lateral ventricle, in a 3D ultrasound volume (Fig. 8.20). Due to the small physical size of the structures and the noise in the ultrasound image, it is hard to detect those structures reliably [4]. This is the major motivation for the development of HDN.

A greedy search strategy is used by HDN to determine the detection order of multiple objects across the image pyramid. The most reliable object is detected first. The next object selected for detection is the one contributing to the largest reduction in ambiguity. For example, Fig. 8.19 shows the selected detection network for fetal brain structures. The pose of cerebellum is detected at 4-mm resolution. The detected pose candidates are propagated to 2-mm resolution and refined within a proper searching range. The cerebellum pose is further refined at 1-mm resolution to obtain the final detection result. Furthermore, the detected cerebellum at 2-mm resolution is exploited to predict the pose of the lateral ventricle at the same resolution. The lateral ventricle pose is further refined at 1-mm resolution. The cisterna magna only needs to be detected once at 1-mm resolution, given an initial prediction based on the cerebellum. This network structure is determined automatically using the greedy search strategy. Even though it may not generate a global optimum solution, its performance is much better than an arbitrarily selected detection order.

Publications

- Carneiro, G., Amat, F., Georgescu, B., Good, S., Comaniciu, D.: Semantic-based indexing of fetal anatomies from 3-D ultrasound data using global/semi-local context and sequential sampling. In: *Proc. IEEE Conf. Computer Vision and Pattern Recognition*, pp. 1–8 (2008)

- Sofka, M., Zhang, J., Zhou, S.K., Comaniciu, D.: Multiple object detection by sequential Monte Carlo and hierarchical detection network. In: *Proc. IEEE Conf. Computer Vision and Pattern Recognition*, pp. 1735–1742 (2010)

8.3 Detection and Segmentation of Anatomical Structures

8.3.1 Heart Chamber Segmentation in CT

This application relies on a four-chamber heart model and is the first one for which the MSL based object detection and segmentation was developed [69, 71]. The segmentation is formulated as a two-step learning problem: anatomical structure localization and boundary delineation. After determining the pose of the heart chambers, we estimate the 3D shape through learning-based boundary delineation (Fig. 8.21).

The method has been tested on the largest dataset (with 323 volumes from 137 patients) reported in the literature. The resulting system is the fastest, with a speed of 4.0 s per volume (on a dual-core 3.2 GHz processor) for automatic segmentation of all four chambers. We achieve the state-of-the-art segmentation errors, ranging from 1.13 to 1.57 mm for different chambers. The Left Ventricle (LV) endocardium segmentation error can be further reduced to 0.84 mm using an optimal smooth surface to tightly enclose the whole LV blood pool extracted using an adaptive thresholding [74].

LV detection is also one of the applications for which we proposed and tested constrained MSL [73]. The natural constraints in all three marginal spaces (translation, rotation, and scaling marginal spaces) are automatically learned from the training set and used during detection to further improve the MSL efficiency.

The heart chamber segmentation module has been integrated into a full body CT segmentation system [46]. Although the original module was trained on contrasted cardiac CT volumes (capturing only the region around the heart), it works very well on full body CT datasets.

Publications

- Zheng, Y., Barbu, A., Georgescu, B., Scheuering, M., Comaniciu, D.: Fast automatic heart chamber segmentation from 3D CT data using marginal space learning and steerable features. In: *Proc. Int'l Conf. Computer Vision*, pp. 1–8 (2007)
- Zheng, Y., Georgescu, B., Barbu, A., Scheuering, M., Comaniciu, D.: Four-chamber heart modeling and automatic segmentation for 3D cardiac CT volumes. In: *Proc. of SPIE Medical Imaging*, vol. 6914, pp. 1–12 (2008)

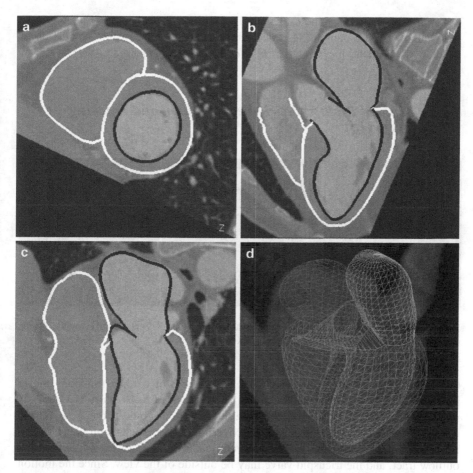

Fig. 8.21 Segmentation of all four heart chambers in a CT volume, including the left ventricle endocardial and epicardial surfaces, left atrium, right ventricle, and right atrium. (**a**)–(**c**) are three orthogonal cuts of the volume and (**d**) is a 3D visualization of the segmented heart mesh model

- Zheng, Y., Barbu, A., Georgescu, B., Scheuering, M., Comaniciu, D.: Four-chamber heart modeling and automatic segmentation for 3D cardiac CT volumes using marginal space learning and steerable features. *IEEE Trans. Medical Imaging* **27**(11), 1668–1681 (2008)
- Zheng, Y., Georgescu, B., Vega-Higuera, F., Comaniciu, D.: Left ventricle endocardium segmentation for cardiac CT volumes using an optimal smooth surface. In: *Proc. of SPIE Medical Imaging*, vol. 7259, pp. 1–11 (2009)
- Zheng, Y., Georgescu, B., Ling, H., Zhou, S.K., Scheuering, M., Comaniciu, D.: Constrained marginal space learning for efficient 3D anatomical structure detection in medical images. In: *Proc. IEEE Conf. Computer Vision and Pattern Recognition*, pp. 194–201 (2009)

- Seifert, S., Barbu, A., Zhou, K., Liu, D., Feulner, J., Huber, M., Suehling, M., Cavallaro, A., Comaniciu, D.: Hierarchical parsing and semantic navigation of full body CT data. In: *Proc. of SPIE Medical Imaging*, pp. 1–8 (2009)

8.3.2 Left and Right Ventricle Segmentation and Tracking in 3D MRI

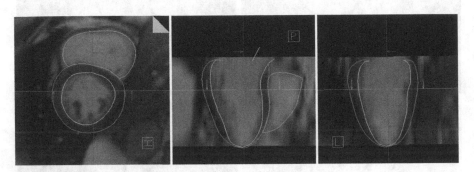

Fig. 8.22 Automatic segmentation of the left and right ventricles in an MRI volume. Three orthogonal views are shown. Image courtesy of Xiaoguang Lu

Cardiac MRI is a main modality for the assessment of cardiac function, due to its good soft-tissue discrimination capability. A stack of 8–10 short-axis slices is scanned. In a typical acquisition, the slice field of view is quite large, however the extension along the long axis is limited, covering only the Left Ventricle (LV) and Right Ventricle (RV). A part of the left ventricular outflow tract, right ventricular outflow tract, and the tricuspid valve may be outside of the view. Since the motion of the LV and RV is highly correlated, Lu et al. [40] proposed to segment them using a joint ventricular model. The ventricles are segmented using the MSL in the first frame, then, their motion is tracked in a cine sequence. Figure 8.22 shows the segmented LV and RV in an MRI volume.

Automatic LV segmentation has applications not only for the cardiac function analysis, but also for automatic view planning for cardiac MRI acquisition. The conventional cardiac MRI acquisition needs to be aligned to a few standard cardiac views, e.g., the short-axis view and various long-axis views (e.g., two-, three-, and four-chamber views). A typical protocol involves sequential acquisition of quite a few localizer volumes. The operator needs to have detailed knowledge of the heart to plan the views at every step, while the patient is in the scanner.

Lu et al. [39] proposed a fully automatic algorithm to prescribe short-axis stack and standard long-axis views from a single low-resolution 3D MRI acquisition. The 3D localizer MRI acquisition results in a low resolution volume (e.g., a typical resolution of $1.6 \times 2 \times 5$ mm^3). The LV is then automatically detected and segmented using the MSL. High-resolution acquisition of the short-axis stack can then be planned. To prescribe the long-axis views, the RV should be detected and segmented too. Alternatively, the anterior and inferior RV insertion points can be detected on a mid-ventricular short-axis slice. Different long-axis views (including two-, three-, and four-chamber views) can then be prescribed using the RV insertion points and LV blood pool center. The entire view planning is fully automatic and takes less than 10 s.

Publications

- Lu, X., Wang, Y., Georgescu, B., Littmann, A., Comaniciu, D.: Automatic delineation of left and right ventricles in cardiac MRI sequences using a joint ventricular model. In: *Proc. Functional Imaging and Modeling of the Heart*, pp. 250–258 (2011)
- Lu, X., Jolly, M.P., Georgescu, B., Hayes, C., Speier, P., Schmidt, M., Bi, X., Kroeker, R., Comaniciu, D., Kellman, P., Mueller, E., Guehring, J.: Automatic view planning for cardiac MRI acquisition. In: *Proc. Int'l Conf. Medical Image Computing and Computer Assisted Intervention*, pp. 479–486 (2011)

8.3.3 Left Ventricle Segmentation and Tracking in 3D Ultrasound

This application detects, segments, and tracks the Left Ventricle (LV) endocardium in a 3D ultrasound volume sequence (Fig. 8.23) [65–67]. It is related to the automatic detection of standard echocardiographic views in 3D ultrasound, as discussed in Sect. 8.2.16.

The tracking module combines the tracking-by-detection and optical flow methods to achieve both failure recovery capability and temporal consistency. We first build a cardiac motion model on a manifold and use the model to provide one-step forward prediction to generate the motion prior. The MSL based detection module also provides robust tracking-by-detection result, which is generated by performing LV detection/segmentation around the predicted position. Tracking-by-detection is robust and can recover from failures; however, the motion consistency is not preserved. Therefore, we also exploit a robust 3D optical flow module, which enforces the motion coherence.

Compared to each individual tracking method, the combined approach achieves the best result with sub-voxel accuracy. The resulting tracking algorithm is completely automatic and computationally efficient. It requires less than 1.5 s to process a 3D volume, which contains 4,925,440 voxels.

The work can be extended to segment and track the LV epicardium and myocardium [58]. Once the motion of the myocardium (enclosed between the endocardium and epicardium surfaces) is tracked accurately, multiple clinically

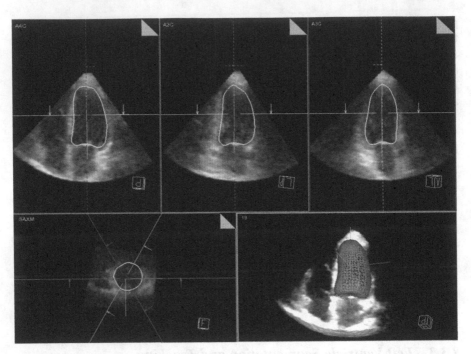

Fig. 8.23 The four canonical views and 3D representations of the left ventricle segmentation result in an ultrasound volume. Image courtesy of Lin Yang. ©2008 IEEE. Reprinted, with permission, from Yang, L., Georgescu, B., Zheng, Y., Meer, P., Comaniciu, D.: 3D ultrasound tracking of the left ventricles using one-step forward prediction and data fusion of collaborative trackers. In: *Proc. IEEE Conf. Computer Vision and Pattern Recognition*, pp. 1–8 (2008)

relevant cardiac function measurements can be calculated, such as the strain and stress of the myocardium, wall thickness, and myocardium regional viability.

Publications

- Yang, L., Georgescu, B., Zheng, Y., Foran, D.J., Comaniciu, D.: A fast and accurate tracking algorithm of left ventricles in 3D echocardiography. In: *Proc. IEEE Int'l Sym. Biomedical Imaging*, pp. 221–224 (2008)
- Yang, L., Georgescu, B., Zheng, Y., Meer, P., Comaniciu, D.: 3D ultrasound tracking of the left ventricles using one-step forward prediction and data fusion of collaborative trackers. In: *Proc. IEEE Conf. Computer Vision and Pattern Recognition*, pp. 1–8 (2008)
- Yang, L., Georgescu, B., Zheng, Y., Wang, Y., Meer, P., Comaniciu, D.: Prediction based collaborative trackers (PCT): A robust and accurate approach toward 3D medical object tracking. *IEEE Trans. Medical Imaging* **30**(11), 1921–1932 (2011)

- Wang, Y., Georgescu, B., Comaniciu, D., Houle, H.: Learning-based 3D myocardial motion flow estimation using high frame rate volumetric ultrasound data. *In: Proc. IEEE Int'l Sym. Biomedical Imaging*, pp. 1097–1100 (2010)

8.3.4 Whole-Heart Segmentation in CT

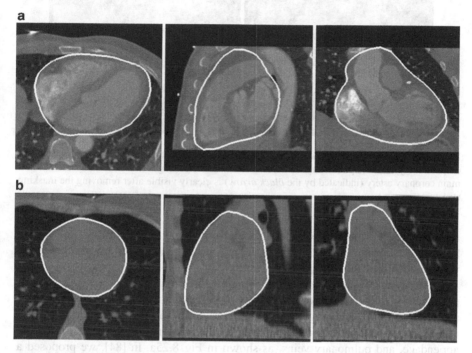

Fig. 8.24 Whole-heart segmentation for (**a**) contrasted and (**b**) non-contrasted CT scans. From left to right: transaxial, sagittal, and coronal views

Segmenting the heart as a whole from CT data, also called heart isolation [17], has clinical value in several applications, e.g., 3D volume visualization of coronary arteries, radiotherapy planning, and automatic calculation of the calcium score. The whole heart segmentation reported in [75] exploits the efficiency of the MSL, being designed for both contrasted and non-contrasted CT scans (Fig. 8.24). To handle the challenges caused by large shape variations and weak image boundary, an optimal mean shape is calculated from the training set to improve the shape initialization accuracy.

The method has been quantitatively evaluated on 589 volumes from 288 patients (including 485 contrasted and 104 non-contrasted volumes). We achieve a mean mesh segmentation error of 1.75 mm for contrasted data and 2.10 mm for non-contrasted data. For the application on coronary artery visualization, the sternum

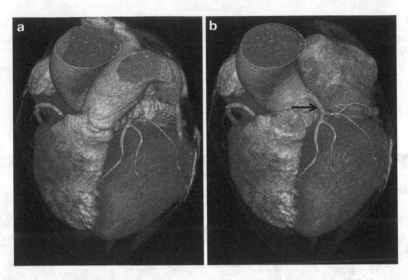

Fig. 8.25 3D volume visualization of the whole-heart segmentation results. (**a**) Before removal of pulmonary arteries, pulmonary veins, and left atrial appendage. (**b**) After removal. The left main coronary artery (indicated by the *black arrow*) is clearly visible after removing the masking structures

and rib cage are explicitly excluded in a post-processing step to further improve the boundary delineation accuracy. On average, our approach takes 1.5 s to process a volume, including the post-processing step.

A 3D volume visualization of the segmented heart provides an intuitive way for physicians to diagnose the coronary artery disease. Although most coronary arteries are clearly visible after segmenting the heart from surrounding tissues, the left main coronary artery may be still blocked by the pulmonary artery trunk, left atrial appendage, and pulmonary veins, as shown in Fig. 8.25a. In [84], we proposed a method to further segment and remove those extra structures. The pulmonary artery trunk and left atrial appendage are segmented using the MSL and then removed from the volume. Due to the limited field of view, the proximal left and right pulmonary arteries are often only partially present. Without a consistent presentation, the left and right pulmonary arteries are segmented using controlled region growing from the segmented pulmonary artery trunk. Similarly, controlled region growing is also used to segment the pulmonary veins starting from the segmented left atrium chamber body. For visualization purpose, the segmentation accuracy on critical regions needs to have a voxel-level accuracy. The segmentation is carefully refined to achieve a clean visualization without cutting the coronary arteries and bypass arteries, as shown in Fig. 8.25.

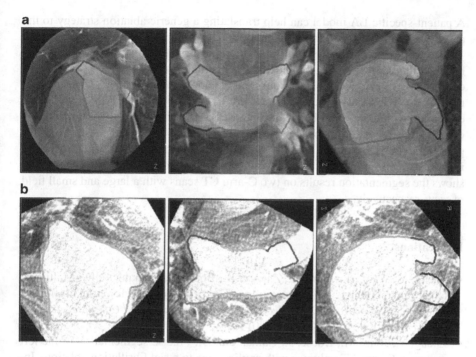

Fig. 8.26 The segmentation of left atrium chamber body, left atrial appendage, and pulmonary veins on (**a**) a large volume and (**b**) a small volume. Three orthogonal views are shown for each volume

Publications

- Zheng, Y., Georgescu, B., Vega-Higuera, F., Zhou, S.K., Comaniciu, D.: Fast and automatic heart isolation in 3D CT volumes: Optimal shape initialization. In: *Proc. MICCAI Workshop on Machine Learning in Medical Imaging*, pp. 84–91 (2010)
- Zhong, H., Zheng, Y., Funka-Lea, G., Vega-Higuera, F.: Segmentation and removal of pulmonary arteries, veins and left atrial appendage for visualizing coronary and bypass arteries. In: *Proc. Workshop on Medical Computer Vision* (In conjunction with CVPR), pp. 24–30 (2012)

8.3.5 Segmentation of Left Atrium, Pulmonary Vein, and Left Atrial Appendage in C-arm CT

Automatic segmentation of the Left Atrium (LA), left atrial appendage, and Pulmonary Veins (PV) has important applications in pre-operative assessment and intra-operative guidance for the catheter based ablation to treat atrial fibrillation.

A patient-specific LA model can help translating a generic ablation strategy to the patient's specific anatomy, thus making the ablation more effective for each patient.

Due to the large variations in the PV drainage patterns, we developed a part-based method to handle the complexity of the structures about the LA [82, 83]. We define six parts, namely, the left atrium chamber body, left atrial appendage, and four major PVs. Statistical shape constraints are enforced during the MSL based pose estimation to improve the detection robustness. After detection and segmentation of all parts, we merge them together to generate a consolidated mesh [76]. The potential extra right middle PVs are extracted using graph cuts inside a region of interest defined by the two already segmented RIPV and RSPV [64]. Figure 8.26 shows the segmentation results on two C-arm CT scans with a large and small field of view, respectively.

Publications

- Zheng, Y., Wang, T., John, M., Zhou, S.K., Boese, J., Comaniciu, D.: Multi-part left atrium modeling and segmentation in C-arm CT volumes for atrial fibrillation ablation. In: *Proc. Int'l Conf. Medical Image Computing and Computer Assisted Intervention*, vol. 3, pp. 487–495 (2011)
- Zheng, Y., John, M., Boese, J., Comaniciu, D.: Precise segmentation of the left atrium in C-arm CT volumes with applications to atrial fibrillation ablation. In: *Proc. IEEE Int'l Sym. Biomedical Imaging*, pp. 1421–1424 (2012)
- Yang, D., Zheng, Y., John, M.: Graph cuts based left atrium segmentation refinement and right middle pulmonary vein extraction in C-arm CT. In: *Proc. of SPIE Medical Imaging*, pp. 1–9 (2013)
- Zheng, Y., Yang, D., John, M.: Multi-part modeling and segmentation of left atrium in C-arm CT for image-guided ablation of atrial fibrillation. *IEEE Trans. Medical Imaging*, (2014) In Press

8.3.6 Aorta Segmentation in CT/C-arm CT

Segmentation of the aorta with a focus on the aortic root plays an important role in pre-operative intervention planning and intra-operative visual guidance for Transcatheter Aortic Valve Implantation (TAVI). For instance, the size of the aortic annulus needs to be measured accurately to properly size a prosthetic valve.

This work is related to the aortic valve landmark detection as presented in Sect. 8.2.13. In [77, 78], we described a part-based aorta segmentation, which can handle structural variations in case the aortic arch and descending aorta are missing in the volume. The whole aorta model is split into four parts: aortic root, ascending aorta, aortic arch, and descending aorta. Discriminative learning is applied to separately train a detector for each part, exploiting the domain knowledge embedded in an expert-annotated dataset. Compared to cardiac CT, the C-arm CT

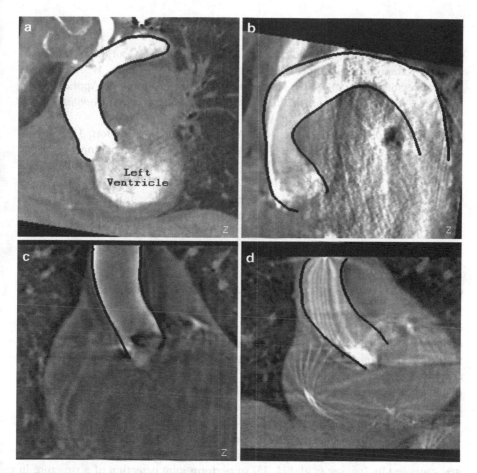

Fig. 8.27 Automatic aorta segmentation in C-arm CT on a few example volumes. (**a**) Good contrast, however, with severe valve regurgitation. (**b**) Fair image quality. (**c**) Contrast agent is almost washed out due to bad timing of the C-arm CT scan. (**d**) Streak artifacts generated by catheters

data generally have much lower image quality (also larger variations) as shown in Fig. 8.27. However, our system works well on such challenging and heterogeneous datasets.

A fourfold cross-validation is performed on 319 C-arm CT volumes from 276 patients [78]. The mean segmentation error of the aorta is 1.08 mm, with a standard deviation of 0.56 mm, while the entire detection/segmentation procedure takes around 0.8 s.

A similar technique can be used to detect, segment, and track the ascending aorta in cardiac CT volume sequences [19].

Publications

* Zheng, Y., John, M., Liao, R., Boese, J., Kirschstein, U., Georgescu, B., Zhou, S.K., Kempfert, J., Walther, T., Brockmann, G., Comaniciu, D.: Automatic aorta segmentation and valve landmark detection in C-arm CT: Application to aortic valve implantation. In: *Proc. Int'l Conf. Medical Image Computing and Computer Assisted Intervention*, vol. 1, pp. 476–483 (2010)
* Zheng, Y., John, M., Liao, R., Nottling, A., Boese, J., Kempfert, J., Walther, T., Brockmann, G., Comaniciu, D.: Automatic aorta segmentation and valve landmark detection in C-arm CT for transcatheter aortic valve implantation. *IEEE Trans. Medical Imaging* **31**(12), 2307–2321 (2012)
* Grbic, S., Ionasec, R.I., Zheng, Y., Zaeuner, D., Georgescu, B., Comaniciu, D.: Aortic valve and ascending aortic root modeling from 3D and 3D+t CT. In: *Proc. of SPIE Medical Imaging*, pp. 1–8 (2010)

8.3.7 Heart Valve Segmentation in 3D Ultrasound and CT

The characterization of the function of valve leaflets plays an important role for the diagnosis of the valve disease, such as valve stenosis, regurgitation, or congenital malformations. Ionasec et al. [23] presented a detailed physiological model of the aortic valve, where the MSL provided the valve pose estimate and a learning based boundary detector was used to guide the boundary refinement. The heart contains four valves and the same technique can be extended to model and segment the mitral valve [24,54], pulmonary valve, and tricuspid valve [18] (Figs. 8.28 and 8.29).

A 3D dynamic sequence (3D+t) is often captured to analyze the motion of a heart valve. Joint spatio-temporal MSL, also called trajectory spectrum learning, was proposed by Ionasec et al. [24,25] to perform joint detection of a structure in the whole sequence simultaneously. Unlike the independent detection method, the temporal context of the anatomy is also considered, and, unlike the tracking method, all frames are treated equally. Exploiting the periodicity of the valve motion, Fourier analysis is performed on the trajectory of a 3D landmark point and a few low frequency components are retained to compactly represent the landmark's trajectory. This is similar to nonrigid MSL [72], where we use the statistical shape model to concentrate the shape variations to a few major deformation modes. Similarly to nonrigid MSL, the steerable features framework is extended to capture the motion information in the spatio-temporal MSL. Refer to [24,25] for more details.

Publications

* Ionasec, R.I., Georgescu, B., Gassner, E., Vogt, S., Kutter, O., Scheuering, M., Navab, N., Comaniciu, D.: Dynamic model-driven quantitative and visual

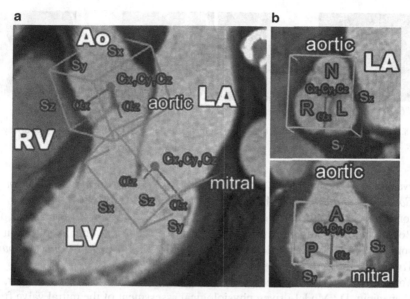

Fig. 8.28 Bounding boxes for aortic and mitral valves encoding their individual translation (c_x, c_y, c_z), rotation $(\bar{\alpha}_x, \bar{\alpha}_y, \bar{\alpha}_z)$ and scale (s_x, s_y, s_z). (**a**) Three chamber view, (**b**) aortic and mitral valves seen from the aorta and left atrium respectively, towards the LV. The letters L, R, and N indicate the left, right, and non-coronary aortic leaflets, respectively. Similarly, the letters A and P indicate the anterior and posterior mitral leaflets, respectively. Image courtesy of Razvan Ionasec. ©2010 IEEE. Reprinted, with permission, from Ionasec, R.I., Voigt, I., Georgescu, B., Wang, Y., Houle, H., Vega-Higuera, F., Navab, N., Comaniciu, D.: Patient-specific modeling and quantification of the aortic and mitral valves from 4D cardiac CT and TEE. *IEEE Trans. Medical Imaging* **29**(9), 1636–1651 (2010)

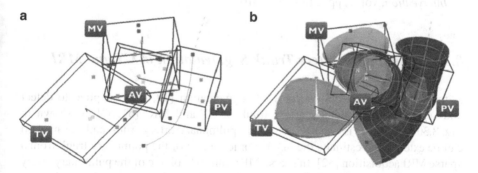

Fig. 8.29 A complete model for heart valves consisting of Aortic Valve (AV), Mitral Valve (MV), Pulmonary Valve (PV), and Tricuspid Valve (TV). (**a**) Estimated similarity transformation illustrated as a bounding box, together with anatomical landmarks. (**b**) Complete mesh surface model. Image courtesy of Sasa Grbic

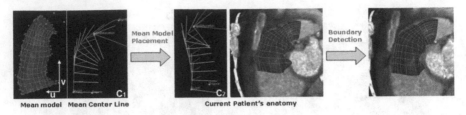

Fig. 8.30 Pulmonary artery trunk detection/segmentation in a CT volume. Image courtesy of Dime Vitanovski

evaluation of the aortic valve from 4D CT. In: *Proc. Int'l Conf. Medical Image Computing and Computer Assisted Intervention*, vol. 1, pp. 686–694 (2008)

- Ionasec, R.I., Wang, Y., Georgescu, B., Voigt, I., Navab, N., Comaniciu, D.: Robust motion estimation using trajectory spectrum learning: Application to aortic and mitral valve modeling from 4D TEE. In: *Proc. Int'l Conf. Computer Vision*, pp. 1601–1608 (2009)
- Voigt, I., Ionasec, R.I., Georgescu, B., Houle, H., Huber, M., Hornegger, J., Comaniciu, D.: Model-driven physiological assessment of the mitral valve from 4D TEE. In: *Proc. of SPIE Medical Imaging*, pp. 1–11 (2009)
- Ionasec, R.I., Voigt, I., Georgescu, B., Wang, Y., Houle, H., Vega-Higuera, F., Navab, N., Comaniciu, D.: Patient-specific modeling and quantification of the aortic and mitral valves from 4D cardiac CT and TEE. *IEEE Trans. Medical Imaging* **29**(9), 1636–1651 (2010)
- Grbic, S., Ionasec, R., Vitanovski, D., Voigt, I., Wang, Y., Georgescu, B., Navab, N., Comaniciu, D.: Complete valvular heart apparatus model from 4D cardiac CT. In: *Proc. Int'l Conf. Medical Image Computing and Computer Assisted Intervention*, vol. 1, pp. 218–226 (2010)

8.3.8 Pulmonary Artery Trunk Segmentation in CT and MRI

A technique similar to the aortic root segmentation [19, 77] is applied to detect and segment the pulmonary artery trunk in CT and MRI [51, 53], as shown in Fig. 8.30. The MSL is used to detect the pulmonary artery trunk and the method can be extended to estimate the 4D dynamic motion of the pulmonary trunk from a sparse MRI acquisition [52]. In sparse MRI, one 3D volume of the pulmonary artery trunk at the end-diastolic phase is captured, together with two dynamic acquisitions of the 2D long axis and short axis views. Since the 3D information is only available from the end-diastolic phase and temporal information is only available from two 2D views, it is not straightforward to recover the full 3D dynamics of the pulmonary artery trunk. In [52], during the training phase, 3D dynamic CT data are also scanned and the intrinsic distance function mapping sparse MRI to CT is learned. During the detection phase, the learned distance measurement is used to predict the full dynamics from sparse MRI.

For coronary artery analysis using cardiac CT, the whole heart is often segmented from the surrounding tissue to generate a 3D volume visualization of the coronary arteries (refer to Sect. 8.3.4). However, the visualization of the left main coronary artery may be blocked by the pulmonary arteries, pulmonary veins, and left atrial appendage. In addition to removing pulmonary veins and left atrial appendage, in [84], the pulmonary artery trunk together with the proximal left and right pulmonary arteries are segmented using the MSL and then removed from the volume so that the left main coronary artery is clearly visible on the 3D volume visualization (see Fig. 8.24).

Publications

- Vitanovski, D., Ionasec, R.I., Georgescu, B., Huber, M., Taylor, A.M., Hornegger, J., Comaniciu, D.: Personalized pulmonary trunk modeling for intervention planning and valve assessment estimated from CT data. In: *Proc. Int'l Conf. Medical Image Computing and Computer Assisted Intervention*, vol. 1, pp. 17–25 (2009)
- Vitanovski, D., Tsymbal, A., Ionasec, R.I., Georgescu, B., Huber, M., Taylor, A., Schievano, S., Zhou, S.K., Hornegger, J., Comaniciu, D.: Cross-modality assessment and planning for pulmonary trunk treatment using CT and MRI imaging. In: *Proc. Int'l Conf. Medical Image Computing and Computer Assisted Intervention*, vol. 1, pp. 460–467 (2010)
- Vitanovski, D., Tsymbal, A., Ionasec, R., Georgescu, B., Zhou, S.K., Hornegger, J., Comaniciu, D.: Learning distance function for regression-based 4D pulmonary trunk model reconstruction estimated from sparse MRI data. In: *Proc. of SPIE Medical Imaging*, pp. 1–7 (2011)
- Zhong, H., Zheng, Y., Funka-Lea, G., Vega-Higuera, F.: Segmentation and removal of pulmonary arteries, veins and left atrial appendage for visualizing coronary and bypass arteries. In: *Proc. Workshop on Medical Computer Vision* (In conjunction with CVPR), pp. 24–30 (2012)

8.3.9   Esophagus Segmentation in CT

A critical complication of catheter based atrial fibrillation ablation is atrio-esophageal fistula, where the esophagus is mistakenly penetrated by the ablation catheter. The air from the esophagus can enter the left atrium, creating a life threatening situation. The segmentation of the esophagus helps during intervention planning to define an optimal ablation strategy to avoid the region close to the esophagus. Overlaying the segmented esophagus model onto the fluoroscopic

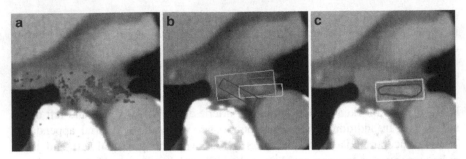

Fig. 8.31 Workflow of esophagus segmentation in CT. (**a**) Detected position candidates (*dark dots*). (**b**) Detected candidates of oriented bounding boxes. (**c**) Segmented esophagus. The results are shown on a 2D slice for easy visualization, although 3D segmentation is performed. Image courtesy of Johannes Feulner

image sequence also provides valuable visual guidance during the intervention. Furthermore, in lymph node detection, the segmented esophagus can be excluded from the search [16], therefore reducing false positive detections.

Recently, Feulner et al. [12,14,15] presented an automatic method for esophagus segmentation in CT. The intersection of the esophagus on each axial CT slice is approximated as an ellipse. Five parameters of an ellipse are estimated through MSL. After independent ellipse detection, each slice keeps multiple candidates (as shown in Fig. 8.31b) and the best candidate is selected using a Markov Random Field (MRF) model. An initial esophagus surface mesh is then generated, followed by boundary refinement using a learning based boundary detector. A mean surface segmentation error of 1.80 mm is achieved on 144 datasets.

Publications

- Feulner, J., Zhou, S.K., Cavallaro, A., Seifert, S., Hornegger, J., Comaniciu, D.: Fast automatic segmentation of the esophagus from 3D CT data using a probabilistic model. In: *Proc. Int'l Conf. Medical Image Computing and Computer Assisted Intervention*, vol. 1, pp. 255–262 (2009)
- Feulner, J., Zhou, S.K., Huber, M., Cavallaro, A., Hornegger, J., Comaniciu, D.: Model-based esophagus segmentation from CT scans using a spatial probability map. In: *Proc. Int'l Conf. Medical Image Computing and Computer Assisted Intervention*, vol. 1, pp. 95–102 (2010)
- Feulner, J., Zhou, S.K., Hammon, M., Seifert, S., Huber, M., Comaniciu, D., Hornegger, J., Cavallaro, A.: A probabilistic model for automatic segmentation of the esophagus in 3-D CT scans. *IEEE Trans. Medical Imaging* **30**(6), 1252–1264 (2011)

8.3.10   Liver Segmentation in CT

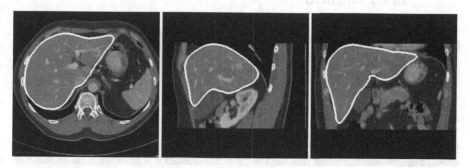

Fig. 8.32 Typical liver segmentation result in a CT volume. From left to right: transaxial, sagittal, and coronal views of the same volume

The task of liver segmentation (Fig. 8.32) from an abdominal CT volume benefited from the development of the constrained MSL and nonrigid MSL [32, 72, 73]. The segmentation needs to work robustly on CT volumes scanned by different imaging protocols, contrasted and non-contrasted, various resolutions and field-of-views, coming from patients with different diseases.

Constrained MSL helped reducing the liver detection time from more than 6 s to less than 0.5 s. In addition, nonrigid MSL combined with constrained MSL reduced the shape initialization error by 11 %.

The liver segmentation system has been tested on a challenging dataset containing 226 volumes. We achieve a final mesh surface error of 1.45 mm, based on a threefold cross-validation, which compares favorably with the state-of-the-art. Our overall system runs as fast as 10 s per volume, while other state-of-the-art solutions take at least 1 min [44], often up to 15 min [21, 27], to process a volume.

Publications

- Ling, H., Zhou, S.K., Zheng, Y., Georgescu, B., Suehling, M., Comaniciu, D.: Hierarchical, learning-based automatic liver segmentation. In: *Proc. IEEE Conf. Computer Vision and Pattern Recognition*, pp. 1–8 (2008)
- Zheng, Y., Georgescu, B., Ling, H., Zhou, S.K., Scheuering, M., Comaniciu, D.: Constrained marginal space learning for efficient 3D anatomical structure detection in medical images. In: *Proc. IEEE Conf. Computer Vision and Pattern Recognition*, pp. 194–201 (2009)
- Zheng, Y., Georgescu, B., Comaniciu, D.: Marginal space learning for efficient detection of 2D/3D anatomical structures in medical images. In: *Proc. Information Processing in Medical Imaging*, pp. 411–422 (2009)

8.3.11   Segmentation of Prostate, Bladder, and Rectum in CT and MRI

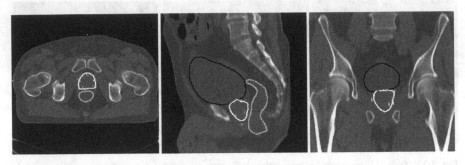

Fig. 8.33 Segmentation of prostate (*white*), bladder (*black*), and rectum (*gray*) in a pelvic CT scan. From left to right: transaxial, sagittal, and coronal views of the same volume. Image courtesy of Chao Lu

Pelvic region analysis plays an important role in diagnosis and treatment planning for prostate cancer and bladder cancer. Segmentation of the prostate, as well as the bladder and rectum, from a three dimensional CT volume often serves as the first step in image-based radiotherapy studies and continuously attracts research attention. Although intensive research has been performed, accurate segmentation of 3D soft tissue structures in the pelvic region is still a challenging problem, due to the large variations in organ shapes and in the texture pattern inside and along organ boundaries (Fig. 8.33).

An automatic system to segment the prostate, bladder, and rectum is presented in [33]. The MSL is employed to estimate the pose of all three organs. The main contribution of this work is on the accurate and robust delineation of the weak boundary. A novel information theoretic scheme based on the Jensen-Shannon divergence is incorporated into the boundary inference process to drive the mesh to the best fit of the image, thus improving the segmentation accuracy. The proposed approach has been tested on a challenging dataset containing 188 volumes from diverse sources. It not only produces excellent segmentation accuracy, but also runs about 80 times faster than previously published solutions [9].

The MSL has been also applied to segment the prostate in MR images [3]. A major challenge of MR image segmentation is to handle large intensity variations caused by difference in scanners and imaging settings. Therefore, the input image is first normalized to achieve a globally consistent intensity distribution, while the artifacts caused by the endorectal coil are further normalized using Poisson image editing. To provide accurate shape initialization, three nonrigid deformation parameters based on principal component analysis are estimated using nonrigid MSL [72]. The whole prostate surface is split into six regions, each region benefiting from its own boundary detector.

The system has been tested on the MICCAI PROMISE-12 Challenge dataset of T2 weighted MR images. Its segmentation accuracy has been ranked the second

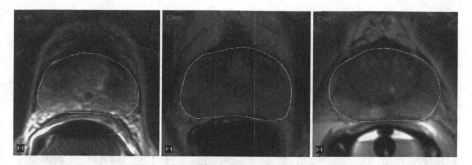

Fig. 8.34 Prostate segmentation results on three MRI volumes. For each volume, the middle transaxial slice is shown. Image courtesy of Neil Birkbeck

with a score only slightly lower than the first, while the segmentation was much faster than all other algorithms. It took about 3 s to segment one volume, while the algorithm with a slightly higher accuracy required 8 min. Figure 8.34 shows the segmentation results on three PROMISE-12 volumes.

Publications

- Lu, C., Zheng, Y., Birkbeck, N., Zhang, J., Kohlberger, T., Tietjen, C., Boettger, T., Duncan, J.S., Zhou, S.K.: Precise segmentation of multiple organs in CT volumes using learning-based approach and information theory. In: *Proc. Int'l Conf. Medical Image Computing and Computer Assisted Intervention*, vol. 2, pp. 462–469 (2012)
- Birkbeck, N., Zhang, J., Zhou, S.K.: Region-specific hierarchical segmentation of MR prostate using discriminative learning. In: *MICCAI Grand Challenge: Prostate MR Image Segmentation*, pp. 4–11 (2012)

8.3.12   Lung Segmentation in CT

Lung segmentation in thoracic CT is an important prerequisite for monitoring the progression and treatment of pulmonary diseases. Healthy lung segmentation is often regarded as an easy task due to lung's much darker image intensity compared to surrounding tissues. Therefore, simple low-level image segmentation methods, e.g., thresholding or region growing, often produce satisfactory results. However, due to pulmonary diseases such as pulmonary fibrosis, a pathological lung may have a similar intensity to the neighboring heart and diaphragm, making automatic segmentation far more difficult.

Sofka et al. [47] proposed to use stable landmarks on the lung surface to further improve shape initialization accuracy. Figure 8.35a shows the system diagram of the

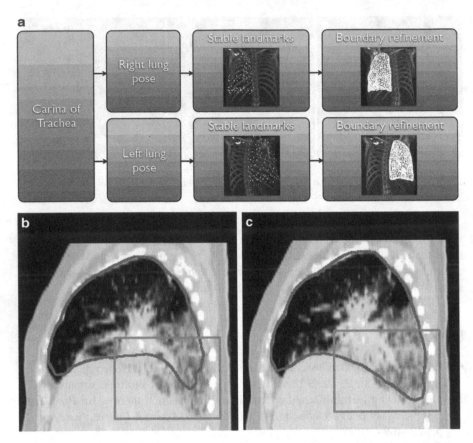

Fig. 8.35 Pathological lung segmentation in CT data. (**a**) System diagram. Lung segmentation results without (**b**) and with (**c**) further shape initialization using stable landmarks. Image courtesy of Michal Sofka

approach. Instead of estimating the pose of the left and right lung independently, the carina of trachea is detected and used to predict the initial pose of both lungs. The MSL is then applied to refine the pose estimate and an initial shape of the lung surface is generated. During the training phase, a few stable landmarks are selected on the lung surface, based on their detectability, and one detector is trained for each stable landmark. During the detection phase, the position of each landmark is inferred from the initial lung surface, followed by refinement using its own detector. The detected landmarks are used to align the lung shape model to generate more accurate shape initialization before final boundary delineation. As shown in Fig. 8.35c, with further shape initialization using stable landmarks, more accurate segmentation is achieved, especially around the pathological area.

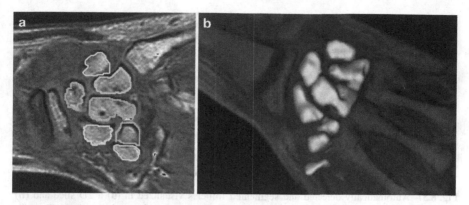

Fig. 8.36 Automatic detection and segmentation of wrist bones in an MRI volume. (**a**) Segmented wrist bones on a slice. (**b**) Enhanced 3D visualization of wrist bones after segmentation. Image courtesy of Alexander Schwing

Publication

- Sofka, M., Wetzl, J., Birkbeck, N., Zhang, J., Kohlberger, T., Kaftan, J., Declerck, J., Zhou, S.K.: Multi-stage learning for robust lung segmentation in challenging CT volumes. In: *Proc. Int'l Conf. Medical Image Computing and Computer Assisted Intervention*, vol. 3, pp. 667–674 (2011)

8.3.13   Wrist Bone Segmentation in 3D MRI

Physical examinations of wrist carpal bones play an important role for assessing arthritis and bone erosion. Humans typically have eight such small angular bones arranged in two rows in each of the left and right wrists (Fig. 8.36). Their manual segmentation in MRI to evaluate and follow the course of the disease is a tedious process.

Koch et al. [30] proposed a fully automatic machine learning based approach. The MSL is used to detect the bounding box of each bone; however, random forests are used for classification, instead of the probabilistic boosting-tree. The voxel intensity inside the detected bounding box is approximated as a Gaussian mixture model whose parameters are estimated using the Expectation and Maximization (EM) algorithm. A graph cut-based segmentation is employed to derive the final boundaries. The single-node cost term in the graph cut formulation is based on a likelihood function using the estimated Gaussian mixture model. The method covers both T1 and T2 weighted MR images.

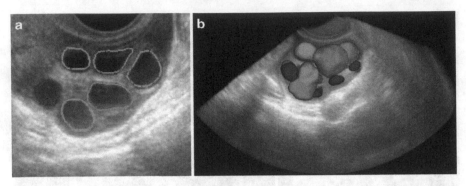

Fig. 8.37 Automatically detected and segmented follicles visualized in (**a**) a 2D slice and (**b**) 3D. Image courtesy of Terrence Chen. ©2009 IEEE. Reprinted, with permission, from Chen, T., Zhang, W., Good, S., Zhou, K.S., Comaniciu, D.: Automatic ovarian follicle quantification from 3D ultrasound data using global/local context with database guided segmentation. In: *Proc. Int'l Conf. Computer Vision*, pp. 795–802 (2009)

Publication

- Koch, M., Schwing, A.G., Comaniciu, D., Pollefeys, M.: Fully automatic segmentation of wrist bones for arthritis patients. In: *Proc. IEEE Int'l Sym. Biomedical Imaging*, pp. 636–640 (2011)

8.3.14   Ovarian Follicle Detection/Segmentation in 3D Ultrasound

2D ultrasound is traditionally used to monitor ovarian follicular development and quantify the size and number of follicles during the in vitro fertilization cycles. Three major axes of ovarian follicles are measured manually in clinical practice. Such measure is error-prone, due to the irregular shape of follicles, and cumbersome due to extensive manual manipulations to count and measure each individual follicle. Automatic measurement in 3D ultrasound data has not only the potential to decrease the examination time, but also to provide more accurate 3D volume measurement of each follicle (Fig. 8.37).

Chen et al. presented a system to automatically detect and segment the ovarian follicles in 3D ultrasound [7]. Since the follicles are bounded inside an ovary, the bounding box of the ovary is first detected using the MSL and the position and size of follicles are estimated inside this box.

There may be up to 30 follicles inside an ovary and similar to [29], Chen et al. observed the sample concentration problem of the MSL, the detected pose candidates concentrating on a few larger and darker follicles. Cluster analysis and non-maximum suppression are used to reduce the number of pose candidates and

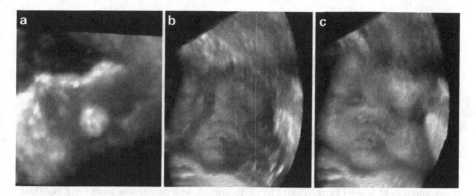

Fig. 8.38 Example of fetal face detection and carving. (**a**) Original pose of a loaded volume. (**b**) The face is detected and aligned to the front view. (**c**) Carved volume after removing stuffs at front of the face. Image courtesy of Shaolei Feng. ©2009 IEEE. Reprinted, with permission, from Feng, S., Zhou, S., Good, S., Comaniciu, D.: Automatic fetal face detection from ultrasound volumes via learning 3D and 2D information. In: *Proc. IEEE Conf. Computer Vision and Pattern Recognition*, pp. 2488–2495 (2009)

make their distribution more uniform. The final segmentation is achieved through graph cuts. Extensive evaluations conducted on 501 volumes containing 8,108 follicles show that the method is able to detect and segment ovarian follicles with high robustness and accuracy, being much faster than the current ultrasound manual workflow.

Publication

- Chen, T., Zhang, W., Good, S., Zhou, K.S., Comaniciu, D.: Automatic ovarian follicle quantification from 3D ultrasound data using global/local context with database guided segmentation. In: *Proc. Int'l Conf. Computer Vision*, pp. 795–802 (2009)

8.3.15 Fetal Face Detection and Segmentation in 3D Ultrasound

Feng et al. [11] presented an application of the MSL for the automatic detection and segmentation of a fetal face in 3D ultrasound. The detected face can be used to guide a sonographer to steer the ultrasound probe in searching for a pleasant view to generate a photo for the expecting parents. The extra tissue in front of the fetal face, e.g., placenta, hands and feet of the fetus, can be carved to avoid the face occlusion in the generated photo (Fig. 8.38).

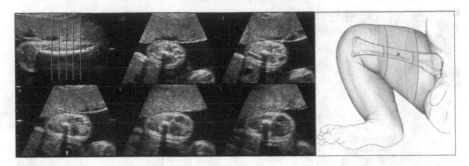

Fig. 8.39 Segmentation of a fetal limb in 3D ultrasound to estimate the fractional limb volume. Image courtesy of Shaolei Feng. ©2012 SPIE. Reprinted, with permission, from Feng, S., Zhou, K.S., Lee, W.: Automatic fetal weight estimation using 3D ultrasonography. In: *Proc. of SPIE Medical Imaging*, vol. 8315, pp. 1–7 (2012)

If done manually, it takes minutes for an expert sonographer to find a satisfactory view. Using the constrained MSL, the fetal face is detected and segmented within 1 s, by combining both 3D face surface detection and 2D face profile detection. The use of the 2D face profile is motivated by the acquisition workflow: most often sonographers navigating the transducer to capture first the face profile.

Publication

- Feng, S., Zhou, S., Good, S., Comaniciu, D.: Automatic fetal face detection from ultrasound volumes via learning 3D and 2D information. In: *Proc. IEEE Conf. Computer Vision and Pattern Recognition*, pp. 2488–2495 (2009)

8.3.16   Fetal Limb Segmentation in 3D Ultrasound

A couple of ultrasound exams are recommended to monitor the development and healthiness of a fetus. As an important clinical measurement, fetal weight often needs to be estimated during an ultrasound exam. The estimation typically involves a few simple geometric measurements (e.g., the femur length, abdominal circumference, circumference and diameter of the head) in 2D ultrasound [5]. One limitation of these measurements is that with the exception of abdominal circumference, they do not include soft tissue development for the assessment of general fetal nutritional status. Recently, fractional limb volume has been introduced for more accurate fetal weight estimation. In [10], the MSL based segmentation is employed to automatically segment a limb; therefore, the fetal weight can be estimated automatically and accurately in about 2 s (Fig. 8.39).

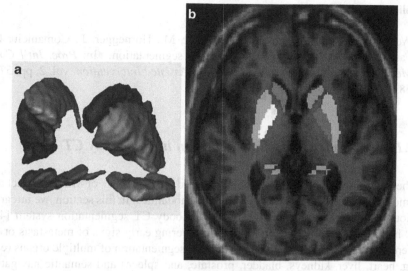

Fig. 8.40 The segmented eight subcortical structures rendered in (**a**) 3D and (**b**) overlaid to an axial slice of a T1-weighted MR image. Image courtesy of Michael Wels

Publication

- Feng, S., Zhou, K.S., Lee, W.: Automatic fetal weight estimation using 3D ultrasonography. In: *Proc. of SPIE Medical Imaging*, vol. 8315, pp. 1–7 (2012)

8.3.17 Multiple Subcortical Brain Structure Segmentation in 3D MRI

Many scientific questions in neurology, like the revelation of degenerative disease mechanisms require quantitative volumetric analysis of subcortical gray matter structures in large populations of patients and healthy controls. The MSL has been used to automatically detect and segment the following subcortical gray matter structures: caudate nucleus, hippocampus, globus pallidus, and putamen (Fig. 8.40) [60]. Each anatomy has one instance in the left and right brain hemisphere, respectively, resulting in eight structures in total. The resulting system is robust to process brain MRI images from a variety of scanners and the whole processing time is 13.9 s on average, faster than most of the approaches in the literature.

Publication

- Wels, M., Zheng, Y., Carneiro, G., Huber, M., Hornegger, J., Comaniciu, D.: Fast and robust 3-D MRI brain structure segmentation. In: *Proc. Int'l Conf. Medical Image Computing and Computer Assisted Intervention*, vol. 2, pp. 575–583 (2009)

8.3.18 Multiple Organ Segmentation in Full Body CT

In the previous sections, we have demonstrated the capability of MSL to detect and segment various organs in all major imaging modalities. In this section, we integrate various components together to build a full body CT segmentation system [46]. Full body CT scanning is common for discovering early signs of metastasis or for differential diagnosis. Automatic parsing and segmentation of multiple organs (e.g., lung, heart, liver, kidneys, bladder, prostate, and spleen) and semantic navigation inside the body can help the clinician to efficiently obtain an accurate diagnosis (Fig. 8.41).

Seifert et al. [46] proposed a fast segmentation solution, in which networks of 1D and 3D landmarks are trained to quickly parse the 3D CT data and estimate which organs and landmarks are present, as well as their most probable locations. Using this approach, the segmentation of six organs as well as the detection of 19 body landmarks can be obtained in about 20 s with high accuracy.

Later on, Kohlberger et al. [31] proposed a level set based segmentation refinement procedure to further improve the consistency and accuracy of the boundary. The level set function guarantees that the extracted meshes are free of overlap. The refinement procedure is initialized and performed in a narrow band around the Active Shape Model (ASM) [8] results to speed up the computation and avoid segmentation leakage. Using the level set based refinement, Kohlberger et al. reported a reduction of the mesh surface segmentation error by 20–40 % for different organs.

Publications

- Seifert, S., Barbu, A., Zhou, K., Liu, D., Feulner, J., Huber, M., Suehling, M., Cavallaro, A., Comaniciu, D.: Hierarchical parsing and semantic navigation of full body CT data. In: *Proc. of SPIE Medical Imaging*, pp. 1–8 (2009)
- Kohlberger, T., Zhang, J., Sofka, M., Birkbeck, N., Wetal, J., Kaftan, J., Declerck, J., Zhou, S.K.: Automatic multi-organ segmentation using learning-based segmentation and level set optimization. In: *Proc. Int'l Conf. Medical Image Computing and Computer Assisted Intervention*, vol. 3, pp. 338–345 (2011)

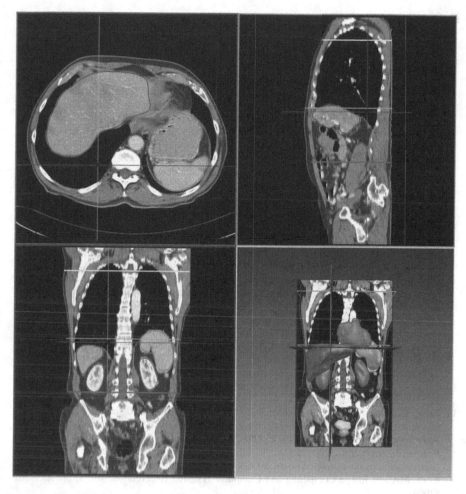

Fig. 8.41 Segmentation of multiple organs in a full body CT volume

8.4 Conclusions

In this chapter we reviewed the applications of Marginal Space Learning (MSL) for the detection and segmentation of anatomical structures in medical images. All applications demonstrate the robustness and efficiency of the MSL. In most applications it achieves state-of-the-art accuracy, while often being an order of magnitude faster than other approaches. The MSL is also flexible enough to work with all major medical imaging modalities, including X-ray, ultrasound, CT, and MRI.

References

1. Barbu, A., Sühling, M., Xu, X., Liu, D., Zhou, S.K., Comaniciu, D.: Automatic detection and segmentation of lymph nodes from CT data. IEEE Trans. Medical Imaging **31**(2), 240–250 (2012)
2. Barbu, A., Suehling, M., Xu, X., Liu, D., Zhou, S.K., Comaniciu, D.: Automatic detection and segmentation of axillary lymph nodes. In: Proc. Int'l Conf. Medical Image Computing and Computer Assisted Intervention, vol. 1, pp. 28–36 (2010)
3. Birkbeck, N., Zhang, J., Zhou, S.K.: Region-specific hierarchical segmentation of MR prostate using discriminative learning. In: MICCAI Grand Challenge: Prostate MR Image Segmentation, pp. 4–11 (2012)
4. Carneiro, G., Amat, F., Georgescu, B., Good, S., Comaniciu, D.: Semantic-based indexing of fetal anatomies from 3-D ultrasound data using global/semi-local context and sequential sampling. In: Proc. IEEE Conf. Computer Vision and Pattern Recognition, pp. 1–8 (2008)
5. Carneiro, G., Georgescu, B., Good, S., Comaniciu, D.: Detection of fetal anatomies from ultrasound images using a constrained probabilistic boosting tree. IEEE Trans. Medical Imaging **27**(9), 1342–1355 (2008)
6. Chen, T., Wang, Y., Durlak, P., Comaniciu, D.: Real time assistance for stent positioning and assessment by self-initialized tracking. In: Proc. Int'l Conf. Medical Image Computing and Computer Assisted Intervention, vol. 1, pp. 405–413 (2012)
7. Chen, T., Zhang, W., Good, S., Zhou, K.S., Comaniciu, D.: Automatic ovarian follicle quantification from 3D ultrasound data using global/local context with database guided segmentation. In: Proc. Int'l Conf. Computer Vision, pp. 795–802 (2009)
8. Cootes, T.F., Taylor, C.J., Cooper, D.H., Graham, J.: Active shape models—their training and application. Computer Vision and Image Understanding **61**(1), 38–59 (1995)
9. Feng, Q., Foskey, M., Chen, W., Shen, D.: Segmenting CT prostate images using population and patient-specific statistics for radiotherapy. Medical Physics **37**(8), 4121–4132 (2010)
10. Feng, S., Zhou, K.S., Lee, W.: Automatic fetal weight estimation using 3D ultrasonography. In: Proc. of SPIE Medical Imaging, vol. 8315, pp. 1–7 (2012)
11. Feng, S., Zhou, S., Good, S., Comaniciu, D.: Automatic fetal face detection from ultrasound volumes via learning 3D and 2D information. In: Proc. IEEE Conf. Computer Vision and Pattern Recognition, pp. 2488–2495 (2009)
12. Feulner, J., Zhou, S.K., Cavallaro, A., Seifert, S., Hornegger, J., Comaniciu, D.: Fast automatic segmentation of the esophagus from 3D CT data using a probabilistic model. In: Proc. Int'l Conf. Medical Image Computing and Computer Assisted Intervention, vol. 1, pp. 255–262 (2009)
13. Feulner, J., Zhou, S.K., Hammon, M., Hornegger, J., Comaniciu, D.: Lymph node detection and segmentation in chest CT data using discriminative learning and a spatial prior. Medical Image Analysis **17**(2), 254–270 (2013)
14. Feulner, J., Zhou, S.K., Hammon, M., Seifert, S., Huber, M., Comaniciu, D., Hornegger, J., Cavallaro, A.: A probabilistic model for automatic segmentation of the esophagus in 3-D CT scans. IEEE Trans. Medical Imaging **30**(6), 1252–1264 (2011)
15. Feulner, J., Zhou, S.K., Huber, M., Cavallaro, A., Hornegger, J., Comaniciu, D.: Model-based esophagus segmentation from CT scans using a spatial probability map. In: Proc. Int'l Conf. Medical Image Computing and Computer Assisted Intervention, vol. 1, pp. 95–102 (2010)
16. Feulner, J., Zhou, S.K., Huber, M., Hornegger, J., Comaniciu, D., Cavallaro, A.: Lymph node detection in 3-D chest CT using a spatial prior probability. In: Proc. IEEE Conf. Computer Vision and Pattern Recognition, pp. 2926–2932 (2010)
17. Funka-Lea, G., Boykov, Y., Florin, C., Jolly, M.P., Moreau-Gobard, R., Ramaraj, R., Rinck, D.: Automatic heart isolation for CT coronary visualization using graph-cuts. In: Proc. IEEE Int'l Sym. Biomedical Imaging, pp. 614–617 (2006)
18. Grbic, S., Ionasec, R., Vitanovski, D., Voigt, I., Wang, Y., Georgescu, B., Navab, N., Comaniciu, D.: Complete valvular heart apparatus model from 4D cardiac CT. In: Proc. Int'l Conf. Medical Image Computing and Computer Assisted Intervention, vol. 1, pp. 218–226 (2010)

19. Grbic, S., Ionasec, R.I., Zheng, Y., Zaeuner, D., Georgescu, B., Comaniciu, D.: Aortic valve and ascending aortic root modeling from 3D and 3D+t CT. In: Proc. of SPIE Medical Imaging, pp. 1–8 (2010)

20. Heimann, T., Mountney, P., John, M., Ionasec, R.: Learning without labeling: Domain adaptation for ultrasound transducer localization. In: Proc. Int'l Conf. Medical Image Computing and Computer Assisted Intervention, vol. 3, pp. 49–56 (2013)

21. Heimann, T., Münzing, S., Meinzer, H.P., Wolf, I.: A shape-guided deformable model with evolutionary algorithm initialization for 3D soft tissue segmentation. In: Proc. Information Processing in Medical Imaging, pp. 1–12 (2007)

22. Hennemuth, A., Boskamp, T., Fritz, D., Kühnel, C., Bock, S., Rinck, D., Scheuering, M., Peitgen, H.O.: One-click coronary tree segmentation in CT angiographic images. In: Proc. Computer Assisted Radiology and Surgery, pp. 317–321 (2005)

23. Ionasec, R.I., Georgescu, B., Gassner, E., Vogt, S., Kutter, O., Scheuering, M., Navab, N., Comaniciu, D.: Dynamic model-driven quantitative and visual evaluation of the aortic valve from 4D CT. In: Proc. Int'l Conf. Medical Image Computing and Computer Assisted Intervention, vol. 1, pp. 686–694 (2008)

24. Ionasec, R.I., Voigt, I., Georgescu, B., Wang, Y., Houle, H., Vega-Higuera, F., Navab, N., Comaniciu, D.: Patient-specific modeling and quantification of the aortic and mitral valves from 4D cardiac CT and TEE. IEEE Trans. Medical Imaging 29(9), 1636–1651 (2010)

25. Ionasec, R.I., Wang, Y., Georgescu, B., Voigt, I., Navab, N., Comaniciu, D.: Robust motion estimation using trajectory spectrum learning: Application to aortic and mitral valve modeling from 4D TEE. In: Proc. Int'l Conf. Computer Vision, pp. 1601–1608 (2009)

26. John, M., Liao, R., Zheng, Y., Nottling, A., Boese, J., Kirschstein, U., Kempfert, J., Walther, T.: System to guide transcatheter aortic valve implantations based on interventional 3D C-arm CT imaging. In: Proc. Int'l Conf. Medical Image Computing and Computer Assisted Intervention, vol. 1, pp. 375–382 (2010)

27. Kainmueller, D., Lange, T., Lamecker, H.: Shape constrained automatic segmentation of the liver based on a heuristic intensity model. In: MICCAI Workshop on 3D Segmentation in the Clinic: A Grand Challenge, pp. 1–10 (2007)

28. Kelm, B.M., Wels, M., Zhou, S.K., Seifert, S., Suehling, M., Zheng, Y., Comaniciu, D.: Spine detection in CT and MR using iterated marginal space learning. Medical Image Analysis 17(8), 1283–1292 (2013)

29. Kelm, B.M., Zhou, S.K., Suehling, M., Zheng, Y., Wels, M., Comaniciu, D.: Detection of 3D spinal geometry using iterated marginal space learning. In: Proc. MICCAI Workshop Medical Computer Vision — Recognition Techniques and Applications in Medical Imaging, pp. 96–105 (2010)

30. Koch, M., Schwing, A.G., Comaniciu, D., Pollefeys, M.: Fully automatic segmentation of wrist bones for arthritis patients. In: Proc. IEEE Int'l Sym. Biomedical Imaging, pp. 636–640 (2011)

31. Kohlberger, T., Zhang, J., Sofka, M., Birkbeck, N., Wetal, J., Kaftan, J., Declerck, J., Zhou, S.K.: Automatic multi-organ segmentation using learning-based segmentation and level set optimization. In: Proc. Int'l Conf. Medical Image Computing and Computer Assisted Intervention, vol. 3, pp. 338–345 (2011)

32. Ling, H., Zhou, S.K., Zheng, Y., Georgescu, B., Suehling, M., Comaniciu, D.: Hierarchical, learning-based automatic liver segmentation. In: Proc. IEEE Conf. Computer Vision and Pattern Recognition, pp. 1–8 (2008)

33. Lu, C., Zheng, Y., Birkbeck, N., Zhang, J., Kohlberger, T., Tietjen, C., Boettger, T., Duncan, J.S., Zhou, S.K.: Precise segmentation of multiple organs in CT volumes using learning-based approach and information theory. In: Proc. Int'l Conf. Medical Image Computing and Computer Assisted Intervention, vol. 2, pp. 462–469 (2012)

34. Lu, L., Barbu, A., Wolf, M., Liang, J., Bogoni, L., Salganicoff, M., Comaniciu, D.: Simultaneous detection and registration for ileo-cecal valve detection in 3D CT colonography. In: Proc. European Conf. Computer Vision, pp. 465–478 (2008)

35. Lu, X., Chen, T., Comaniciu, D.: Robust discriminative wire structure modeling with applications to stent enhancement in fluoroscopy. In: Proc. IEEE Conf. Computer Vision and Pattern Recognition, pp. 1121–1127 (2011)

36. Lu, X., Georgescu, B., Jolly, M.P., Guehring, J., Young, A., Cowan, B., Littmann, A., Comaniciu, D.: Cardiac anchoring in MRI through context modeling. In: Proc. Int'l Conf. Medical Image Computing and Computer Assisted Intervention, vol. 1, pp. 383–390 (2010)
37. Lu, X., Georgescu, B., Littmann, A., Mueller, E., Comaniciu, D.: Discriminative joint context for automatic landmark set detection from a single cardiac MR long axis slice. In: Proc. Functional Imaging and Modeling of the Heart, pp. 457–465 (2009)
38. Lu, X., Georgescu, B., Zheng, Y., Otsuki, J., Bennett, R., Comaniciu, D.: AutoMPR: Automatic detection of standard planes from three dimensional echocardiographic data. In: Proc. IEEE Int'l Sym. Biomedical Imaging, pp. 1279–1282 (2008)
39. Lu, X., Jolly, M.P., Georgescu, B., Hayes, C., Speier, P., Schmidt, M., Bi, X., Kroeker, R., Comaniciu, D., Kellman, P., Mueller, E., Guehring, J.: Automatic view planning for cardiac MRI acquisition. In: Proc. Int'l Conf. Medical Image Computing and Computer Assisted Intervention, pp. 479–486 (2011)
40. Lu, X., Wang, Y., Georgescu, B., Littmann, A., Comaniciu, D.: Automatic delineation of left and right ventricles in cardiac MRI sequences using a joint ventricular model. In: Proc. Functional Imaging and Modeling of the Heart, pp. 250–258 (2011)
41. Lu, X., Xue, H., Jolly, M.P., Guetter, C., Kellman, P., Hsu, L.Y., Arai, A., Zuehlsdorff, S., Littmann, A., Georgescu, B., Guehring, J.: Simultaneous detection of landmarks and key-frame in cardiac perfusion MRI using a joint spatial-temporal context model. In: Proc. of SPIE Medical Imaging, pp. 1–7 (2011)
42. Mountney, P., Ionasec, R., Kaizer, M., Mamaghani, S., Wu, W., Chen, T., John, M., Boese, J., Comaniciu, D.: Ultrasound and fluoroscopic images fusion by autonomous ultrasound probe detection. In: Proc. Int'l Conf. Medical Image Computing and Computer Assisted Intervention, vol. 2, pp. 544–551 (2012)
43. Park, J., Feng, S., Zhou, K.S.: Automatic computation of 2D cardiac measurements from B-mode echocardiography. In: Proc. of SPIE Medical Imaging, vol. 8315, pp. 1–11 (2012)
44. Ruskó, L., Bekes, G., Németh, G., Fidrichf, M.: Fully automatic liver segmentation for contrast-enhanced CT images. In: MICCAI Workshop on 3D Segmentation in the Clinic: A Grand Challenge, pp. 143–150 (2007)
45. Schwing, A., Zheng, Y.: Reliable extraction of the mid-sagittal plane in 3d brain mri via hierarchical landmark detection. In: Proc. IEEE Int'l Sym. Biomedical Imaging, pp. 1–4 (2014)
46. Seifert, S., Barbu, A., Zhou, K., Liu, D., Feulner, J., Huber, M., Suehling, M., Cavallaro, A., Comaniciu, D.: Hierarchical parsing and semantic navigation of full body CT data. In: Proc. of SPIE Medical Imaging, pp. 1–8 (2009)
47. Sofka, M., Wetzl, J., Birkbeck, N., Zhang, J., Kohlberger, T., Kaftan, J., Declerck, J., Zhou, S.K.: Multi-stage learning for robust lung segmentation in challenging CT volumes. In: Proc. Int'l Conf. Medical Image Computing and Computer Assisted Intervention, vol. 3, pp. 667–674 (2011)
48. Sofka, M., Zhang, J., Zhou, S.K., Comaniciu, D.: Multiple object detection by sequential Monte Carlo and hierarchical detection network. In: Proc. IEEE Conf. Computer Vision and Pattern Recognition, pp. 1735–1742 (2010)
49. Tek, H., Gulsun, M.A., Laguitton, S., Grady, L., Lesage, D., Funka-Lea, G.: Automatic coronary tree modeling. The Insight Journal pp. 1–8 (2008)
50. Tzoumas, S., Wang, P., Zheng, Y., John, M., Comaniciu, D.: Robust pigtail catheter tip detection in fluoroscopy. In: Proc. of SPIE Medical Imaging, vol. 8316, pp. 1–8 (2012)
51. Vitanovski, D., Ionasec, R.I., Georgescu, B., Huber, M., Taylor, A.M., Hornegger, J., Comaniciu, D.: Personalized pulmonary trunk modeling for intervention planning and valve assessment estimated from CT data. In: Proc. Int'l Conf. Medical Image Computing and Computer Assisted Intervention, vol. 1, pp. 17–25 (2009)
52. Vitanovski, D., Tsymbal, A., Ionasec, R., Georgescu, B., Zhou, S.K., Hornegger, J., Comaniciu, D.: Learning distance function for regression-based 4D pulmonary trunk model reconstruction estimated from sparse MRI data. In: Proc. of SPIE Medical Imaging, pp. 1–7 (2011)

53. Vitanovski, D., Tsymbal, A., Ionasec, R.I., Georgescu, B., Huber, M., Taylor, A., Schievano, S., Zhou, S.K., Hornegger, J., Comaniciu, D.: Cross-modality assessment and planning for pulmonary trunk treatment using CT and MRI imaging. In: Proc. Int'l Conf. Medical Image Computing and Computer Assisted Intervention, vol. 1, pp. 460–467 (2010)
54. Voigt, I., Ionasec, R.I., Georgescu, B., Houle, H., Huber, M., Hornegger, J., Comaniciu, D.: Model-driven physiological assessment of the mitral valve from 4D TEE. In: Proc. of SPIE Medical Imaging, pp. 1–11 (2009)
55. Wang, C., Smedby, O.: An automatic seeding method for coronary artery segmentation and skeletonization in CTA. The Insight Journal pp. 1–8 (2008)
56. Wang, P., Zheng, Y., John, M., Comaniciu, D.: Catheter tracking via online learning for dynamic motion compensation in transcatheter aortic valve implantation. In: Proc. Int'l Conf. Medical Image Computing and Computer Assisted Intervention, vol. 2, pp. 17–24 (2012)
57. Wang, Y., Chen, T., Wang, P., Rohkohl, C., Comaniciu, D.: Automatic localization of balloon markers and guidewire in rotational fluoroscopy with application to 3D stent reconstruction. In: Proc. European Conf. Computer Vision, pp. 428–441 (2012)
58. Wang, Y., Georgescu, B., Comaniciu, D., Houle, H.: Learning-based 3D myocardial motion flow estimation using high frame rate volumetric ultrasound data. In: Proc. IEEE Int'l Sym. Biomedical Imaging, pp. 1097–1100 (2010)
59. Wels, M., Kelm, B.M., Tsymbal, A., Hammon, M., Soza, G., Suehling, M., Cavallero, A., Comaniciu, D.: Multi-stage osteolytic spinal bone lesion detection from CT data with internal sensitivity control. In: Proc. of SPIE Medical Imaging, vol. 8315, pp. 1–8 (2012)
60. Wels, M., Zheng, Y., Carneiro, G., Huber, M., Hornegger, J., Comaniciu, D.: Fast and robust 3-D MRI brain structure segmentation. In: Proc. Int'l Conf. Medical Image Computing and Computer Assisted Intervention, vol. 2, pp. 575–583 (2009)
61. Wu, D., Liu, D., Puskas, Z., Lu, C., Wimmer, A., Tietjen, C., Soza, G., Zhou, S.K.: A learning based deformable template matching method for automatic rib centerline extraction and labeling in CT images. In: Proc. IEEE Conf. Computer Vision and Pattern Recognition, pp. 980–987 (2012)
62. Wu, W., Chen, T., Barbu, A., Wang, P., Strobel, N., Zhou, S.K., Comaniciu, D.: Learning-based hypothesis fusion for robust catheter tracking in 2D X-ray fluoroscopy. In: Proc. IEEE Conf. Computer Vision and Pattern Recognition, pp. 1097–1104 (2011)
63. Wu, W., Chen, T., Strobel, N., Comaniciu, D.: Fast tracking of catheters in 2D fluoroscopic images using an integrated CPU-GPU framework. In: Proc. IEEE Int'l Sym. Biomedical Imaging, pp. 1184–1187 (2012)
64. Yang, D., Zheng, Y., John, M.: Graph cuts based left atrium segmentation refinement and right middle pulmonary vein extraction in C-arm CT. In: Proc. of SPIE Medical Imaging, pp. 1–9 (2013)
65. Yang, L., Georgescu, B., Zheng, Y., Foran, D.J., Comaniciu, D.: A fast and accurate tracking algorithm of left ventricles in 3D echocardiography. In: Proc. IEEE Int'l Sym. Biomedical Imaging, pp. 221–224 (2008)
66. Yang, L., Georgescu, B., Zheng, Y., Meer, P., Comaniciu, D.: 3D ultrasound tracking of the left ventricles using one-step forward prediction and data fusion of collaborative trackers. In: Proc. IEEE Conf. Computer Vision and Pattern Recognition, pp. 1–8 (2008)
67. Yang, L., Georgescu, B., Zheng, Y., Wang, Y., Meer, P., Comaniciu, D.: Prediction based collaborative trackers (PCT): A robust and accurate approach toward 3D medical object tracking. IEEE Trans. Medical Imaging 30(11), 1921–1932 (2011)
68. Zhang, W., Mantlic, F., Zhou, S.K.: Automatic landmark detection and scan range delimitation for topogram images using hierarchical network. In: Proc. of SPIE Medical Imaging, vol. 7623, pp. 1–8 (2010)
69. Zheng, Y., Barbu, A., Georgescu, B., Scheuering, M., Comaniciu, D.: Fast automatic heart chamber segmentation from 3D CT data using marginal space learning and steerable features. In: Proc. Int'l Conf. Computer Vision, pp. 1–8 (2007)

70. Zheng, Y., Barbu, A., Georgescu, B., Scheuering, M., Comaniciu, D.: Four-chamber heart modeling and automatic segmentation for 3D cardiac CT volumes using marginal space learning and steerable features. IEEE Trans. Medical Imaging **27**(11), 1668–1681 (2008)
71. Zheng, Y., Georgescu, B., Barbu, A., Scheuering, M., Comaniciu, D.: Four-chamber heart modeling and automatic segmentation for 3D cardiac CT volumes. In: Proc. of SPIE Medical Imaging, vol. 6914, pp. 1–12 (2008)
72. Zheng, Y., Georgescu, B., Comaniciu, D.: Marginal space learning for efficient detection of 2D/3D anatomical structures in medical images. In: Proc. Information Processing in Medical Imaging, pp. 411–422 (2009)
73. Zheng, Y., Georgescu, B., Ling, H., Zhou, S.K., Scheuering, M., Comaniciu, D.: Constrained marginal space learning for efficient 3D anatomical structure detection in medical images. In: Proc. IEEE Conf. Computer Vision and Pattern Recognition, pp. 194–201 (2009)
74. Zheng, Y., Georgescu, B., Vega-Higuera, F., Comaniciu, D.: Left ventricle endocardium segmentation for cardiac CT volumes using an optimal smooth surface. In: Proc. of SPIE Medical Imaging, vol. 7259, pp. 1–11 (2009)
75. Zheng, Y., Georgescu, B., Vega-Higuera, F., Zhou, S.K., Comaniciu, D.: Fast and automatic heart isolation in 3D CT volumes: Optimal shape initialization. In: Proc. MICCAI Workshop Machine Learning in Medical Imaging, pp. 84–91 (2010)
76. Zheng, Y., John, M., Boese, J., Comaniciu, D.: Precise segmentation of the left atrium in C-arm CT volumes with applications to atrial fibrillation ablation. In: Proc. IEEE Int'l Sym. Biomedical Imaging, pp. 1421–1424 (2012)
77. Zheng, Y., John, M., Liao, R., Boese, J., Kirschstein, U., Georgescu, B., Zhou, S.K., Kempfert, J., Walther, T., Brockmann, G., Comaniciu, D.: Automatic aorta segmentation and valve landmark detection in C-arm CT: Application to aortic valve implantation. In: Proc. Int'l Conf. Medical Image Computing and Computer Assisted Intervention, vol. 1, pp. 476–483 (2010)
78. Zheng, Y., John, M., Liao, R., Nottling, A., Boese, J., Kempfert, J., Walther, T., Brockmann, G., Comaniciu, D.: Automatic aorta segmentation and valve landmark detection in C-arm CT for transcatheter aortic valve implantation. IEEE Trans. Medical Imaging **31**(12), 2307–2321 (2012)
79. Zheng, Y., Lu, X., Georgescu, B., Littmann, A., Mueller, E., Comaniciu, D.: Automatic left ventricle detection in MRI images using marginal space learning and component-based voting. In: Proc. of SPIE Medical Imaging, pp. 1–12 (2009)
80. Zheng, Y., Lu, X., Georgescu, B., Littmann, A., Mueller, E., Comaniciu, D.: Robust object detection using marginal space learning and ranking-based multi-detector aggregation: Application to automatic left ventricle detection in 2D MRI images. In: Proc. IEEE Conf. Computer Vision and Pattern Recognition, pp. 1343–1350 (2009)
81. Zheng, Y., Tek, H., Funka-Lea, G., Zhou, S.K., Vega-Higuera, F., Comaniciu, D.: Efficient detection of native and bypass coronary ostia in cardiac CT volumes: Anatomical vs. pathological structures. In: Proc. Int'l Conf. Medical Image Computing and Computer Assisted Intervention, vol. 3, pp. 403–410 (2011)
82. Zheng, Y., Wang, T., John, M., Zhou, S.K., Boese, J., Comaniciu, D.: Multi-part left atrium modeling and segmentation in C-arm CT volumes for atrial fibrillation ablation. In: Proc. Int'l Conf. Medical Image Computing and Computer Assisted Intervention, vol. 3, pp. 487–495 (2011)
83. Zheng, Y., Yang, D., John, M., Comaniciu, D.: Multi-part modeling and segmentation of left atrium in C-arm CT for image-guided ablation of atrial fibrillation. IEEE Trans. Medical Imaging (2014). In Press
84. Zhong, H., Zheng, Y., Funka-Lea, G., Vega-Higuera, F.: Segmentation and removal of pulmonary arteries, veins and left atrial appendage for visualizing coronary and bypass arteries. In: Proc. Workshop on Medical Computer Vision (In conjunction with CVPR), pp. 24–30 (2012)

Chapter 9
Conclusions and Future Work

9.1 Summary of Contributions

This book is centered around the efficient detection and segmentation of 2D and 3D
anatomical structures in medical images. Following are our key contributions.

1. **Marginal Space Learning**
   To localize a 3D object, one needs to estimate nine pose parameters, three for
   position, three for orientation, and three for anisotropic scaling. We present
   a simple but elegant method for the efficient estimation of the pose parameters, called Marginal Space Learning (MSL). The MSL partitions the pose
   estimation problem into a sequence of problems formulated in lower dimension
   spaces, but of increasingly higher dimensionality, called marginal spaces. Thus,
   the pose of a 3D object is estimated in three steps: position estimation, position-
   orientation estimation, and position-orientation-scale estimation. Each search
   space is efficiently pruned, by preserving after each step only a small number of
   candidate hypotheses. In this way, the number of testing hypotheses is reduced
   by six orders of magnitude, compared to the exhaustive full space search.

2. **Steerable Features**
   Efficient learning based detection methods always rely on efficient image
   features. Global features, such as Haar wavelet features, are effective to capture
   the global information (e.g., orientation and scale) of an object. To capture the
   orientation information of a hypothesis, we should rotate either the volume or
   the feature templates. It is time consuming to rotate a 3D volume and there
   is no efficient way to rotate the Haar wavelet feature templates. We introduce
   the steerable features, which can efficiently capture the position, orientation,
   and scale information of a pose hypothesis. We sample points from the volume
   under a sampling pattern and compute at each point local features such as voxel
   intensity and gradient. The novelty of the steerable features is that they embed
   the position, orientation, and scale information into the distribution of sampling
   points, while each individual feature is locally defined. Instead of aligning the

Y. Zheng and D. Comaniciu, *Marginal Space Learning for Medical Image Analysis:*   257
Efficient Detection and Segmentation of Anatomical Structures,
DOI 10.1007/978-1-4939-0600-0_9, © Springer Science+Business Media New York 2014

volume to a pose hypothesis, we steer the sampling pattern. The steerable features can be extended to incorporate nonrigid deformation parameters or temporal information for the joint spatio-temporal estimation.

3. **Comparison of Marginal Space Learning and Full Space Learning in 2D**
   The MSL can be extended to detect the bounding box of five degrees of freedom corresponding to 2D objects. We perform a thorough comparison experiment on left ventricle detection in 2D MRI images of the MSL and Full Space Learning (FSL), which exhaustively searches the original full pose parameter space. Experiments show the MSL significantly outperforms the FSL, on both training and test sets. The MSL is about eight times faster than FSL and reduces the box detection error by 78 %. Due to its superior performance, MSL is also often used to detect 2D objects in medical imaging.

4. **Constrained Marginal Space Learning**
   We present two methods to further constrain the search by exploiting the correlation among object pose parameters, one for the position space and the other for the orientation and scale spaces. The position search space is constrained by the minimum margin calculated from the training set. To constrain the search of the orientation or scale space, we present an example-based strategy by focusing the search to regions with high probability. Using the constrained MSL, we improve the detection speed often by an order of magnitude, resulting in a system that can process one volume in under a second for various 3D object detection tasks.

5. **Quaternion Formulation for Orientation Space**
   The original MSL used Euler angles to represent the orientation of a 3D object. However, the Euler angle representation has some intrinsic limitations, e.g., multiple configurations yielding the same orientation, lacking a good distance measure between two orientations, and difficulty to uniformly sample the orientation space to generate testing hypotheses. We adapt the quaternion formulation to overcome all these limitations. Quaternions provide an elegant conceptual framework, being much easier to use and calculate the true distance between two orientations.

6. **Optimal Mean Shape**
   For nonrigid object segmentation, a mean shape is aligned to the estimated object pose as the initial shape for the subsequent shape boundary evolution. We present an approach to derive a mean shape that can optimally represent the shape population of the training set. The optimal mean shape minimizes the residual errors after compensating the translation, rotation, and scaling of the object. Using the optimal mean shape, we calculate the transformation that aligns the mean shape towards each individual training shape. These transformation parameters provide the pose ground truth that MSL can learn to estimate.

7. **Nonrigid Marginal Space Learning**
   The original MSL only estimates a rigid transformation (translation, rotation, and anisotropic scaling) of an object. To provide a more accurate shape initialization for a nonrigid object, we present nonrigid MSL, which directly estimates nonrigid deformation parameters.

8. **Part-Based Object Detection and Segmentation**
   To better cope with complex objects of high degree of anatomical variation, we introduce part-based object representations that help us maintaining a globally consistent shape. Many anatomical structures can be naturally split into different parts (e.g., the aorta is composed of aortic root, ascending aorta, aortic arch, and descending aorta). Although the global object may exhibit large variations, the object parts are less prone to distortions and therefore can be detected and segmented more reliably. Different applications may demand different methods to split the object into parts, enforce constraints during part detection, and aggregate the results of part detectors. We demonstrated the robustness and accuracy of part-based object detection and segmentation in several applications.

9. **Learning-Based Boundary Detector**
   We present a generic nonrigid object detection and segmentation framework, for which the MSL is used to provide an accurate shape initialization. To further improve the boundary delineation, a learning based boundary detector is designed to guide the boundary evolution within the Active Shape Model framework.

10. **Review of 35 MSL-Based Medical Imaging Applications**
    Last but not least, we perform a thorough literature review of the MSL-based applications related to diverse medical image analysis tasks. A total of 35 applications are discussed, covering the detection and segmentation of interventional devices and organs in major imaging modalities, including Fluoroscopy, Ultrasound, Computed Tomography, and Magnetic Resonance Imaging.

9.2 Future Work

We discuss in this section a few potential directions and challenges for future work in medical image analysis.

1. **Comprehensive Detection and Characterization of Pathological Structures**
   The MSL provides a great starting point to detect, segment and characterize anatomical structures for which multiple training examples exist. The more examples we provide, the more reliable the end results are. Unfortunately, the disease space exhibits a large complexity and often it is difficult to gather and learn examples about all potential manifestations of a certain disease. More than that, the area of congenital diseases is extremely difficult to characterize statistically, due to the often exceptions in the associated topology of the anatomical structures (e.g., aortic valve with only two leaflets, heart with only two chambers).

Fig. 9.1 Blood flow
computation in the heart
using the segmented
patient-specific cardiac
geometry and pressure
measurements. Image
courtesy of Viorel Mihalef

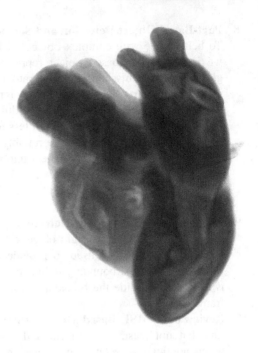

2. **Reproducible Image Quantification**

   In this book we constantly provided evaluations on large image databases,
   containing hundreds and sometimes thousands of anatomical structure examples.
   To our knowledge, this provides already a step forward in terms of formal testing
   of algorithms in medical imaging. Nevertheless, much more needs to be done.
   The question of reproducibility of the quantification results is critical for medical
   imaging, especially for longitudinal studies. How depended is a measurement on
   the selected scanning protocol, on the imaging technician, and on the particular
   behavior of the image interpretation algorithm? The assessment of a certain
   therapy response relies heavily on image quantification. For example, the earlier
   we can confidently assess a change in the observed tumor, the better; a more
   informed action can be taken, with potential life saving consequences.

3. **Real-Time Image Quantification for Minimally Invasive Procedures**

   With the advances in minimally invasive interventions and surgeries, the role of
   medical imaging increases. The medical imaging scanners, endoscopes, laparo-
   scopes, and video cameras are becoming a clinician's new eyes. The information
   provided by these devices has to be robustly fused, visualized and interpreted, in
   real-time. The constant emergence of new image-guided procedures brings great
   benefits to the patients, by minimizing the trauma linked to the surgery. At the
   same time, new challenges of speed and robustness are demanded for automatic,
   real-time image interpretation and quantification.

4. **System Medicine**

   On the longer term, the challenge is to support medicine to become more
   predictive, based on evidence and a better understanding of the human body

and disease spectrum through imaging. We evolve from only characterizing the geometry and parts of a certain organ to model the organ as a complete system, and characterize its function and evolution under certain therapy. Future patient-specific models, whose parameters are estimated by solving inverse problems from images, will help predicting the success of a certain therapy and selecting the best one for the patient in question, thus minimizing the risk and maximizing the outcome.

For example, Fig. 9.1 shows the patient-specific blood flow in the heart computed from the extracted geometric model presented in Chap. 7, enhanced with the heart valve models discussed in Sect. 8.3.7 of Chap. 8. Using such models we will be able to understand and predict the behavior of the heart as a system following a certain intervention (e.g., the implant of a prosthetic valve). Such scenario will bring immense benefits to the patient by helping to select the right treatment, will help reducing the cost of healthcare by making the medicine more precise, and will create new demands for medical imaging and the quantification of the image content.

Index

Printed in the United States
By Bookmasters